COGNITIVE VULNERABILITY TO EMOTIONAL DISORDERS

COGNITIVE VULNERABILITY TO EMOTIONAL DISORDERS

Edited by

Lauren B. Alloy
Temple University

John H. Riskind
George Mason University

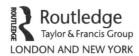

Routledge
Taylor & Francis Group
LONDON AND NEW YORK

First published in 1996 by Lawrence Erlbaum Associates
10 Industrial Avenue, Mahwah, New Jersey 07430

This edition published in 2012 by Routledge
27 Church Road, Hove, East Sussex BN3 2FA
711 Third Avenue, New York, NY 10017, USA

Routledge is an imprint of the Taylor & Francis Group, an informa business

Cover design by Kathryn Houghtaling Lacey
Sculpture: "Medusa in the New Age" by Adrienne L. Romer

Library of Congress Cataloging-in-Publication Data

Cognitive vulnerability to emotional disorders / edited by Lauren B. Alloy, John H. Riskind.
    p.   cm.
Includes bibliographical references and index.
ISBN 0-8058-3828-7 (cloth)
ISBN 0-8058-5774-5 (pbk)
    1. Affective disorders—Risk factors.   2. Anxiety—Risk factors.   3. Eating disorders—
Risk factors.   4. Emotions and cognition.   5. Cognitive styles.   I. Alloy, Lauren B.
II. Riskind, John H.

RC537.C6324   2005
616.85'2—dc22   2005047279
                                                                            CIP

Contents

Preface

In modern life, anxiety disorders, together with depressive disorders, rank at the top of the most devastating forms of mental illness in Western society. These disorders affect as many as 46 million individuals in the United States alone (Kessler et al., 1994). In response, there is a rapidly proliferating literature on these emotional disorders, as well as on the group of closely related eating disorders.

Cognitive models of psychopathology have become prominent in contemporary attempts to understand the causes, mechanisms, and effective treatments for psychological problems. In these models, factors such as appraisals, attributions, and cognitive styles are important. Cognitive theories assume that mental processes—such as interpretation, attention, or memory—are intermediary events that intercede between environmental stimuli and emotional responses. Cognitive theories have received increasing attention not only in the clinical and psychiatric literatures, but also in the social and personality, experimental, cognitive, and developmental ones.

If emotional disorders such as anxiety and depression are, indeed, influenced by cognitive factors, it is important to understand the ways that these factors may contribute to cognitive vulnerability. Some individuals are clearly more susceptible than others to developing emotional disorders, and to experiencing chronic problems or recurrences. What, then, makes them susceptible? This is, in essence, a question about cognitive vulnerability, and one of the most vibrant research efforts in psychopathology is now devoted to exploring it. The literature is rapidly burgeoning on cognitive vulnerability to not only depression but emotional disorders such as bipolar, panic, OCD, and eating disorders; new developments are constantly being reported.

Thus, we felt the lack of, and need for, a book that would present and synthesize the latest knowledge about cognitive factors in vulnerability to emotional disorders.

Most work on cognition addresses *concurrent cognitions or biases* (about which there is a huge literature). Work on vulnerability is different. It concerns the *cognitive antecedents* of these, and the disorders in which they are implicated. Understanding cognitive vulnerabilities is important for understanding how disorders develop, how they are maintained, and how they can be prevented and treated.

Cognitive vulnerabilities are faulty beliefs, long-previously developed cognitive patterns, or structures that are hypothesized to set the stage for later psychological problems. They are in place long before the earliest signs or symptoms of disorder first appear. These vulnerabilities are generally purported to create specific liabilities to particular psychological disorders after individuals encounter stressful events, and to maintain the problems after their onset. Only by addressing these vulnerabilities can long-term therapeutic improvements be maintained, and the risk of recurrences or relapse be reduced.

We have structured this book to make it easy for readers to focus on particular interests. They can read about specific disorders (e.g., depression or bipolar disorder, suicide, obsessive-compulsive or panic disorder), read about groups of disorders (e.g., mood disorders or anxiety disorders), or read about emotional disorders in general. The book is organized in what we hope is a highly accessible way within a common overarching conceptual framework. All the chapters build on a model of cognitive vulnerability that is described in the first chapter. This model explains the relationships between developmental factors, cognitive vulnerabilities as risk factors for later disorder, the nature of specific vulnerabilities for specific disorders, and the difference between distal antecedents of disorders (e.g., depressive inferential styles, dysfunctional attitudes) and proximal cognitive factors (e.g., schema activation, or inferences). It synthesizes the commonalities evidenced by a number of different cognitive clinical approaches to emotional disorders. The first chapter also provides an overview of the major issues bearing on design and methods, and how these must be guided by theory.

The remainder of the book is divided into three sections, on mood disorders, anxiety disorders, and eating disorders, respectively. Each section contains a series of chapters summarizing the latest formulation of the role of cognitive vulnerabilities in a particular disorder, by a leading expert who describes emerging theory and research, and also identifies areas where work remains to be done, since cognitive vulnerability is still less studied than other aspects of cognitive function in emotional disorder. Each section concludes with an integrative chapter, also by a leading expert, which offers incisive commentary, theoretical synthesis, and insightful suggestions for further systematic research.

Part I concentrates on mood disorders, both depressive and bipolar. Chapters by Alloy, Abramson, Safford, and Gibb, and Ingram, Miranda, and Segal, describe major recent findings and theoretical issues concerning cognitive vulnerability to depression; chapters by Alloy, Reilly-Harrington, Fresco, and Flannery-Schroeder, and Pettit and Joiner, describe recent developments on research on cognitive vulnerability to bipolar disorder and suicide, respectively. A chapter by Traill and Gotlib sums up and synthesizes. Part II focuses on the major anxiety disorders. A chapter by Riskind and Williams describes work on a common cognitive vulnerability to anxiety disorders that differentiates them from depression. Other chapters by Schmidt and Woolaway-Bickel on panic disorder, Rachman, Shafran, and Riskind on OCD, Ledley, Fresco, and Heimberg on social anxiety, and Feeny and Foa on PTSD, describe recent findings and theoretical issues concerning specific anxiety disorders. Wells and Matthews sum up and synthesize. Part III is devoted to bulimia and anorexia nervosa, which are closely related to anxiety and depression and may share some of the same underlying causal processes. Chapters by Abramson, Bardone-Cone, Vohs, Joiner, and Heatherton on bulimia, and by Garner and Magana on anorexia nervosa discuss current work; a chapter by Keel sums up and synthesizes.

We are excited about this book and hope that it will be helpful to all who seek to understand the cognitive-behavioral basis of mood, anxiety, and eating disorders in the service of more effective prevention and treatment. Our field of inquiry has expanded rapidly and witnessed much recent progress; we hope also that the book will stimulate further research.

REFERENCE

Kessler, R. C., McGonagle, K. A., Zhao, S., Nelson, C. G., Hughes, C. R., Eshleman, S., Witchen, H. U., & Kendler, K. S. (1994). Lifetime and 12-month prevalence of DSM-III-R psychiatric disorders in the United States: Results from the National Comorbidity Survey. *Archives of General Psychiatry, 51*, 8–49.

Cognitive Vulnerability to Emotional Disorders: Theory and Research Design/Methodology

John H. Riskind
George Mason University

Lauren B. Alloy
Temple University

Emotional disorders have adversely affected human lives since the earliest recorded history. As long ago as 400 BC, Hippocrates identified "melancholia" and "mania." Today, emotional disorders rank at the top of any list of the most devastating mental illnesses in Western society (e.g., Rovner, 1993). As many as 46 million individuals in the United States alone suffer from depression and anxiety disorders (Kessler et al., 1994). The enormous impact on society (e.g., health costs and disability, job loss, health problems) has prompted a great deal of effort to search for their causes. This quest has been inspired by a variety of conceptual paradigms—psychoanalytic (Freud, 1964), biological (Meehl, 1962), attachment (Ainsworth, 1982; Bowlby, 1969), environmental life stress (Monroe & Simons, 1991), and learning approaches (Lewinsohn, 1974; Mowrer, 1939).

The cognitive revolution of the 1950s and 1960s became a formidable force in psychology. One of its results was the introduction of a cognitive paradigm for understanding the causes of emotional disorders. Cognitive theorists maintained that cognition, or more specifically, maladaptive cognition, plays a central role in the etiology of emotional disorders (e.g., Beck, 1967; Kelly, 1955; Seligman, 1975). The emergence of cognitive perspectives, and their forerunners (e.g., Ellis, 1970; Kelly, 1955; Rotter, 1954), represented a dramatic shift from other conceptual paradigms in the conceptualization and treatment of emotional disorders. As a good illustration, consider the radical changes that swept the depression literature in the late 1960s. Shattering the traditional assumption that depression was simply affective and biological, Beck's cognitive model was based on the idea that systematic cognitive distortions in thinking about the self, world, and future help to catalyze and maintain depression and other emotional disorders. Seligman's (e.g., 1975) work on the phenomenon of learned helplessness eventually led to ways to fuse Beck's cognitive clinical observations with an experimental tradition in studying depression (e.g., Abramson, Seligman, & Teasdale, 1978). During the past three decades, experimental cognitive traditions that deal with attention, memory, and information processing have been extended to depression, anxiety, and other disorders (e.g., Mathews & MacLeod, 1994; J. M. G. Williams, Watts, MacLeod, & Mathews, 1988).

This chapter reviews some of the basic issues relating to theory and to the design and methods of cognitive vulnerability research on emotional disorders. It first discusses basic tenets of cognitive models of emotional disorder, including the concept of cognitive mediation and vulnerability–stress interaction, and common features of a prototypical cognitive vulnerability model. It also examines important issues that remain for further investigation (e.g., comorbidity, developmental pathways, the interaction of cognitive and biological vulnerabilities). It then describes issues concerned with the interface of theory and research design, including the crucial role of theory in determining the proper design of research studies. Actual design options and methods used in cognitive vulnerability research, and their strengths and limitations, are also discussed. Finally, there is a brief summary and concluding comments.

BASIC TENETS OF COGNITIVE MODELS
OF EMOTIONAL DISORDER

The most basic tenet of cognitive clinical models is that cognitions mediate the relation between events that people experience and the emotions that they feel. A passage from Dickens aptly illustrates this keystone of cognitive models of emotional disorders and other psychopathology. It clearly conveys the fact that individuals can radically differ from each other in the ways that they privately explain and understand different characteristics of the same stimulus event:

> "Oh, you cruel, cruel boy, to say I am a disagreeable wife!," cried Dora. "Now, my dear Dora, you must know that I never said that!" "You said I wasn't comfortable!" said Dora. "I said the housekeeping was not comfortable!" "It's exactly the same thing!" cried Dora. And she evidently thought so, for she wept most grievously. (Dickens, 1979, p. 616)

The basic precept of cognitive models of emotional disorder, then, is that a person's emotional responses to a situation are influenced by the interpretation (or appraisal) the person makes of its meaning (e.g., Fridja, 1987; Lazarus, 1991; Ortony, Clore, & Collins, 1988; Roseman, Spindel, & Jose, 1990). People's appraisals are not simple mirrorlike reflections of the elements of objective reality. Hence, it is not only a particular situation that determines the way people feel or emotionally respond, but also the special meaning that is subjectively constructed by the person that is important. It is just as important that the situation (absolute reality) does not directly determine how the person feels or responds. The same guiding principle applies to stimuli that are perceived within the interior of the person (e.g., physical sensations, thoughts, emotions) as to stimuli that are found in the external environment.

Cognitive models are also based on the general idea that there is a continuity of normal and abnormal cognitive processes. For instance, Beck (1991) stated that "the [cognitive] model of psychopathology proposes that the excessive dysfunctional behavior and distressing emotions or inappropriate affect found in various psychiatric disorders are exaggerations of normal adaptive processes" (p. 370). Thus, it is quite simple to apply the presuppositions of cognitive models to emotional disorders such as depression and panic disorder, or related ones such as eating disorders. For example, triggering events such as a social rejection or a small increase in body weight are construed by some individuals as a small setback; others perceive them as no less than decisive evidence of utter failure and personal defect. In addition, some people exhibit relatively characteristic or stable patterns in the ways in which they appraise emotion-provoking stimuli (e.g., Abramson et al., 1978; Riskind, Williams, Gessner, Chrosniak, & Cortina, 2000; Weiner, 1985). The bottom line is that habitual differences in the manner in which people interpret particular kinds of events can affect their future risk for developing particular kinds of emotional disorders.

The cognitive factors conceived to be important in emotional disorders can include both *distal* phenomena that were present before the disorder, and *proximal* phenomena that occur very close to, or even during, the episode of disorder and its symptoms (Abramson, Metalsky, & Alloy, 1989). Distal cognitive factors are normally relatively enduring cognitive predispositions to respond to stressful situations in maladaptive ways (e.g., dysfunctional attitudes or explanatory styles). They are higher in generality (or abstraction) as well as more distal to future episodes of disorders than proximal cognitions, which are more transitory or specific thoughts or mental processes that occur very close to, or even during, the episode of disorder. And, proximal cognitions (e.g., specific thoughts or images) are typically produced when individuals process the meaning of a stressful event in any situation through the filter of the underlying cognitive vulnerability.

Cognitive Vulnerability–Stress Paradigm

Today, most cognitive models presuppose that the outcomes resulting from cognitive vulnerabilities depend on interactions with environmental precipitants. Some good examples of precipitants include stressful life events, early childhood traumas, faulty parenting, or medical injuries. In other words, the models incorporate a *vulnerability–stress* paradigm in which it is recognized that psychological disorders are caused by an interaction between predisposing (constitutional or learned) and precipitating (environmental) factors. These factors can trigger the development of emotional disorders or psychological problems for certain individuals (e.g., see Alloy, Abramson, Raniere, & Dyller, 1999), but the specific degree and even direction of the response can differ enormously from one person to another. For example, some individuals seem to be relatively "resilient" and often overcome the difficulties that accompany stressful events (e.g., Hammen, 2003); others seem overwhelmed by even minor problems. Thus, precipitating events are particularly likely to produce emotional disorders among individuals who have a preexisting cognitive vulnerability to the disorders.

Most individuals in stressful situations do not develop clinically significant disorders. Moreover, the specific disorder that emerges for different individuals is not determined just by the precipitating stress alone (i.e., precipitating stresses do not just occur in conjunction with any one clinical disorder). For example, stressful events are elevated in depression (Brown & Harris, 1978; Paykel, 1982), bipolar disorder and mania (see chap. 4, this vol.; Johnson & Roberts, 1995), anxiety disorders (Last, Barlow, & O'Brien, 1984; Roy-Byrne, Geraci, & Uhde, 1986), and even schizophrenia (Zuckerman, 1999). In light of these findings, cognitive vulnerability–stress models are offered to help account for not only *who* is vulnerable to developing emotional disorder (e.g., individuals with a particular cognitive style), and *when* (e.g., after a stress), but to *which* disorders they are vulnerable (e.g., depression, eating disorder, etc.).

The earliest vulnerability–stress models (e.g., Meehl, 1962) emphasized constitutional *biological* traits (e.g., genetic traits) as vulnerabilities. But, this approach was quickly expanded in terms of cognitive vulnerabilities, personality factors, and interpersonal strategies (e.g., Abramson et al., 1989; Blatt & Zuroff, 1992; D. A. Clark, Beck, & Alford, 1999; Ingram, Miranda, & Segal, 2001; Joiner, Alfano, & Metalsky, 1992; Rachman, 1997; Riskind, 1997; Robins, 1990). Researchers in the cognitive tradition favor the term *vulnerability* to *diathesis*, because the former term embraces the idea of learned and modifiable predispositions, instead of immutable genetic or biological traits (e.g., Just, Abramson, & Alloy, 2001).

Beck's (1967, 1976) theory was the earliest to expound a *cognitive vulnerability–stress interaction*. Beck postulated that whether or not individuals possess an enduring cognitive predisposition to emotional disorders depends on if they have acquired maladaptive knowledge structures or schemata during the course of childhood. These schemata are internal frameworks, constructed of attitudes, beliefs, and concepts that individuals use when they interpret past, present, and future experiences. Because they influence the ways in which they interpret and initially experience events, schemata moderate the idiosyncratic subjective meaning and thus the impact of stressful events. These cognitive schemata promote maladjustment when they are poorly grounded in social reality or are otherwise dysfunctional. Hence, individuals with maladaptive schemata are more likely to make dysfunctional interpretations of stressful events that increase vulnerability to emotional disorders. Once they have made such appraisals (e.g., of failures as personal defects), a series of changes in mental processes are initiated that can culminate—by way of changes in the contents of thinking and information processing—in depression or anxiety. Thus, in Beck's cognitive model, emotional disorders result from a combination of predisposing, environmental, and developmental factors that lead individuals to engage in dysfunctional thinking and information processing.

COMMON FEATURES OF COGNITIVE VULNERABILITY MODELS: A FRAMEWORK ENCAPSULATING RELATIONSHIPS

The conceptual framework presented in Fig. 1.1 depicts several distinct features of the prototypical cognitive vulnerability model of emotional disorders and other psychological problems. Such cognitive models generally share the assumption that there are a series of causal chains by which enduring vulnerabilities develop and (with relevant stressor combinations) become converted into the emotional disorders or problems. These causal chains commence with earlier life experiences (e.g., faulty attachment relationships, childhood traumas, modeling) that lead individuals by means of developmental pathways to develop cognitive vulnerabilities. Once cognitive vulnerability factors have coalesced and are put into play or are activated, they alter the individual's responses and are seen as serving schematic processing functions (e.g., D. A. Clark, Beck, & Alford, 1999). That is, the cognitive vulnerabilities represent a mental mechanism that shapes the individual's selective processing, attention, and memory,

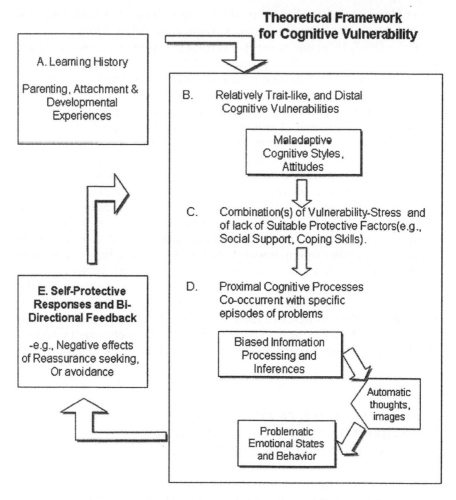

FIG. 1.1.   Theoretical framework for cognitive vulnerability.

and molds changes in the concomitant contents of the individual's think-ing (i.e., the ideation, imagery, or "automatic" thoughts").

Although a vulnerability–stress interaction is a central feature of cogni-tive vulnerability models, there are many possible variations. First, the triggering conditions that are hypothesized to precipitate symptoms or episodes of disorder may be both "public" and "private" events. Public events include achievement failures, disruptions of interpersonal relation-ships, or collectively evident threats to well-being. Private events include unusual bodily sensations, unwanted thoughts, or traumatic memories.

Thus, the putative cognitive vulnerability that influences the risk of emotional disorder can be represented by a depressive inferential style (see chap. 2, this vol.), a cognitive network of negative self-referent cognition (chap. 3, this vol.), a looming cognitive style (chap. 7, this vol.), or a tendency to catastrophically misinterpret the meaning of experienced bodily sensations (see chap. 8, this vol.). In this conceptual framework, the output is represented by the emotional disorder or symptoms that result from the interaction between the precipitating event and cognitive vulnerability.

A critical element of many cognitive models is that specific biases of information processing and proximal cognitions are assumed to differ with different disorders (Beck & D. A. Clark, 1997; J. M. G. Williams et al., 1988). For example, the bias in social phobia is for information relevant to the threat of public humiliation, and is accompanied by proximal thoughts like "I'll make a fool of myself" (see chap. 10, this vol.). The specific bias in panic disorder is for information relevant to unusual bodily sensations that might signal impending heart attacks or other feared calamities, and is accompanied by thoughts such as "I'm having a heart attack" (see chap. 8, this vol.). Such "disorder-specific" information-processing biases are presumably instigated when cognitive vulnerabilities (the distal factors) are put into play or engaged that were present long before the symptoms or episode. Hence, the specific vulnerability hypothesis of cognitive models is that the vulnerabilities to different disorders can dramatically differ. The mental processing biases can in turn be seen as penetrating a range of basic information processes (e.g., selective attention, encoding, and retrieval in memory, interpretation).

The stages of processing and specific subject matter that are implicated, however, depend on the particular cognitive models and disorders. For example, in some models, the primary disorder-specific bias in anxiety is in selective attention for threatening stimuli, whereas the primary bias in depression is in the elaboration in memory of negative information during encoding (e.g., J. M. G. Williams et al., 1988). In general, the basic idea of disorder-specific content and biases has been an impetus for considerable research on cognition in emotional disorders.

Several additional factors may also influence the net effects of the cognitive vulnerability, by reason of having power to either inhibit or intensify reactions to precipitating stresses. As Fig. 1.1 shows, some factors (e.g., social support, an intimate relation with a spouse or lover, effective coping mechanisms) are often seen in cognitive models as operating as *protective factors* that work against the development of disorders (e.g., Brown & Harris, 1978; S. Cohen & Wills, 1985; Panzarella, Alloy, & Whitehouse, 2004). For example, even when cognitively vulnerable individuals are exposed to stress, the presence of certain protective factors may shield them from disorders, or reduce the likelihood they will develop psychological problems. Such factors can be either transitory, "providential" factors (e.g., fortuitous, but temporary, social support during stress), or quite stable (e.g., lifelong relationships). Sometimes they can be unidentified by researchers or even unknown. In contrast, *exacerbating factors* are additional stresses or factors that worsen an emotional disorder after it has already been acquired. Examples include stressful life events (e.g., further medical illnesses, psychological problems, or negative affect expressed by others) that impinge on individuals subsequent to the onset of their emotional disorders.

It seems that individuals become more supersensitive or defenseless to the impact of negative events, and therefore cope less well, once a psychological disorder such as a depressive episode (Hammen, 1991) has been acquired. Such an observation invites comparisons to the weakened state of people who are medically ill. Taken collectively, this line of reasoning suggests that even when individuals have equivalent vulnerability–stress combinations, they can still differ in their trajectories of disorder owing to differences in protective and exacerbating factors.

Finally, as Fig. 1.1 indicates, vicious cycles involving bidirectional causal links (and feedback loops) with disorder-related behaviors can also contribute to the onset, maintenance, or recurrence of disorders. Under the pressure of the stress and intense symptoms, for example, cognitively vulnerable individuals tend to engage in various maladaptive *self-protective* or *compensatory behaviors*. In instances of depression, individuals often have a heightened inclination to engage in reassurance seeking from others (Joiner, Alfano, & Metalsky, 1992). Individuals who are depressed also contribute to the occurrence of self-generated life events (e.g., creating interpersonal conflicts or excessive demands) that can maintain and exaggerate their depression (Hammen, 2003). In instances of anxiety disorders, individuals often engage in cognitive avoidance strategies that can include worry, thought suppression, or wishful thinking (see chap. 7, this vol.). Here, avoidance behaviors can be relatively subtle, such as looking away from the faces of others to avoid seeing imagined rejection. In this way, compensatory avoidance behaviors often insidiously enforce and maintain the erroneous beliefs as well as the symptoms of the emotional disorder (e.g., beliefs about the likelihood of rejection; see D. M. Clark & Wells, 1995).

According to cognitive models, emotional disorders persist as long as the cognitive components of the disorders are active, and improve when they are altered (see chap. 9, this vol.). Furthermore, temporary relief is produced by changes in proximal cognitive components of the disorder, whereas durable improvement requires changes of the underlying cognitive vulnerability factors.

COMPLEX THEORETICAL ISSUES FOR RESEARCH ON COGNITIVE VULNERABILITY TO EMOTIONAL DISORDERS

This section examines several complex theoretical issues and open conceptual questions that confront cognitive vulnerability models. (Other issues have methodological implications that are discussed at the end of the Research Design section.)

Specificity of Cognitive Vulnerability Factors

There is an important distinction for cognitive models between specific and nonspecific causal factors in emotional disorders. *Specific* causal factors are relatively unique or focal factors in that they influence and predict the development of a particular disorder, but they do not apply equally to all psychopathology in general. For example, some cognitive vulnerability factors may apply to just a single form of anxiety disorder (e.g., just to OCD). In contrast, others may extend to the whole spectrum of anxiety disorders, but not apply to depression or other psychopathology (e.g., chap. 7, this vol.; N. L. Williams, Shahar, Riskind, & Joiner, 2004). Alternatively, *nonspecific* (or common) causal factors potentially cut across a range of different disorders (e.g., depression, anxiety, bipolar disorders, even schizophrenia) and, in this way, have relatively low discriminatory power (Ingram, 1990; see also D. A. Clark, 1997). Two examples appear to include the experience of uncontrollability (Chorpita & Barlow, 1998) or disturbances in self-focused attention (Ingram, 1990). Such factors can play an important, but nonspecific, role in many disorders, but they do not adequately explain what is distinct, special, or unique about particular disorders.

The theme of causal specificity may apply to the whole configuration of distal and proximal causes. For example, cognitive vulnerability factors, compensatory behaviors, or even precipitating stresses (e.g., Finlay-Jones & Brown, 1981) may be either specific or nonspecific. The search for specific and nonspecific causal factors in cognitive vulnerability models of emotional disorders continues to be a major impetus for research.

Relation Between Cognitive Vulnerability and the Classification of Psychopathology

Emotional disorders can be characterized or classified at different levels of abstraction, and the most appropriate level for focus may depend on the question or circumstances at issue. Consider the case of generalized anxiety disorder and panic disorder. Both are anxiety disorders (at a high level), and for some purposes it may be legitimate to collectively group them as a "single" disorder. Indeed, this was the case (i.e., in the diagnosis of "anxiety neurosis") in classification systems not long ago. The shifts in the diagnostic classification of the two disorders can be interpreted as demonstrating that there are both similarities and differences between these disorders in their underlying causal mechanisms. For example, an underlying core of "inappropriate fear" would seem a common element of anxiety disorders, yet its manifestations vary in different disorders. For example, the core state of fear is persisting and low grade in generalized anxiety disorder, and its manifestations may be muted or curbed by the presence of a largely abstracted and verbal worry process (see chap. 7, this vol.). In contrast, the fear state seems to erupt into a full-blown and uncurbed crescendo in panic disorder. Taken collectively, there is clearly a need to understand both the similarities and dissimilarities in the causes of various emotional disorders.

Relations Between Noncognitive Factors and Cognitive Vulnerability

Additional factors potentially related to vulnerability to emotional disorders—such as personality and demographic variables, developmental experiences, or interpersonal patterns—can be logically placed within the cognitive paradigm. For example, personality characteristics such as negative affectivity or neuroticism can be seen as the consequences of the activation of underlying negative schemata (e.g., Jolly & Kramer, 1994). Factors, such as the availability of social support or of intimate relationships with spouses (or lovers), can be seen as moderating the impact of cognitive vulnerability and stress, because they help to highlight to people that they have positive aspects to their self-identities, world, or future prospects. Hence, having access to social support could perhaps "buffer" vulnerable individuals from the possible detrimental effects of stress by preventing them from succumbing to hopelessness (Dobkin, Panzarella, Fernandez, Alloy, & Cascardi, 2004; Panzarella et al., 2004). For example, in social support, the imparting of more adaptive inferences about the causes, meaning, and consequences of negative life events is particularly helpful. Similarly, factors such as gender or gender-roles can be interpreted within the cognitive paradigm in terms of their relation to dysfunctional rumination patterns that affect a person's focus of attention (e.g., Nolen-Hoeksema, Morrow, & Fredrickson, 1993). Likewise, factors such as physical illness or age could be hypothesized to influence mental or coping resources (e.g., Baumeister & Heatherton, 1996) for counteracting ingrained cognitive biases or neutralizing proximal dysfunctional cognitions when they arise. In these ways, it is often possible to specify testable mental mechanisms or processes by which "noncognitive" variables interact with the cognitive system.

Cognitive models are often based on empirical phenomena or observations that were originally conceptualized in other terms. For example, Lewinsohn's (1974) behavioral theory of depression reinterpreted the psychoanalytic concepts of "loss" and "dependency," respectively, in terms of the ideas of "loss of reinforcement" and "lack of social skills." Current cognitive theories of depression reinterpreted the same phenomena in terms of cognitive processes such as "depressive" inference patterns (see chap. 2, this vol.) or memory structures (see chap. 3, this vol.). Another good example is the "looming vulnerability" model of anxiety (see chap. 7, this vol.). Here, ethological observations of fearful responses to forward moving objects are seen as a "low order" instance of a more general theme and hypothesized effect of inner mental representation of rapidly intensifying danger in humans. As a consequence, cognition includes a broad set of phenomena, and the cognitive clinical paradigm is flexible enough, without much stretching, to include new ideas. Furthermore, by bringing in new observations (e.g., from psychoanalytic, behavioral, ethological, experimental cognitive research), we can broaden our knowledge by making statements of cognitive theory that are not merely explanatory, but also expansive.

Biological Factors and Cognitive Vulnerability–Stress Interactions

In the absence of a relevant cognitive vulnerability, it is also plausible that biologically vulnerable individuals are relatively unlikely to develop an emotional disorder, just like the mere presence of hydrogen molecules is unlikely to coalesce into water (H_2O) without oxygen. For example, it is often suggested that seasonal affective disorder (SAD) or premenstrual syndrome (PMS) are largely biological. However, a common clinical impression of individuals with these disorders is that they often have more generalized cognitive vulnerabilities to depression. Unwanted changes in seasonal patterns of light, or of bodily symptoms due to PMS, may serve as "stresses" in cognitive vulnerability–stress interactions.

It is possible that cognitive vulnerabilities and biological diatheses mutually moderate each other's effects on the development of future emotional disorders. For example, genetic diathesis–stress interactions may be better predictors when individuals have cognitive vulnerabilities. The "stress" produced by psychosocial stressors (i.e., the appraisal of the meaning of the stresses) is dependent on individuals' cognitive vulnerabilities. By the same token, cognitive vulnerability–stress interactions may be more potent predictors of future disorder when individuals have a higher familial genetic risk for the given disorder(s).

Consequently, it could be useful in the future to include assessments of cognitive and biological vulnerability, as well as stress, within the same studies of emotional disorder. For example, a well-known study by Kendler, Neale, Kessler, and Heath (1992) found that anxiety and mood disorders seemed to originate from the same genes, but partly different environments. Had Kendler et al. assessed cognitive vulnerabilities, they might have discovered that anxiety and mood disorders arise from the "same genes, but different cognitive vulnerabilities."

Effects of Multiple Cognitive Vulnerabilities
on Total Risk, Severity, and Comorbidity

Another pair of questions that remains open is whether there are any additional effects due to multiple cognitive vulnerabilities on both the risk or severity of episodes of given disorders or their symptoms and the risk of comorbidity of disorders? In the first case, research has suggested that as psychosocial risk factors (e.g., family dysfunction, child abuse) accumulate, they impose an increasingly greater cumulative "risk burden" on individuals, such that they are more liable to develop psychological problems or disorder. Perhaps there is a comparable cumulative risk burden for multiple cognitive vulnerabilities. For example, do depression-prone individuals have a higher risk for developing depression because they have a *compound vulnerability* (i.e., both dysfunctional attitudes and depressive inferential styles), than if they were to have just one of the cognitive vulnerabilities alone, or even than their summation of effects (e.g., see Riskind, Rholes, Brannon, & Burdick, 1989; Robinson & Alloy, 2003)? Alternatively, is the effect of having two separate cognitive vulnerabilities no greater than the simple effect of having only one alone (i.e., there is a threshold, beyond which there is no additional effect)? In this connection, it seems clear that we can sometimes predict disorder by rather complex interactive combinations of cognitive factors (e.g., see chap. 13, this vol.).

In the second case, from the perspective of cognitive theories, how does the *comorbidity* of emotional disorders develop (Alloy, Kelly, Mineka, & Clements, 1990)? For example, across clinical and nonclinical studies, it is well known that anxiety and depression appear in a comorbid form (e.g., Gotlib, 1984; Zinbarg & Barlow, 1996). In addition, it is known that symptoms of anxiety and depression are often more severe when they co-occur than when they occur separately (see Riskind et al., 1991). If it can be assumed that cognitive vulnerability factors can vary with relative independence of each other across individuals, then it can be inferred that a subset of individuals with *compound vulnerabilities* may be identified (i.e., they combine cognitive vulnerabilities to different disorders) that are far likelier to develop comorbid emotional disorders. Preliminary support for this general proposition is offered by a recent study (not reported here) that assessed both depressive explanatory style and looming maladaptive style, and examined their main effects and interactions (Riskind & Williams, 2000). As expected, individuals who had the compound vulnerability exhibited more severe symptoms of anxiety and depression than would be expected from the simple summation of their separate effects. Thus, the study of cognitive vulnerability factors holds out promise for understanding the psychological antecedents of comorbid emotional disorders.

Disorder-Specific Developmental Pathways?

The conceptual framework in Fig. 1.1 assumes that people's antecedent childhood experiences can help to mold the nature of the cognitive vulnerabilities they later develop. Indeed, there is evidence that early life experiences and developmental events can lead to cognitive vulnerabilities (e.g., see chap. 2, this vol.; Gibb, Alloy, Abramson, & Marx, 2003; Ingram, 2003; Ingram, Bailey, & Siegle, 2004; Riskind et al., 2004; Rogers, Reinecke, & Setzer, 2004; Safford, Alloy, Crossfield, Morocco, & Wang, 2004; Williams & Riskind, 2004). Examples include faulty attachment relationships, parental psychopathology, emotional or physical abuse, negative life stress, physical illnesses, parental modeling, and parental interpretations to children of the meaning of children's experienced events (e.g., see chap. 2, this vol.). But, a crucial question remains: *Why* do similar developmental events seem to lead to presumably different cognitive vulnerabilities (e.g., to depression vs. anxiety)?

It seems quite probable that some developmental factors (e.g., childhood events) are likely to be common rather than specific factors in emotional disorders (echoing the point about common versus specific cognitive vulnerabilities themselves). If developmental variables were to constitute such common factors, they would be expected to play a general, but nonspecific, role in the pathogenesis of many disorders.

Moreover, certain sets of developmental factors (e.g., faulty attachments, or peer rejection), on the one hand, and of parental feedback, on the other, may sometimes *interact* to codetermine the developmental outcomes. If parental (or other adult) feedback is an especially powerful determinant of children's interpretations of events, then it would follow that such feedback has a formidable role in determining the outcome of a developmental event for specific vulnerabilities. For example, the odds that children develop a depressive cognitive vulnerability (e.g., from faulty attachment experiences) could be far higher when their interpretations of the experiences are coupled with depressogenic parental feedback (e.g., "you are worthless and hopeless"). In contrast, the odds that they develop a specific anxiety-related cognitive vulnerability may be far higher when their special meaning is guided by the occurrence of anxiety-producing parental interpretations of the same events (e.g., "displeasing others will cause rejection").

Additionally, and not necessarily incompatible with the aforementioned, it is possible that the variability in the particular factual details of childhood experiences may also help account for differences in the vulnerabilities that are developed. For example, children could be more prone to develop depression-related cognitive patterns if they have been subjected to *unremitting* or relatively constant parental abuse or criticism. In contrast, they might be more prone to develop anxiety-related patterns if they have been subjected to more *variable* parental negative events, and/or if some positive protective factors are present. Therefore, more work on these developmental questions is clearly warranted.

THE ROLE OF THEORY IN DESIGN SELECTION: THE INTERFACE OF THEORY AND RESEARCH METHODS

Thus far, the chapter has examined theoretical features of cognitive vulnerability models and some vital questions that remain open for cognitive models. This section discusses the role that theory plays in the process of design selection and the necessity of tailoring the research design selected to the research questions and specific logic of the cognitive models of interest. First, it examines several questions related to the kinds of causal relations specified, the nature of the vulnerability–stress combination, and the role of cognitive priming. Then it distinguishes several specific logical criteria needed to support a hypothesized vulnerability factor.

Hypothesized Causal Relations in Cognitive Vulnerability–Stress Models

The types of causal relations postulated by a cognitive model are central to selecting an appropriate research design. In addition to the distinction between distal and proximal causes, the appropriate design is also influenced by whether the hypothesized causal role is necessary, sufficient, or contributory. In terms of the latter roles, a necessary cause is an etiological factor that is an essential condition (either in the present or the past) for the disorder to occur. In the absence of the etiological factor, the disorder cannot occur, although the factor by itself does not require the disorder to occur (i.e., the factor is necessary but not sufficient). A sufficient cause is an etiological factor that guarantees the occurrence of the disorder, although the factor may not be necessary for the disorder (e.g., the factor is sufficient but not necessary). A contributory cause increases the statistical likelihood that the disorder will occur by playing a supporting causal role, but is neither necessary nor sufficient for the occurrence of the disorder (Abramson et al., 1989). As previously noted, the distinction between specific and nonspecific causal factors is also important, and has been a major impetus for the emphasis that many recent cognitive models have given to disorder-specific cognitions.

Another chief element of the causal relations in cognitive models has to do with the cognitive vulnerability–stress combination (e.g., Abramson, Alloy, & Hogan, 1997; Alloy et al., 1999; Monroe & Simons, 1991). On the one hand, some cognitive models may hypothesize that the cognitive vulnerability and stress combine in an additive fashion as a straightforward summation. On the other hand, in other models there is true statistical interaction. Here, the cognitive vulnerability and stress are assumed to combine in a true interactive synergism that predicts outcomes beyond the separate additive effects of the vulnerability and stress. For instance, a combination of a high level of cognitive vulnerability and high stress is more likely to lead to an episode of the emotional disorder in question than either factor (or their additive combination) alone. The specific manner in which these factors are postulated to combine determines the appropriate statistical analyses that are needed, as well as the levels of the cognitive vulnerability–stress combination that must be sampled (or experimentally manipulated) to test the model (see Alloy et al., 1999).

Still another element relevant to the hypothesized causal relations lies in the distinction between moderating and mediating factors (Baron & Kenny, 1986; Holmbeck, 1997). A *moderator* is a third variable that codetermines outcomes by affecting the relation between the independent variable (e.g., the cognitive vulnerability or stress or both) and the dependent variable (disorder). In essence, a moderator statistically interacts with the vulnerability or stress (or both) and affects the direction or strength of the relation between the vulnerability–stress combination and disorder. For example, suppose that gender is a moderator. This would mean that the direction and/or strength of the cognitive vulnerability–stress combination would depend on whether participants were male or female. It is also possible that there are even moderator variables that can lead certain cognitive vulnerability factors, under rather limited conditions, to play a protective rather than a vulnerability role.

In contrast, a *mediator* is a third variable assumed to account for the relation between an independent variable (e.g., the distal cognitive vulnerability and proximal stress, or their combination) and the dependent variable (e.g., the disorder). The mediator can be seen as the transitional process or intermediary mental mechanism by which the cognitive vulnerability–stress combination becomes converted into an episode of disorder. For example, as shown in Fig. 1.1, biases in mental processes of memory or attention could be seen as a third variable that mediates the relation between a cognitive vulnerability and the onset of disorder. In essence, moderators specify the conditions under which a vulnerability–stress combination will lead to a disorder. In contrast, mediators specify how or why the vulnerability–stress combination leads to disorder.

The two previous roles become more complicated when third variables simultaneously act as both moderators and mediators (i.e., moderating mediators). To illustrate, a disorder-specific processing bias is hypothesized to play a mediator role in the causal chains by which certain cognitively vulnerable individuals (e.g., with a depressive inferential style) develop an emotional disorder (see Fig. 1.1). At the same time, the disorder-specific processing bias is a third variable that can be hypothesized to play a moderator role in that other cognitively vulnerable individuals who lack the disorder-specific processing bias do not show an equal probability of developing the disorder. In this more complex case, a third variable (e.g., a disorder-specific processing bias) serves to both moderate and mediate the impact of a cognitive vulnerability on the development of a disorder (see Baron & Kenny, 1986, on moderated mediators).

Activation of Cognitive Vulnerabilities

A preceding section briefly alluded to the idea that the degree to which a cognitive vulnerability is in play can be important in cognitive models. Indeed, several models have emphasized that cognitive vulnerabilities can vary dramatically in the degree to which they are engaged and "put into play" in processing at different times (e.g., Ingram, Miranda, & Segal, 1998). During periods when such vulnerabilities are in an inactive or latent state, a cognitive priming task such as a relevant mood-induction or activating provocation task (Riskind & Rholes, 1984) could be required to detect them. Thus, there is an analogy between a cardiac stress test (which is used to reveal a hidden coronary dysfunction) and a cognitive priming task (which is used to reveal a hidden cognitive vulnerability). This being so, it may sometimes be necessary to bring out a latent vulnerability with the aid of an appropriate priming test (for evidence, see chap. 3, this vol.).

Together with a priming task, it may sometimes help in detecting cognitive vulnerabilities to reduce thought suppression. For example, some research shows that an imposed cognitive load (e.g., being asked to retain a sequence of numbers in mind) can help reveal dysfunctional beliefs that are suppressed (Wenzlaff, 1993). Research also suggests that whereas under no load conditions, individuals are apparently able to correct for underlying biases, under cognitive load conditions, they may evidence biases to make negative judgments about other people (Weary, Tobin, & Reich, 2001).

Future research is clearly needed to determine the extent to which the notion of cognitive priming, perhaps in conjunction with an imposed cognitive load, is valuable when attempting to detect different cognitive vulnerabilities (see Alloy et al., 1999). In this regard, certain kinds of cognitive vulnerabilities (e.g., the depressive inferential style, see chap. 2, this vol.) could be chronically accessible (i.e., "pre-potent") because of their frequent use in daily thinking, and hence not require a priming procedure to be observed. The extent to which the detection of different kinds of cognitive vulnerabilities require specific priming for their detection needs further work.

Logical Criteria Necessary for Support of a Putative Cognitive Vulnerability

The main logical criteria that must be satisfied to establish strong empirical support for a hypothesized cognitive vulnerability have not been identified. There are four such criteria. First, the temporal precedence and stability of the vulnerability independent of the symptoms of the disorder must be established (e.g., Alloy et al., 1999; Ingram et al., 1998). That is, the putative vulnerability must temporally precede the initial onset of the disorder, or, in the case of a vulnerability factor for the course of a disorder, it must precede episodes or symptom exacerbations of the disorder (i.e., it has *predictive validity*). Second, it must exhibit some degree of stability independent of the symptoms of the disorder. That is, the vulnerability must be shown to be more than just a transient state manifestation or consequence of the changing symptoms of the disorder.

Third, and of equal importance, alternative explanations of results must be eliminated as plausible options. This aim is achieved in part by establishing that the predicted relationships are not due to potential third variables or confounds (J. Cohen & P. Cohen, 1983; Cook & Campbell, 1979). In this regard, further confidence in the validity of the putative vulnerability is also achieved by providing supplementary evidence that the vulnerability factor plays a causal role in the development of symptoms or onset of disorder (i.e., obtaining evidence for its *construct validity*). That is, confidence in the putative vulnerability is increased by evidence that it is attended by a set of causal mechanisms and causal chains hypothesized by the model (e.g., seen in the figure). Along these lines, important evidence on these issues is supplied by a network of findings showing predicted differences in personality characteristics, information processing, coping patterns, and so forth of individuals who are high or low in cognitive vulnerability (see chap. 2, this vol., for an excellent example). For example, results that can be interpreted as demonstrating the developmental antecedents or mediating processing deficits that are the specific predicted outcomes for the cognitive theory (but not a "rival" third factor) can support the construct validity of the putative cognitive vulnerability.

A fourth, and final, criterion for causal status should also be mentioned. If a theory of interest claims that the vulnerability factor is specific or near-exclusively applicable to a certain disorder, then it must further be shown that the factor is largely applicable to the disorder of interest and not to other disorders (i.e., it has *discriminant validity*). Hence, evidence that the putative vulnerability to a disorder has temporal precedence and stability, while supporting a causal role, does not provide a sufficient basis to establish that the vulnerability factor has specificity. The upshot is that to establish that cognitive factors are specific causes, it is also imperative to directly test the specificity of the predicted outcomes.

ISSUES IN RESEARCH DESIGN

In making choices about suitable research designs for testing a cognitive model, a researcher may be motivated by various factors, including the feasibility of implementing different design options. This section first describes the ideal design in a best case scenario. It then considers some design options and the relative trade-offs of different choices in terms of their strengths and limitations.

Design in a Best Case Scenario

In most research, the strongest test of the causal hypotheses of a cognitive vulnerability model is provided by a true experimental design. The unique importance of experimental designs is that independent variables are directly manipulated, and extraneous factors, including individual differences that are present prior to the study, are controlled. For example, in "clinical trials" or therapy-outcome studies, different treatment conditions (e.g., cognitive therapy versus pharmacotherapy) represent the manipulated independent variable(s), and participants with some disorder (e.g., all with major depressive disorder) are randomly assigned to the different treatment groups or conditions. The effects of the randomly assigned independent variables (e.g., treatment conditions) are then assessed on measures of the dependent variables (e.g., scores on depression inventories). In true experimental designs, the experimental control over sources of error permits a relatively strong basis for assuming that experimental treatments cause group differences. The strong basis for causal inference reflects the fact that the experimental groups are most probably equivalent on all variables (e.g., individual differences between the participants that were present before the experiment) except those that are experimentally manipulated.

The ideal research design also incorporates additional elements that help to rule out possible sources of error. For example, the *internal validity* of experimental manipulations (or of what they are intended to manipulate) is established by means of manipulation checks (e.g., assessments of the fidelity of therapy treatment to a therapy manual). Additionally, "pretest–posttest designs" can be used to ensure that the experimental groups are, indeed, equated on the dependent variables of interest (e.g., depression) before the experimental treatments. "Posttest only" designs that lack pretest measures are open to the threat that their internal validity is compromised because of differences between the groups that were present, due to chance, before assignment to the treatments. In the best case scenario, the ideal research design is entirely experimental, and uses additional elements and experimental controls to rule out possible sources of error.

Needless to say, it is hard to imagine that a researcher would randomly assign participants to different conditions to experimentally manipulate their level of cognitive vulnerability (e.g., high vs. low) and stress (high vs. low). For example, for both ethical as well as pragmatic reasons, researchers would not attempt to randomly assign young children to conditions that manipulate their attachment relationships (e.g., "good" versus "bad") to test their probability of developing future emotional disorders. Thus, cognitive vulnerability researchers almost inevitably rely on other research designs, including analogue, quasi-experimental, and correlational research designs (Alloy et al., 1999).

Analogue and Quasi-Experimental Studies

Given that true experimental designs are usually impossible to implement in research on human cognitive vulnerability, some cognitive vulnerability research uses analogue and quasi-experimental designs. Analogue studies (which can use laboratory animals or nonclinical human participants as proxies for actual clinical patients) can sometimes have value for testing parts of cognitive vulnerability theories. For example, experimental manipulations in *animal analogue* studies have been used to test potential causal variables featured in the learned helplessness model of depression in humans (e.g., see Seligman, 1975). Likewise, experimental manipulations in analogue studies with humans have tested cognitive models of depression by randomly assigning normal (i.e., nondisordered) participants to different mood induction conditions (e.g., depression vs. elation vs. neutral) and assessing mood changes or changes in cognitive biases (e.g., Riskind, 1989). As detailed elsewhere (Abramson & Seligman, 1977), analogue studies must meet certain criteria if they are to have validity as analogues for human psychological problems. In particular, they must establish close similarities between the analogue model (e.g., learned helplessness) and the clinical disorder (e.g., human depression), and between essential features of the disorder (e.g., the motivational and cognitive deficits in depression) and the features of the analogue model (e.g., behavioral and learning deficits in helpless animals). In other words, these studies must establish the construct validity of both the experimental manipulations (e.g., helplessness) and of the dependent variables as models for the disorder of interest. Under conditions when these criteria are met, analogue studies can provide a useful type of convergent evidence for the "construct validity" of the causal mechanisms hypothesized by a cognitive vulnerability model.

A quasi-experimental design can offer another option for testing cognitive vulnerability models. These designs contain some elements of experimental control (e.g., there is, by definition, at least one experimental manipulation), yet they are not wholly experiments because they do not assign participants on a random basis to one of the independent variables (referred to as the "quasi-experimental variable"). For example, responses of high risk (cognitively vulnerable) and low risk (nonvulnerable) individuals might be compared on an experimental laboratory task of memory that manipulates a "within-subjects" factor (e.g., the positive or negative valence of information). Such quasi-experimental designs are, to be sure, generally interpretable and wholly defensible as designs that permit causal inferences for some purposes. For example, the designs are adequate for testing causal inferences "within" the high (or low) cognitive vulnerability group, in that half of the participants are randomly assigned to serve as a control for the other half of the participants who receive a different manipulation or intervention.

At the same time, when any of the statistical analyses involve the quasi-experimental "between-group" variable of interest (e.g., the cognitive vulnerability), the design does not permit an unambiguous test of causal hypotheses. The crux of the difficulty is created by the fact that the participants are "self-selected" into the quasi-experimental groups, rather than randomly assigned. That is, the quasi-experimental groups (e.g., of cognitive vulnerability) may be inadvertently different in neuroticism, gender, other psychopathology, or any other number of third variables that are correlated with the quasi-experimental variable.

One of the main solutions that researchers using quasi-experimental designs often implement to minimize this difficulty is to use a participant matching approach. In one of the two main variants of participant matching, a researcher ensures that when the groups as a whole are compared on the third variables, they are shown not to differ ("samplewide matching"). In the second main variant, each group participant is paired (matched) on a case-by-case basis with a participant in another group who is matched with similar characteristics ("case-by-case matching"). For example, each participant in a cognitive vulnerability group can be paired with another participant who is matched on potential confounding third variables such as gender, educational level, or another demographic detail. In addition to these variants, a further common solution is to use statistical methods such as hierarchical regression analysis or analysis of covariance to remove the effects of potential confounding variables. But none of these solutions can replace the advantages of direct experimental control and random assignment.

Correlational Designs: Cross-Sectional, Look-Back, and Prospective

Still other design options that can be used to study cognitive vulnerability include "cross-sectional," "remitted disorder," and "retrospective or follow-back" designs (Alloy et al., 1999). First, cross-sectional (case control) studies compare a group with a disorder of interest to a normal control group (and, perhaps, groups with other disorders) on characteristics such as their respective scores on cognitive vulnerability measures. Such studies can be seen as preliminary tests or sources of hypotheses of potential vulnerability factors. Even so, they are wholly inadequate for establishing the temporal precedence or stability of a vulnerability independent of the symptoms of the disorder. That is, such designs are saddled with the alternative possibility that scores for the putative cognitive vulnerability are simply correlates, consequences, or "scars" of the disorder, rather than antecedent causes or risk factors of the disorder (Just et al., 2001; Lewinsohn, Steinmetz, Larson, & Franklin, 1981).

Similar difficulties interfere with the causal inferences that can be drawn from "remitted disorder" designs in which previously symptomatic individuals are examined in a remitted state to see whether a hypothesized cognitive vulnerability is present. Such designs can be useful for circumscribed purposes, such as for testing if the presence of cognitive vulnerability factors following an episode of disorder predicts relapses or recurrences of the disorder. Even so, these cannot be used to determine if the cognitive vulnerability factors of interest were actually present before the episode, or if they are really an outcome of the disorder (Just et al., 2001).

Retrospective and follow-back designs are types of longitudinal studies that "look backward" (instead of forward) over time. In retrospective studies, participants are asked to recall information about their cognitive vulnerabilities (or past stresses) before their first episodes. The main problem with these designs is that the recall of participants can be influenced by forgetting, cognitive biases, or even the presence of a current disorder (or early beginnings of disorder; Alloy et al., 1999). For example, if depressed individuals are asked to recall past life experiences, they might exhibit biased recall of stressful events or past dysfunctional attitudes as a consequence of their current depressive moods. In follow-back studies, which are more unbiased in these respects, objective records of participants are located that existed before the onset of disorder (e.g., medical records, personal diaries) and are then compared for group differences. This being said, for present purposes, an especially relevant form of follow-back studies applies *content analysis* techniques (Peterson, Seligman, Yurko, Martin, & Friedman, 1998) to extract cognitive vulnerability patterns (e.g., depressive attributional patterns) from verbatim material. For example, cognitive vulnerabilities may potentially be assessed by verbatim material from diaries, letters, or narratives written by participants years or even decades before. The primary reason for preferring follow-back studies over other "look backward" designs is that the "study" groups examined are compared on objective data, or at least on data that are coded objectively, independent of the experimenters' knowledge of the diagnostic status of the groups. An occasional problem such studies face, however, is that there have been changes over time in the methods or procedures by which the original objective data were recorded.

Beware, however, when using most of the preceding designs ("look backward," remitted disorder, cross-sectional designs) because, in testing cognitive models, individuals in the disorder groups may have developed clinical disorders for highly heterogeneous etiological reasons. For example, the origins of the depressive disorders for some individuals may reside in a biological diathesis or dysfunctional interpersonal patterns, not the hypothesized cognitive vulnerability. Hence, if researchers were simply to compare individuals with or without the emotional disorders, then they may be examining superficially similar disorders that are in fact generated by quite different causal processes. So subjects may present with emotional disorders that have seemingly similar *phenotypes*, but different underlying causes or *genotypes* (see chap. 2, this vol., on hopelessness depression). If it should turn out that no differences in the hypothesized cognitive vulnerability are obtained, then the null results represent an ambiguous basis for inference. For example, it might simply be that an incorrect "subtype" of disorder was selected (not the one with the putative cognitive vulnerability). The main work so far to emphasize this general proposition is on depression. Moreover, a variety of depression theories have advanced "specific symptom" hypotheses about distinct constellations of symptoms associated with specific vulnerability factors (e.g., chap. 2, this vol.; also see Blatt & Zuroff, 1992; Beck, Epstein, & Harrison, 1983). By the same token, it could also prove important for many other emotional disorders or their subtypes to distinguish them by their putative causal processes or underlying genotypes.

Given the normal inability to implement true experimental studies of the development of emotional disorder, it seems safe to say that prospective ("look-forward"), longitudinal studies are the preferred design. Thus, in the "real" best case, a prospective design is used in which the potential cognitive vulnerability is assessed in participants prior to the onset of an episode (or symptoms) of the disorder of interest. In such a design, the cognitive vulnerability is assessed before the measurement at a later point in time of the symptoms or diagnoses of the disorder. On the basis of these features, prospective designs can help to establish both the vulnerability factor's temporal precedence and independence from symptoms (Alloy et al., 1999). Still, these are not the only benefits of a prospective design. For example, an additional reason to prefer prospective studies is that high risk participants have not yet experienced the clinical disorder. Thus, this design removes the potentially confounding effects of the previous presence of the disorders (e.g., of medication, hospitalization). Moreover, possible experimenter bias is eliminated because the researcher does not know who will eventually develop the disorder. It is also worth noting that prospective studies can also be used to establish if the hypothesized cognitive vulnerability applies with specificity to the clinical disorder of interest and not other disorders (i.e., discriminant validity).

Finally, the most preferred form of prospective, longitudinal design is the *behavioral high risk design* (Alloy et al., 1999). In this kind of study, participants are selected who are presently nondisordered but who have behavioral (or cognitive) characteristics postulated to make them vulnerable to possibly developing a particular disorder. These "high risk" participants are then followed prospectively over multiple points in time, along with a comparison group of individuals who score low on the hypothesized risk factor. The behavioral high risk design has the advantage of allowing the researcher to establish the precedence and stability of the hypothesized cognitive vulnerability factor in individuals who do not presently possess the disorder of interest. Another benefit is that the design allows the researcher to examine the role of other factors (e.g., stress, protective factors) in influencing which high risk participants later develop the emotional disorder. Nevertheless, care is still required in such behavioral high risk studies and in selecting participants. For example, it is necessary to ensure the retention of participants because of the possibility of differences in attrition (mortality) between groups that can undermine the validity of results.

Taken collectively, in addition, the generalizability or "external validity" of all these study designs must be examined with care. In other words, it can be an open question as to whether the results generalize or transfer from the specific study sample to other parts of the population. Thus, other studies may be necessary to show that the study generalizes to dissimilar regional, ethnic, socioeconomic segments of the population (for more on sampling strategies, such as heterogeneous sampling, see Alloy et al., 1999).

To summarize the main ideas of this section on design, the ideal design for testing cognitive vulnerability models (i.e., the true experimental study) cannot usually be implemented to examine the development of emotional disorders. Methodological limitations result in highly uncertain conclusions. Behavioral high risk studies provide a good compromise, and are clearly the best designs currently available. However, ultimately, evidence from multiple designs may provide the most compelling convergent validity for the effects of cognitive vulnerabilities. Thus, other research designs can provide useful supplemental support for the construct validity of the hypothesized cognitive vulnerability (e.g., for proposed information-processing biases).

DIFFICULT CONCEPTUAL/METHODOLOGICAL ISSUES IN COGNITIVE VULNERABILITY RESEARCH

Researchers who study cognitive vulnerability to emotional disorders confront several difficult conceptual issues that have bearing on their choices of research design (for more detail, see Alloy, et al., 1999). A complex issue is that most vulnerability models assume the independence of measurements of cognitive vulnerability, stress, and disorder. But, these assumptions are not always warranted. That is, there can be direct effects of emotional disorders on behavior, effects of cognitive vulnerability to disorders on stress, and so on (e.g., see Monroe & Simons, 1991). As an illustration, hopelessness and self-critical thinking can interfere with interpersonal or problem-solving skills or lead depressed individuals to quit jobs or get fired (Hammen, 1991, 2003), and reassurance seeking can lead to rejection by others (Joiner et al., 1992). As Alloy et al. (1999) indicated, these difficult issues pose significant methodological challenges for the researcher.

Finally, several statistical issues can also play critical roles in both the design and analysis of cognitive vulnerability studies. For example, the statistical power of a study (i.e., whether the sample size is large enough to provide a sensitive test of the intended predictions) must be examined to see if it is adequate. In studies of extreme groups (e.g., high risk vs. low risk), there is the potential for statistical regression toward the mean, the nature of which can seriously bias the results.

This chapter has examined general conceptual and methodological issues of psychological vulnerability from the perspective of cognitive theories of emotional disorder. The extension of cognitive vulnerability models to emotional disorders unquestionably represents a uniquely significant advance in their study. This chapter has presented a general conceptual framework of a "prototypical" cognitive vulnerability model that distinguishes distal from proximal causes, developmental events from precipitating events, and specific from nonspecific causes. This framework also recognizes that other protective factors may reduce the likelihood that vulnerable individuals will develop emotional disorders, whereas other exacerbating factors can intensify or prolong disorder. So although there are many complex issues involved in cognitive vulnerability research, it is certain to be an intellectually rewarding and challenging endeavor.

The remaining chapters strongly attest to both the vigor of recent research on cognitive vulnerability processes, and to the role of these processes in determining the likelihood that people will develop emotional disorders. Ultimately, the work presented within this volume has practical as well as theoretical implications. For example, it points to the practical promise of cognitive models in helping to enhance the assessment and diagnosis, treatment, and prevention of emotional disorders (e.g., D. A. Clark, Steer, & Beck, 1994; Dozois & Dobson, 2004). In terms of the overarching cognitive paradigm, the chapters herein extend our current understanding of the psychological mechanisms involved in emotional disorders, as well as amplify our recognition that a great deal of research still remains to be done.

REFERENCES

Abramson, L. Y., Alloy, L. B., & Hogan, M. E. (1997). Cognitive/personality subtypes of depression: Theories in search of disorders. *Cognitive Therapy and Research, 21*, 247–265.

Abramson, L. Y., Metalsky, G. I., & Alloy, L. B. (1989). Hopelessness depression: A theory-based subtype of depression. *Psychological Review, 96*, 358–372.

Abramson, L. Y., & Seligman, M. E. P. (1977). Modeling psychopathology in the laboratory: History and rationale. In J. Maser & M. E. P. Seligman (Eds.), *Psychopathology: Experimental models* (pp. 1–26). San Francisco: Freeman.

Abramson, L. Y., Seligman, M. E., & Teasdale, J. D. (1978). Learned helplessness in humans: Critique and reformulation. *Journal of Abnormal Psychology, 87*, 49–74.

Ainsworth, M. D. S. (1982). *The place of attachment in human behavior.* New York: Basic Books.

Alloy, L. B., Abramson, L. Y., Raniere, D., & Dyller, I. M. (1999). Research methods in adult psychopathology. In P. C. Kendall, J. N. Butcher, & G. N. Holmbeck (Eds.), *Handbook of research methods in clinical psychology* (2nd ed., pp. 466–498). New York: Wiley.

Alloy, L. B., Kelly, K. A., Mineka, S., & Clements, C. M. (1990). Comorbidity of anxiety and depression disorders: A helplessness–hopelessness perspective. In J. D. Maser & C. R. Cloninger (Eds.), *Comorbidity of mood and anxiety disorders* (pp. 499–543). Washington, DC: American Psychiatric Association Press.

Baron, R. M., & Kenny, D. A. (1986). The moderator-mediator variable distinction in social psychological research: Conceptual, strategic, and statistical considerations. *Journal of Personality and Social Psychology, 51*, 1173–1182.

Baumeister, R. F., & Heatherton, T. F. (1996). Self-regulation failure: An overview. *Psychological Inquiry, 7*, 1–15.

Beck, A. T. (1967). *Depression: Clinical, experimental, and theoretical aspects.* New York: Harper & Row.

Beck, A. T. (1976). *Cognitive therapy and the emotional disorders.* New York: International Universities Press.

Beck, A. T. (1991). Cognitive therapy: A 30-year retrospective. *American Psychologist, 46*, 368–375.

Beck, A. T., & Clark, D. A. (1997). An information processing model of anxiety: Automatic and strategic processes. *Behaviour Research and Therapy, 35*, 49–58.

Beck, A. T., Epstein, N., & Harrison, R. (1983). Cognitions, attitudes and personality dimensions in depression. *British Journal of Cognitive Psychotherapy, 1*, 1–16.

Blatt, S. J., & Zuroff, D. C. (1992). Interpersonal relatedness and self-definition: Two prototypes for depression. *Clinical Psychology Review, 12*, 527–562.

Bowlby, J. (1969). *Attachment and loss: Attachment.* New York: Basic Books.

Brown, G. W., & Harris, T. O. (1978). *Social origins of depression.* London: Tavistock.

Chorpita, B. F., & Barlow, D. H. (1998). The development of anxiety: The role of control in the early environment. *Psychological Bulletin, 124*, 3–21.

Clark, D. A. (1997). Twenty years of cognitive assessment: Current status and future directions. *Journal of Consulting and Clinical Psychology, 65*, 996–1000.

Clark, D. A., Beck, A. T., & Alford, B. A. (1999). *Scientific foundations of cognitive theory and therapy of depression.* New York: Wiley.

Clark, D. A., Steer, R. A., & Beck, A. T. (1994). Common and specific dimensions of self-reported anxiety and depression: Implications for the cognitive and tripartite models. *Journal of Abnormal Psychology, 103*, 645–654.

Clark, D. M., & Wells, A. (1995). A cognitive model of social phobia. In R. Heimberg, M. Liebowitz, D. A. Hope, & F. R. Schneider (Eds.), *Social phobia: Diagnosis, assessment and treatment* (pp. 69–93). New York: Guilford.

Cohen, J., & Cohen, P. (1983). *Applied multiple regression/correlation analysis for the behavioral sciences* (2nd ed.). Hillsdale, NJ: Lawrence Erlbaum Associates.

Cohen, S., & Wills, T. A. (1985). Stress, social support and the buffering hypothesis. *Psychological Bulletin, 98*, 310–357.

Cook, T. D., & Campbell, D. (1979). *Quasi-experimentation: Design & analysis issues for field settings.* Boston: Houghton Mifflin.

Dickens, C. (1979). *David Copperfield.* Great Illustrated Classics Edition. New York: Dodd, Mead.

Dobkin, R. D., Panzarella, C., Fernandez, J., Alloy, L. B., & Cascardi, M. (2004). Adaptive inferential feedback, depressogenic inferences, and depressed mood: A laboratory study of the expanded hopelessness theory of depression. *Cognitive Therapy and Research, 28*, 487–509.

Dozois, D. J. A., & Dobson, K. S. (Eds.). (2004). *The prevention of anxiety and depression: Theory, research, and practice.* Washington, DC: American Psychological Association.

Ellis, A. (1970). *Reason and emotion in psychotherapy.* New York: Lyle Stuart.

Finlay-Jones, R., & Brown, G. W. (1981). Types of stressful events and the onset of anxiety and depressive disorders. *Psychological Medicine, 11*, 881–889.

Freud, S. (1964). *The standard edition of the complete psychological works of Sigmund Freud* (J. Strachey, Ed.). Oxford, England: Macmillan.

Fridja, N. (1987). *The emotions*. New York: Cambridge University Press.

Gibb, B. E., Alloy, L. B., Abramson, L. Y., & Marx, B. P. (2003). Childhood maltreatment and maltreatment-specific inferences: A test of Rose and Abramson's (1992) extension of the hopelessness theory. *Cognition & Emotion, 17*, 917–931.

Gotlib, I. H. (1984). Depression and general psychopathology in university students. *Journal of Abnormal Psychology, 93*, 19–30.

Hammen, C. (1991). The generation of stress in the course of unipolar depression. *Journal of Abnormal Psychology, 100*, 555–561.

Hammen, C. (2003). Interpersonal stress and depression in women. *Journal of Affective Disorders, 74*, 49–57.

Holmbeck, G. N. (1997). Toward terminological, conceptual, and statistical clarity in the study of mediators and moderators: Examples from the child-clinical and pediatric psychology literatures. *Journal of Consulting and Clinical Psychology, 65*, 599–610.

Ingram, R. E. (1990). Self-focused attention in clinical disorders: Review and a conceptual model. *Psychological Bulletin, 107*, 156–176.

Ingram, R. E. (2003). Origins of cognitive vulnerability to depression. *Cognitive Therapy and Research, 27*, 77–88.

Ingram, R. E., Bailey, K., & Siegle, Z. (2004). Emotional information processing and disrupted parental bonding: Cognitive specificity and avoidance. *Journal of Cognitive Psychotherapy: An International Quarterly*, 53–64.

Ingram, R. E., Miranda, J., & Segal, Z. V. (1998). *Cognitive vulnerability to depression*. New York: Guilford.

Johnson, S. L., & Roberts, J. E. (1995). Life events and bipolar disorder: Implications from biological theories. *Psychological Bulletin, 117*, 434–449.

Joiner, T. E., Alfano, M. S., & Metalsky, G. I. (1992). When depression breeds contempt: Reassurance-seeking, self-esteem, and rejection of depressed college students by their roommates. *Journal of Abnormal Psychology, 101*, 165–173.

Jolly, J. B., & Kramer, T. A. (1994). The hierarchical arrangement of internalizing cognitions. *Cognitive Therapy and Research, 18*, 1–14.

Just, N., Abramson, L. Y., & Alloy, L. B. (2001). Remitted depression paradigms as tests of the cognitive vulnerability hypotheses of depression onset: A critique and conceptual analysis. *Clinical Psychology Review, 21*, 63–83.

Kelly, G. A. (1955). *The psychology of personal constructs*. New York: Norton.

Kendler, K. S., Neale, M. C., Kessler, R. C., & Heath, A. C. (1992). Major depression and generalized anxiety disorder: Same genes, (partly) different environments? *Archives of General Psychiatry, 49*, 716–722.

Kessler, R. C., McGonagle, K. A., Zhao, S., Nelson, C. B., Hughes, M., Eshleman, S., Wittchen, H. U., & Kendler, K. S. (1994). Lifetime and 12-month prevalence of *DSM–III–R* psychiatric disorders in the United States. Results from the national comorbidity survey. *Archives of General Psychiatry, 51*, 8–19.

Last, C. G., Barlow, D. H., & O'Brien, G. T. (1984). Precipitants of agoraphobia: Role of stressful life events. *Psychological Reports, 54*, 567–570.

Lazarus, R. (1991). *Emotion and adaptation*. New York: Oxford University Press.

Lewinsohn, P. M. (1974). A behavioral approach to depression. In R. J. Friedman & M. M. Katz (Eds.), *The psychology of depression: Contemporary theory and research*. New York: Halstead Press.

Lewinsohn, P. M., Steinmetz, J. L., Larson, D. W., & Franklin, J. (1981). Depression-related cognitions: Antecedent or consequence? *Journal of Abnormal Psychology, 90*, 213–219.

Mathews, A., & MacLeod, C. (1994). Cognitive approaches to emotion and emotional disorders. *Annual Review of Psychology, 45*, 25–50.

Meehl, P. E. (1962). Schizotaxia, schizotypy, schizophrenia. *American Psychologist, 17*, 827–838.

Monroe, S. M., & Simons, A. D. (1991). Diathesis–stress theories in the context of life stress research: Implications for the depressive disorders. *Psychological Bulletin, 110*, 406–425.

Mowrer, O. H. (1939). A stimulus-response analysis of anxiety and its role as a reinforcing agent. *Psychological Review, 46*, 553–565.

Nolen-Hoeksema, S., Morrow, J., & Fredrickson, B. L. (1993). Response styles and the duration of episodes of depressed mood. *Journal of Abnormal Psychology, 10*, 20–28.

Ortony, A., Clore, G. L., & Collins, A. (1988). *The cognitive structure of emotions.* New York: Cambridge University Press.

Panzarella, C., Alloy, L. B., & Whitehouse, W. G. (2004). *Expanded hopelessness theory of depression: On the mechanisms by which social support protects against depression.* Manuscript under editorial review.

Paykel, E. S. (Ed.). (1982). *Handbook of affective disorders.* New York: Guilford.

Peterson, C., Seligman, M. E. P., Yurko, K. H., Martin, L. R., & Friedman, H. S. (1998). Catastrophizing and untimely death. *Psychological Science, 9*, 127–130.

Rachman, S. (1997). A cognitive theory of obsessions. *Behavioral Research and Therapy, 35*, 793–802.

Riskind, J. H. (1989). The mediating mechanisms in mood and memory: A cognitive-priming formulation. *Journal of Social Behavior and Personality, 4*, 173–184.

Riskind, J. H. (1997). Looming vulnerability to threat: A cognitive paradigm for anxiety. *Behaviour Research and Therapy, 35*(5), 386–404.

Riskind, J. H., Moore, R., Harman, B., Hohman, A. A., Beck A. T., & Stewart, B. (1991). The relation of generalized anxiety disorder in general and dysthymic disorder in particular. In R. L. Rapee & D. H. Barlow (Eds.), *Chronic anxiety: Generalized anxiety disorder and mixed-anxiety depression* (pp. 153–171). London: Guilford.

Riskind, J. H., & Rholes, W. S. (1984). Cognitive accessibility and the capacity of cognitions to predict future depression: A theoretical note. *Cognitive Therapy and Research, 8*, 1–12.

Riskind, J. H., Williams, N. L. Altman, M. D., Black, D. O., Balaban, M. S., & Gessner, T. L. (2004). Developmental antecedents of the looming maladaptive style: Parental bonding and parental attachment insecurity. *Journal of Cognitive Psychotherapy: An International Quarterly*, 43–52.

Riskind, J. H., Williams, N. L., Gessner, T., Chrosniak, L. D., & Cortina, J. (2000). The looming maladaptive style: Anxiety, danger, and schematic processing. *Journal of Personality and Social Psychology, 79*, 837–852.

Robins, C. J. (1990). Congruence of personality and life events in depression. *Journal of Abnormal Psychology, 99*, 393–397.

Robinson, M. S., & Alloy, L. B. (2003). Negative cognitive styles and stress-reactive rumination interact to predict depression: A prospective study. *Cognitive Therapy and Research, 27*, 275–291.

Rogers, G. M., Reinecke, M. A., & Setzer, N. J. (2004). Childhood attachment experience and adulthood cognitive vulnerability: Testing state dependence and social desirability hypotheses. *Journal of Cognitive Psychotherapy: An International Quarterly*, 793–790.

Roseman, I. J., Spindel, M. S., & Jose, P. E. (1990). Appraisals of emotion-soliciting events: Testing a theory of discrete emotions. *Journal of Personality and Social Psychology, 59*, 899–915.

Rotter, J. B. (1954). *Social learning and clinical psychology.* Englewood Cliffs, NJ: Prentice-Hall.

Rovner, S. (1993). Anxiety disorders are real and expensive. *Washington Post*, p. WH5.

Roy-Byrne, P. B., Geraci, M., & Uhde, T. W. (1986). Life events and the onset of panic disorder. *American Journal of Psychiatry, 143*, 1424–1427.

Safford, S. M., Alloy, L. B., Crossfield, A. G., Morocco, A. M., & Wang, J. C. (2004). The relationship of cognitive style and attachment to depression and anxiety in young adults. *Journal of Cognitive Psychotherapy: An International Quarterly*, 25–42.

Seligman, M. E. P. (1975). *On depression, development, and death*. San Francisco: Freeman.

Weary, G., Tobin, S. J., & Reich, D. A. (2001). Chronic and temporary distinct expectancies as comparison standards: Automatic contrast in dispositional judgments. *Journal of Personality and Social Psychology, 80*, 365–380.

Weiner, B. (1985). An attributional theory of achievement motivation and emotion. *Psychological Review, 92*, 548–573.

Wenzlaff, R. (1993). The mental control of depression: Psychological obstacles to emotional well-being. In D. M. Wegner & J. W. Pennebaker (Eds.), *Handbook of mental control* (pp. 239–257). Englewood Cliffs, NJ: Prentice-Hall.

Williams, J. M. G., Watts, F. N., MacLeod, C., & Mathews, A. (1988). *Cognitive psychology and emotional disorders*. Chichester, England: Wiley.

Williams, N. L., & Riskind, J. H. (2004). Cognitive vulnerability and attachment. *Journal of Cognitive Psychotherapy: An International Quarterly*, 3–6.

Williams, N. L., Shahar, G., Riskind, J. H., & Joiner, T. E. (2004). The looming maladaptive style predicts shared variance in anxiety disorder symptoms: Further support for a cognitive model of vulnerability to anxiety. *Journal of Anxiety Disorders, 19*, 157–175.

Zinbarg, R. E., & Barlow, D. H. (1996). Structure of anxiety and the anxiety disorders: A hierarchical model. *Journal of Abnormal Psychology, 105*, 181–193.

Zuckerman, M. (1999). *Vulnerability to psychopathology: A biosocial model*. Washington, DC: American Psychological Association.

I

MOOD DISORDERS

2

The Cognitive Vulnerability to Depression (CVD) Project: Current Findings and Future Directions

Lauren B. Alloy
Temple University

Lyn Y. Abramson
University of Wisconsin–Madison

Scott M. Safford
Oregon State University

Brandon E. Gibb
Binghamton University

Research has suggested that depression often occurs following stressful life events (see Monroe & Hadjiyannakis, 2002, for a review). However, individuals can vary widely in their responses to such events. Some may develop severe or long-lasting depression, whereas others do not become depressed at all or may experience mild dysphoria. Several factors have been proposed to explain such individual differences in response to life events. For example, the severity of a given negative life event, the amount of social support an individual receives in the face of a traumatic life event, or individual differences in one's biological constitution or psychological characteristics may all modulate reactivity to stressful events. From a cognitive perspective, the meaning or interpretation individuals give to the life events they experience influences whether or not they become depressed and are vulnerable to recurrent, severe, or long-lasting episodes of depression. Two major cognitive theories of depression, the hopelessness theory (Abramson, Metalsky, & Alloy, 1989; Alloy, Abramson, Metalsky, & Hartlage, 1988) and Beck's theory (Beck, 1967, 1987), reflect such vulnerability–stress models, in which variability in individual susceptibility to depression following stressful events is understood in terms of differences in cognitive patterns that affect how those events are interpreted. According to both theories, particular negative cognitive styles increase an individual's likelihood of developing episodes of depression after experiencing a negative life event—specifically, a cognitively mediated subtype of depression (Abramson & Alloy, 1990; Abramson et al., 1989). These theories propose that people who possess "depressogenic" cognitive styles are vulnerable to depression because they tend to generate interpretations of their experiences that have negative implications for themselves and their futures.

In the hopelessness theory (Abramson et al., 1989), people who exhibit a depressogenic inferential style are hypothesized to be vulnerable to developing episodes of depression, particularly a "hopelessness depression" subtype (HD), when they are exposed to negative life events. This depressogenic inferential style is characterized by a tendency to attribute negative life events to stable (likely to persist over time) and global (likely to affect many areas of life) causes, to infer that negative consequences will follow from a current negative event, and to infer that the occurrence of a negative event in one's life means that one is fundamentally flawed or worthless. People who exhibit such an inferential style should be more likely to make negative inferences regarding the causes, consequences, and self-implications of any stressful event they experience, thereby increasing the likelihood that they will develop hopelessness, the proximal sufficient cause of the symptoms of hopelessness depression.

In Beck's cognitive theory of depression (Beck, 1967, 1987; Beck, Rush, Shaw, & Emery, 1979), negative self-schemata involving themes of inadequacy, failure, loss, and worthlessness are hypothesized to contribute vulnerability to depression. These negative self-schemata are often represented as a set of dysfunctional attitudes, such as "If I fail partly, it is as bad as being a complete failure" or "I am nothing if a person I love doesn't love me." When people with such dysfunctional attitudes encounter negative life events, they are hypothesized to develop negatively biased perceptions of their self (low self-esteem), world, and future (hopelessness), which then lead to depressive symptoms. Although hopelessness theory and Beck's theory differ in terms of some of their specifics, both hypothesize that cognitive vulnerability operates to increase risk for depression through its effects on processing or appraisals of personally relevant life experiences. Despite this similarity, however, studies have suggested that the negative attributional style component of cognitive vulnerability as defined by the hopelessness theory and the dysfunctional attitude component of Beck's theory do represent distinct constructs (e.g., Gotlib, Lewinsohn, Seeley, Rohde, & Redner, 1993; Haeffel et al., 2003; Joiner & Rudd, 1996; Spangler, Simons, Monroe, & Thase, 1997).

A powerful strategy for testing these cognitive vulnerability hypotheses is the *behavioral high risk design* (e.g., Alloy, Lipman, & Abramson, 1992;

Depue et al., 1981). Similar to the genetic high risk design, the behavioral high risk design involves studying individuals hypothesized to be at high or low risk for developing a particular disorder, but who do not currently have one. In a behavioral high risk design, however, individuals are selected based on hypothesized psychological, rather than genetic, vulnerability or invulnerability to the disorder. For example, in testing the cognitive theories of depression, researchers would want to select nondepressed individuals who either have or do not have the hypothesized depressogenic cognitive styles. These groups of cognitively high and low risk individuals can then be compared with respect to their likelihood of having had past occurrences of depression (retrospective design) and their likelihood of experiencing depression in the future (prospective design).

Studies using or approximating a behavioral high risk design have provided substantial support for the cognitive theories of depression. For example, Alloy et al. (1992) utilized a retrospective behavioral high risk design to test the attributional vulnerability hypothesis of the hopelessness theory. They examined the occurrence of major depressive disorder (MD) and HD during the previous 2 years in currently nondepressed undergraduates who either did or did not exhibit attributional vulnerability for depression (indicated by an internal, stable, and global attributional style for negative events). Consistent with the hopelessness theory, they found that attributionally vulnerable students were more likely to exhibit past MD and HD, experienced more episodes, and experienced more severe episodes of these disorders than attributionally invulnerable students. In addition, several other studies approximating a prospective behavioral high risk design have reported that people with negative cognitive styles are more likely to develop depressive moods or symptoms when they experience negative life events than are individuals without such negative styles (e.g., Alloy & Clements, 1998; Alloy, Just, & Panzarella, 1997; Metalsky, Halberstadt, & Abramson, 1987; Metalsky & Joiner, 1992; Metalsky, Joiner, Hardin, & Abramson, 1993; Nolen-Hoeksema, Girgus, & Seligman, 1986, 1992).

These positive results stand in contrast to those found when utilizing typical "remitted depression" designs, which generally have found little support for the cognitive vulnerability hypotheses (e.g., Barnett & Gotlib, 1988; Persons & Miranda, 1992; Segal & Ingram, 1994). In these studies, the cognitive styles of individuals who have recovered from depressive episodes are compared to the cognitive styles of individuals with no history of depression. However, there are several problems with using a remitted depression design to test cognitive vulnerability hypotheses (see Alloy, Abramson, & Just, 1995; Just, Abramson, & Alloy, 2001). For example, depressed individuals are a heterogeneous group and the cognitive theories of depression seek to account for only a subgroup of depressives (i.e., only those with a cognitively mediated subtype of depression). Given that only a subset of such previously depressed individuals are likely to have had a cognitively mediated depression, such heterogeneity can result in equivocal findings when comparing a group of remitted depressed individuals to nondepressed individuals, some of whom may also have a cognitive vulnerability, but have not yet had a depressive episode.

Therefore, in keeping with the suggested methodology already presented, the Temple–Wisconsin Cognitive Vulnerability to Depression (CVD) Project uses a prospective behavioral high risk design to test the cognitive vulnerability and other etiological hypotheses of the hopelessness theory and Beck's theory of depression. The CVD project is a collaborative, two-site study that assesses, among other factors, individual's cognitive styles, the occurrence of negative life events, and the occurrence of both depressive symptoms and clinically significant depressive episodes. This chapter reviews the major findings to date from the CVD project.

CVD PROJECT DESIGN

Participant Selection

Participants were selected for inclusion in the CVD project via a two-phase screening procedure. In the first phase, 5,378 freshmen (2,438 at Temple University, TU, and 2,940 at the University of Wisconsin–Madison, UW) completed two measures of cognitive style: the Cognitive Style Questionnaire (CSQ; Alloy et al., 2000), a modified version of the Attributional Style Questionnaire (ASQ; Peterson et al., 1982), which assesses individuals' styles for inferring causes, consequences, and self-characteristics following the occurrence of positive and negative events, and a modified version of the Dysfunctional Attitudes Scale (DAS; Weissman & Beck, 1978). The primary modifications made to the ASQ in designing the CSQ were that more hypothetical events were included (12 positive and 12 negative events), the hypothetical events were changed to more adequately reflect life events likely to be faced by college students, and the dimensions of consequences and self-characteristics are assessed in addition to the attributional dimensions of internality, stability, and globality. The DAS was modified by adding an additional 24 items that specifically assess dysfunctional beliefs in the achievement and interpersonal domains. Individuals scoring in the highest (most negative) or lowest (most positive) quartile on both the DAS and the CSQ composite (stability + globality + consequences + self) for negative events were designated at high (HR) and low (LR) cognitive risk for depression, respectively (for more details, see Alloy & Abramson, 1999; Alloy et al., 2000). Thus, participants in the CVD project were selected based on the presence versus absence of vulnerability to depression as specified by both the hopelessness theory (Abramson et al., 1989) and Beck's (1967, 1987) theory.

In the second phase of the screening process, a randomly selected subsample of HR and LR participants, who were under age 30, were administered an expanded version of the Schedule for Affective Disorders and Schizophrenia–Lifetime (SADS–L) diagnostic interview (Endicott & Spitzer, 1978). The SADS–L was expanded to allow for the *Diagnostic and Statistical Manual* (*DSM–III–R*; American Psychiatric Association, 1987), as well as Research Diagnostic Criteria (RDC; Spitzer, Endicott, & Robins, 1978) diagnoses, and the data were also recoded according to *DSM–IV* (American Psychiatric Association, 1994). Individuals were excluded from participation in the study if they exhibited any current Axis I disorder, current psychotic symptoms, past history of any bipolar-spectrum disorder, or any serious medical illness that would preclude participation in a longitudinal study. Participants who had a past unipolar mood disorder but had remitted for a minimum of 2 months were retained so as not to result in an unrepresentative sample of HR participants. More specifically, including only those HR participants with no prior history of depressive episodes may have yielded an unrepresentative group of HR participants (e.g., those who exhibit other protective factors, such as strong social support, that warded off the onset of depression). The final CVD project sample included 173 HR (83 at TU, 90 at UW) and 176 LR (87 at TU, 89 at UW) participants. Demographic and cognitive style characteristics of the final sample are presented in Table 2.1 (see Alloy & Abramson, 1999, and Alloy et al., 2000, for more details on the final sample's characteristics and representativeness).

Project Assessments

After agreeing to participate in the study, all participants completed a Time 1 assessment that included measures of Axis II personality disorders and dimensions (Personality Disorders Examination, PDE; Loranger, 1988), self-referent information processing (SRIP Task Battery; Alloy, Abramson, Murray, Whitehouse, & Hogan, 1997), cognitive styles (CSQ, DAS, sociotropy-autonomy, self-consciousness), coping styles (rumination vs. distraction), social support, negative life events (with a combination questionnaire and semi-structured interview modeled after Brown and Harris, 1978), and hypothesized mediating cognitions (inferences for actual events and negative views of self, world, and future). After completing the Time 1 assessment, participants were followed longitudinally for 5½ years. For the first 2½ years of the follow-up, participants completed interview and questionnaire assessments every 6 weeks. For the remaining 3 years of the fol-

TABLE 2.1
Final CVD Project Sample: Demographic
and Cognitive Style Characteristics

	High Risk	Low Risk
Temple Site		
N	83	87
DAS mean item score	4.39 (0.55)	2.17 (0.29)
CSQ–Neg. Comp. mean item score	5.05 (0.47)	2.71 (0.43)
Age (years)	18.45 (1.40)	19.57 (2.98)
Average parental education (years)	13.76 (2.47)	13.45 (2.26)
Combined parental income (US$)	48,061 (36,013)	39,882 (25,906)
Sex (% women)	67.5	66.7
Ethnic group (% Caucasian)	68.3	57.7
Wisconsin Site		
N	90	89
DAS mean item score	4.50 (0.44)	2.23 (0.33)
CSQ–Neg. Comp. mean item score	5.15 (0.40)	2.78 (0.37)
Age (years)	18.67 (0.37)	18.77 (1.14)
Average parental education (years)	15.20 (2.17)	15.03 (2.27)
Combined parental income (US$)	82,911 (100,473)	71,782 (53,219)
Sex (% women)	68.9	67.4
Ethnic group (% Caucasian)	95.6	92.1

Note: DAS = Dysfunctional Attitudes Scale. CSQ–Neg. Comp. = Cognitive Style Questionnaire–Composite for Negative Events.

low-up, participants were interviewed and completed questionnaires every 4 months. During each assessment, questionnaires and interviews were used to assess the occurrence of negative life events, inferences for these events, the components of Beck's (1967, 1987) negative cognitive triad (negative view of self, world, and future), coping styles, social support, and the onset and offset of symptoms and *DSM–III–R* and RDC episodes of depression and other psychopathology. Data from these assessments were also used to assess the onset and offset of symptoms and diagnoses of HD (see Table 2.2 for HD diagnostic criteria).

At the end of each year of follow-up, participants completed measures to reassess their inferential styles and dysfunctional attitudes, as well as their coping styles and self-referent information processing. Further, during the first 2½ years of follow-up, participants and their parents completed a number of measures assessing parents' history of psychopathology, parents' cognitive styles, inferential feedback, and parenting styles, as well as participants' childhood life events and reports of childhood maltreatment. Finally, at the end of the 5½-year follow-up, participants completed a second PDE. For further details about the rationale, design, and methodology of the CVD project, see Alloy and Abramson (1999). Given that the majority of the CVD project data from the second 2½ years

TABLE 2.2

CVD Project Criteria for the Diagnosis of Hopelessness Depression

A	Hopelessness must be present for at least 2 weeks for a definite diagnosis or at least 1 week for a probable diagnosis.
B	At least 5 of the following criterial symptoms must be present for at least 2 weeks, overlapping with each other on at least 12 of 14 days for a definite diagnosis, or at least 4 of the following symptoms must be present for at least 1 week, overlapping with each other on at least 6 out of 7 days for a probable diagnosis.
	Criterial symptoms: sadness, retarded initiation of voluntary responses, suicidal ideation/acts, sleep disturbance–initial insomnia, lack of energy, self-blame, difficulty in concentration, psychomotor retardation, brooding/worrying, lowered self-esteem, dependency
C	The onset of hopelessness must precede the onset of the criterial symptoms by at least 1 day and no more than 1 week.

of follow-up have not yet been analyzed, this chapter focuses primarily on findings so far from the first 2½ years of follow-up.

CVD PROJECT FINDINGS

Do Negative Cognitive Styles Confer Vulnerability to Depression?

A primary hypothesis of the cognitive theories of depression is that certain negative cognitive styles confer vulnerability to symptoms and diagnoses of depression. Although cognitive styles are not immutable (Just et al., 2001) and are open to modification (e.g., through cognitive therapy; see DeRubeis & Hollon, 1995), these styles are typically viewed as relatively stable risk factors. Findings from the CVD project have supported the relative stability of cognitive styles. Specifically, the cognitive styles of our participants remained stable from before to during and after intervening episodes of major depression (Berrebbi, Alloy, & Abramson, 2004). In addition, participants' attributions and inferences for particular negative life events they experienced remained stable over the 5-year follow-up (Raniere, 2000). Thus, cognitive styles appear to be a relatively traitlike vulnerability factor.

One method of testing the cognitive theories' vulnerability hypothesis is to examine whether individuals who exhibit negative cognitive styles are more likely to have a history of depression than are individuals with positive cognitive styles. Thus, in the CVD project, HR participants were expected to have higher lifetime prevalence rates of episodic mood disorders (i.e., MD, minor depression [MiD], and HD) than were LR partici-

TABLE 2.3

Lifetime Prevalence of Depressive and Other Disorders as a Function
of Cognitive Risk Controlling for Age, Phase II Screening BDI Scores, and
SADS–L Current Depressive Symptom Scores

Disorder	Low Risk % ($n = 176$)	High Risk % ($n = 173$)	F_{Risk}	ΔR^2	OR (95% CI)
Major depression	17.0	38.7	9.48***	.025	3.01
(DSM–III–R or RDC)	($n = 30$)	($n = 67$)			(1.84–4.94)
Minor depression	11.9	22.0	3.03*	.008	2.11
(DSM–III–R or RDC)	($n = 21$)	($n = 38$)			(1.18–3.77)
Hopelessness depression	11.9	39.9	22.41****	.059	4.87
(Project Diagnosis)	($n = 21$)	($n = 69$)			(2.81–8.44)
Dysthymic disorder	2.3	3.5	0.37	.001	1.56
(DSM–III–R)	($n = 4$)	($n = 6$)			(0.43–5.64)
Intermittent dysthymic disorder	2.3	4.0	0.37	.001	1.84
(RDC)	($n = 4$)	($n = 7$)			(0.53–6.39)
Depression NOS	3.4	6.4	1.19	.003	1.76
(DSM–III–R)	($n = 6$)	($n = 11$)			(0.63–4.95)
Labile personality	1.1	8.1	0.75	.002	7.76
(RDC)	($n = 2$)	($n = 14$)			(1.74–34.67)
Subaffective dsythymic disorder	0.0	3.5	1.55	.004	13.86
(RDC)	($n = 0$)	($n = 6$)			(0.77–248.04)
Any anxiety disorder	7.4	12.1	0.07	.000	1.76
(DSM–III–R or RDC)	($n = 13$)	($n = 21$)			(0.85–3.63)
Any substance use disorder	8.5	8.7	0.00	.000	1.03
(DSM–III–R or RDC)	($n = 15$)	($n = 15$)			(0.49–2.18)
Other psychiatric disorder	4.0	2.3	0.73	.002	0.58
(RDC)	($n = 7$)	($n = 4$)			(0.17–2.01)

Note: BDI = Beck Depression Inventory; SADS–L = Schedule for Affective Disorders and Schizophrenia–Lifetime Interview; OR = Odds Ratio; CI = Confidence Interval. Degrees of freedom are 1,
338 for major depression, hopelessness depression, labile personality, subaffective dsythymic disorder, any anxiety disorder, and other psychiatric disorder. Degrees of freedom are 1,332 for all other
disorders.
*$p < .08$. ***$p < .01$. ****$p < .001$.
Adapted from "The Temple–Wisconsin Cognitive Vulnerability to Depression Project: Lifetime
History of Axis I Psychopathology in Individuals at High and Low Cognitive Risk for Depression"
by L. B. Alloy, L. Y. Abramson, M. E. Hogan, W. G. Whitehouse, D. T. Rose, M. S. Robinson, R. S.
Kim, & J. B. Lapkin, 2000, Journal of Abnormal Psychology, 109, p. 410. Copyright © 2000 by the American Psychological Association. Adapted with permission.

pants. Controlling for current levels of depressive symptoms, HR participants did indeed exhibit higher lifetime rates of *DSM–III–R* and RDC MD
and HD than did LR participants (Alloy et al., 2000), as well as marginally
higher lifetime rates of RDC MiD (see Table 2.3). In fact, HR participants
were approximately three times more likely to have experienced MD and
almost five times more likely to have experienced HD than were LR participants. The HR–LR differences in lifetime prevalence rates of MD and

HD were maintained when other hypothesized risk factors for depression were controlled (i.e., inferential style for positive events, sociotropy, autonomy, self-consciousness, stress-reactive rumination). Interestingly, the risk groups did not differ in lifetime rates of nonepisodic mood disorders (i.e., *DSM–III–R* dysthymic disorder or RDC intermittent depressive disorder). Supporting the specificity of cognitive vulnerability to the depressive disorders, there were also no risk group differences in participants' lifetime histories of anxiety disorders, substance use disorders, or other psychiatric disorders. Following up on these findings, Haeffel et al. (2003) used an unselected sample of undergraduates to "unpack" the generic cognitive vulnerability of the CVD project. Haeffel et al. found that negative inferential styles, but not dysfunctional attitudes, uniquely predicted lifetime history of clinically significant depressive episodes and anxiety comorbid with depression.

Despite the strengths of these findings, they do not adequately address whether negative cognitive styles serve as a vulnerability factor for depression, because the findings are equally supportive of the alternate hypothesis that negative cognitive styles are a consequence or "scar" left by the past experience of depression (see Lewinsohn, Steinmetz, Larson, & Franklin, 1981). Therefore, to adequately test the cognitive vulnerability hypothesis, data from the prospective portion of the CVD project are required. Results from the first 2½ years of follow-up in the CVD project indicate that risk group status predicted both first onsets and recurrences of both MD and HD during this time period (Alloy, Abramson, Whitehouse, et al., in press). Specifically, among individuals with no prior history of depression, HR participants were more likely than were LR participants to experience a first onset of MD, MiD, and HD (see Table 2.4). These findings provide especially important support for the cognitive vulnerability hypothesis because they are based on a truly prospective test, uncontaminated by prior history of depression. In addition, among individuals with a past history of depression, HR participants were more likely to experience recurrences of MD, MiD, and HD than were LR participants (see Table 2.4). Similar to the results of the retrospective analyses, there were no risk group differences in either first onsets or recurrences of anxiety disorders or other disorders. However, in the full sample, HR participants were more likely than LR participants to have an onset of anxiety disorder comorbid with depression, but not an anxiety disorder alone. Further, each of these results was maintained even after statistically controlling for participants' initial levels of depressive symptoms upon entering the study, as assessed by the Beck Depression Inventory (BDI; Beck et al., 1979).

In addition to contributing vulnerability to depression, the cognitive theories hypothesize that negative cognitive styles should confer risk for suicidality, ranging from suicidal ideation to completed suicides, and that

TABLE 2.4
CVD Project Prospective Rates of First Onsets
and Recurrences of Depressive and Anxiety Disorders

Disorder	Low Risk	High Risk	OR	95% CI	p
Prospective Rates of Depressive and Anxiety Disorders: First Onsets (Subsample With No Prior Depression)					
Any major depression	2.7%	16.2%	7.4	1.6–34.8	.01
RDC minor depression	14.4%	45.9%	5.6	2.2–14.1	.001
Any episodic depression	16.2%	45.9%	4.9	2.0–12.2	.001
Hopelessness depression	3.6%	35.1%	11.6	3.3–41.3	.001
Any anxiety disorder	0.9%	6.8%	9.3	0.8–113.3	.09
Prospective Rates of Depressive and Anxiety Disorders: Recurrences (Subsample With Prior Depression)					
Any major depression	9.4%	28.6%	3.8	1.3–11.0	.02
RDC minor depression	32.8%	56.1%	3.1	1.4–7.0	.02
Any episodic depression	34.4%	62.2%	4.4	1.9–10.1	.001
Hopelessness depression	18.8%	50.0%	4.1	1.7–10.0	.002
Any anxiety disorder	4.7%	10.2%	4.0	0.8–21.5	.11

levels of hopelessness should mediate this relation. Findings from the CVD project have supported this hypothesis (Abramson et al., 1998). Specifically, HR participants were more likely than were LR participants to have a prior history of suicidality. HR participants also had higher levels of suicidality across the first 2½ years of follow-up than did LR participants, and this relation was maintained even after statistically controlling for participants' prior history of suicidality and for other risk factors for suicidality (i.e., prior history of *DSM–III–R* and/or RDC MD, RDC MiD, borderline personality dysfunction, antisocial personality dysfunction, and parental history of depression). This relation was mediated by the participants' mean levels of hopelessness across the 2½-year follow-up.

Thus, both retrospective and prospective results from the CVD project have supported the vulnerability hypothesis of the cognitive theories of depression. Specifically, participants with negative cognitive styles were more likely to have had a past episode of MD and HD and were more likely to experience both first onsets and recurrences of MD, MiD, and HD during the 2½-year follow-up than were participants with positive cognitive styles. Importantly, the risk group differences were not due to residual differences between the groups in levels of depressive symptoms. Similarly, participants with negative cognitive styles were more likely to have a past history of suicidality and higher levels of suicidality across the 2½-year follow-up than were participants with positive cognitive styles. The CVD project findings are important because they provide the first demonstration that, as predicted by the cognitive theories of depression, negative cognitive styles confer risk for full-blown, clinically significant depressive disorders and suicidality. The results also provide support for the hypothesis that the subtype of HD exists in nature and conforms to theoretical description.

SPECIFICITY OF NEGATIVE COGNITIVE STYLES TO HOPELESSNESS DEPRESSION

The hopelessness theory (Abramson et al., 1989) proposes that negative cognitive styles confer vulnerability to HD, specifically, rather than to other subtypes of depression. Supporting this hypothesis, studies have found that negative cognitive styles, both alone and interacting with negative life events, are more strongly related to depressive symptoms hypothesized to be part of the HD symptom cluster (see Table 2.2) than to symptoms not part of the HD symptom cluster (Alloy & Clements, 1998; Alloy et al., 1997; Hankin, Abramson, & Siler, 2001; Joiner et al., 2001; Metalsky & Joiner, 1997) or to symptoms of other forms of psychopathology (Alloy & Clements, 1998). In addition, preliminary analyses based on the first 2½ years of prospective follow-up in the CVD project indicated that cognitive risk predicted first onsets and recurrences of HD (as described earlier), but not *DSM* melancholic depression.

RUMINATION AS A MEDIATOR AND MODERATOR OF COGNITIVE VULNERABILITY TO DEPRESSION

According to the response styles theory of depression (Nolen-Hoeksema, 1991), individuals who tend to ruminate in response to dysphoria will be at increased risk for experiencing more severe and prolonged depressions than will individuals who tend to distract themselves from their dysphoria. Rumination refers to "behaviors and thoughts that focus one's attention on one's depressive symptoms and on the implications of these symptoms" (Nolen-Hoeksema, 1991, p. 569), whereas distraction refers to active attempts to ignore depressive symptoms by focusing on pleasant or neutral activities. Several studies have found support for this theory, demonstrating that rumination is associated with a greater likelihood of major depression and longer and more severe episodes of depression (e.g., Just & Alloy, 1997; Morrow & Nolen-Hoeksema, 1990; Nolen-Hoeksema, 2000; Nolen-Hoeksema & Morrow, 1991; Nolen-Hoeksema, Morrow, & Fredrickson, 1993; Nolen-Hoeksema, Parker, & Larson, 1994; Spasojevic & Alloy, 2001). Abramson et al. (2002) described the expected relation between the cognitive vulnerabilities featured in hopelessness and Beck's theories and rumination and hypothesized that rumination would mediate the effects of these cognitive vulnerabilities on the prospective development of depressive episodes. Consistent with this hypothesis, Spasojevic and Alloy (2001) found that a ruminative response style measured at Time 1 of the CVD project mediated the association between cognitive risk status and the development of prospective episodes of MD. Rumination also mediated the effects of other risk factors (past history of depression, maladaptive dependency, and self-criticism) for MD onset during the follow-up period.

Expanding on the response styles theory, Robinson and Alloy (2003) hypothesized that individuals who have negative inferential styles and, additionally, who tend to ruminate about these negative cognitions in response to the occurrence of stressful life events (stress-reactive rumination), may be more likely to develop episodes of depression in the first place. The idea is that negative cognitive styles provide the negative content, but this negative content may be more likely to lead to depression when it is "on one's mind" than when it is not. Accordingly, Robinson and Alloy proposed that stress-reactive rumination would exacerbate the association between negative cognitive styles and the onset of a depressive episode. Consistent with this hypothesis, using CVD project data, they found that stress-reactive rumination when assessed at Time 1 interacted with cognitive risk to predict prospective onsets of MD and HD episodes (see Fig. 2.1). Among the cognitively LR participants, there was no difference found in the likelihood of future onset of depression based on whether or not such individuals tended to evidence stress-reactive rumination. On the other hand, among the cognitively HR participants, individuals who were also high in stress-reactive rumination evidenced a higher prospective incidence of MD and HD than high risk individuals who did not tend to ruminate in response to stressors.

COGNITIVE VULNERABILITY–STRESS INTERACTION AND PROSPECTIVE DEVELOPMENT OF DEPRESSION

Given that the cognitive theories of depression are vulnerability–stress models in which depressogenic cognitive styles are proposed to confer vulnerability to depression when individuals confront negative life events, it is important to evaluate the interaction between cognitive style and the occurrence of negative life events in predicting onset/recurrence of depression. As indicated earlier, several previous studies have found support for the vulnerability–stress hypothesis (Alloy & Clements, 1998; Alloy et al., 1997; Anderson, 1990; Metalsky et al., 1987, 1993; Metalsky & Joiner, 1992; Nolen-Hoeksema et al., 1986, 1992; Panak & Garber, 1992;

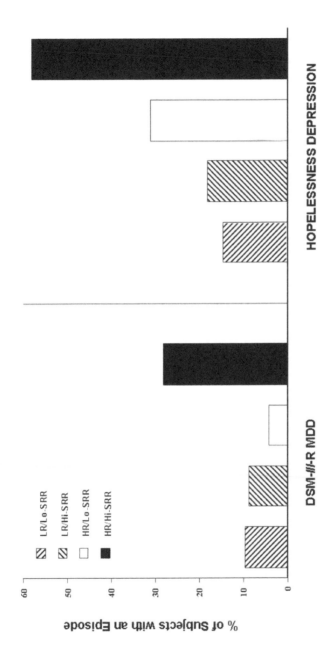

FIG. 2.1. Prospective incidence rate of *DSM–III–R* major depressive disorder (left) and hopelessness depression (right) as a function of cognitive risk group status and Time 1 stress-reactive rumination. LR = Low Risk; HR = High Risk; Lo-SRR = Low Stress-Reactive Rumination; Hi-SRR = High Stress-Reactive Rumination.

Robinson, Garber, & Hilsman, 1995) in predicting depressive symptoms. However, there have been a handful of published studies that have found no support for this hypothesis (Cole & Turner, 1993; Joiner & Wagner, 1995; Tiggemann, Winefield, Winefield, & Goldney, 1991).

To date, little evaluation of the vulnerability–stress hypothesis has been conducted with the CVD project data. Preliminary investigation of this hypothesis using the Temple site data only, in which negative life events were coded as loss and/or danger events using the criterial definitions of Finlay-Jones and Brown (1981), revealed that negative cognitive style, loss events, and danger events all significantly predicted the occurrence of depressive episodes (Safford & Alloy, 1999). However, there were no vulnerability–stress interactions found for episodes of either MD or HD. This particular study evaluated the effects of cognitive style and life events on the first depressive episode experienced during the course of the CVD project, controlling for past history of depression. Further analyses are needed to evaluate if this lack of significant findings is true when both sites' data are used and for all negative life events or just for these two subgroups of life events. In a second preliminary evaluation of the occurrence of depressive episodes across the first 2½ years of follow-up in the CVD project (Robinson, 1997), also using Temple site data only, marginally significant to significant relations were found between the cognitive style × number of negative life events interaction and number of episodes of any depressive disorder, including both minor and major episodes. A third preliminary study of the occurrence of MD and HD episodes across the first 9 months of follow-up in the CVD project using only Temple site data (Panzarella, Alloy, & Whitehouse, in press) found that the interaction between cognitive risk and the number of negative life events predicted onsets of both MD and HD. Moreover, the cognitive vulnerability–stress interaction was further moderated by social support. HR participants with high stress and poor social support had a higher likelihood of developing a MD or HD episode than participants with 0, 1, or 2 of the 3 risk factors. As such, more definitive work remains to be done to evaluate the validity of the vulnerability–stress hypothesis in predicting depressive episodes in the CVD project data from both sites.

Characteristics of Cognitively Vulnerable Individuals

Self-Referent Information Processing. The cognitive theories of depression hypothesize that individuals who are cognitively vulnerable to depression tend to process information about themselves in a negatively biased fashion. For example, Beck (1967, 1987) hypothesized that certain individuals possess negative self-schemata that negatively color their perception, interpretation, and memory of personally relevant experiences.

Similarly, the hopelessness theory (Abramson et al., 1989) proposes that individuals with a negative cognitive style tend to infer negative self-characteristics following the occurrence of negative life events.

Data from the Self-Referent Information Processing (SRIP) Task Battery, administered at the Time 1 assessment of the CVD project, were used to test these hypotheses. Given Beck's hypothesis that individuals with a negative self-schema should demonstrate biased information processing only for depression-relevant stimuli (i.e., stimuli related to themes of incompetence, worthlessness, and low motivation), Alloy et al. (1997) predicted that HR participants would demonstrate information-processing biases for depression-relevant, but not depression-irrelevant, self-referent adjectives. Partial support was obtained for this hypothesis. Specifically, as predicted, compared to LR participants, HR participants showed preferential self-referent processing compared to LR participants for negative depression-relevant material (e.g., words like "failure," "passive," and "useless") as evidenced by relatively greater endorsement, faster processing, greater accessibility, better recall, and higher predictive certainty of this material. In addition, HR participants were less likely to process positive depression-relevant stimuli (e.g., words such as "resourceful," "energetic," and "important") than were LR participants. Finally, although contrary to prediction, there were risk group differences for the depression-irrelevant material on two of the tasks. Specifically, LR participants were more likely than HR participants to judge positive depression-irrelevant stimuli as self-descriptive (e.g., words like "thoughtful") and believed they were more likely to engage in future positive depression-irrelevant behaviors (e.g., giving up a seat on a bus for an elderly lady). However, the group differences were larger for depression-relevant than for depression-irrelevant stimuli even on these tasks. Importantly, all of the risk group differences were maintained even after participants' levels of depressive symptoms were statistically controlled. These findings are unique in demonstrating that the information-processing biases previously demonstrated in depressed individuals (see Ingram, Miranda, & Segal, 1998; Segal, 1988) also extend to nondepressed individuals at high cognitive risk for depression.

We also examined whether the negative self-referent processing exhibited by HR individuals mediated or moderated the predictive association between cognitive risk and prospective onsets of depressive episodes (Steinberg, Oelrich, Alloy, & Abramson, 2004). A composite of the five dependent measures from the SRIP Task Battery partially mediated the cognitive risk effects for prediction of HD episodes, but not MD or MiD episodes. This finding is interesting because HD is hypothesized specifically to be a cognitively mediated subtype of depression. In addition, the negative SRIP composite interacted with cognitive risk to predict first onsets, but not recurrences, of MD and HD. Individuals who both exhibited negative cognitive styles and negative information processing about themselves were at increased risk for a first onset of depression compared to individuals with either of these risk factors alone.

Cognitive Vulnerability and Personality Characteristics. In addition to evaluating negative information processing about the self in individuals prone to depression, it is also important to evaluate the relation between cognitive vulnerability to depression and other personality characteristics and disorders. For example, it has been proposed that individuals with negative cognitive styles might be at increased risk for Axis II personality dysfunction (Smith et al., 2004). In support of this hypothesis, previous studies have indicated that comorbidity between depression and personality disorders is high, ranging from 30% to 70% (see Farmer & Nelson-Gray, 1990). In addition, depressed inpatients with comorbid personality disorders, especially borderline personality disorder, have been found to be more likely to exhibit negative cognitive styles than are depressed inpatients without comorbid personality disorders (Rose, Abramson, Hodulik, Halberstadt, & Leff, 1994). Finally, many personality disorders are partially defined by cognitive patterns that are consistent with definitions of depressogenic cognitive style (Beck et al., 1990). For example, the Cluster C personality disorders (Avoidant, Dependent, and Obsessive-Compulsive) were found to be associated with feelings of incompetence, helplessness, and weakness.

Although the relative specificity of depressogenic cognitive styles has been demonstrated for Axis I psychopathology (e.g., Alloy et al., 2000; Alloy, Abramson, Whitehouse, et al., in press), it has been proposed that such cognitive specificity would not be likely to occur for Axis II personality disorders (Smith et al., 2004). This hypothesized nonspecificity is due to the fact that personality disorders are frequently comorbid with each other and all three of the personality clusters have been associated with depression (Farmer & Nelson-Gray, 1990). In addition, all of the personality clusters are associated with cognitive, behavioral, and interpersonal characteristics consistent with those likely to be found in individuals who are cognitively vulnerable to depression (Smith et al., 2004). In contrast to this proposed nonspecificity between negative cognitive styles and the various personality disorders, there is some evidence that negative cognitive style and HD may be more specifically related to borderline and dependent personality functioning than to other personality disorders (Akhavan, 2000).

To further examine the relation between cognitive style and personality dysfunction, the Personality Disorder Examination (PDE; Loranger, 1988) was administered to all participants at the beginning and end of the CVD project. The PDE interview provides *DSM–III–R* categorical personality disorder diagnoses as well as dimensional scores for each disorder. In analyses of personality dysfunction, as assessed by the PDE at Time 1 of the CVD project, the cognitively high risk group had significantly more diagnosable personality disorders than the low risk group (5.4 vs. 1.7%; Smith et al., 2004). Although these percentages are low for both groups, it must be kept in mind that participants in the CVD project were quite young (mean age = 19 years) and, therefore, relatively unlikely to have full-blown personality disorder. For example, Loranger (1988) indicated that it is difficult to accurately diagnose personality disorder in individuals younger than age 25. Therefore, the fact that HR individuals were more than twice as likely to have a diagnosable personality disorder at such a young age is a significant finding. In addition, although there were not enough participants with diagnosable personality disorders to examine the rates of each personality disorder category separately, all three personality clusters were represented in those diagnosed.

When evaluating personality dysfunction using the dimensional scores, the HR group was rated higher than the LR group for Cluster A paranoid and schizotypal dimensions, Cluster B borderline, histrionic, and narcissistic dimensions, and Cluster C avoidant, dependent, obsessive-compulsive, and passive-aggressive dimensions. Schizoid, antisocial, and sadistic personality dysfunction were the only personality dimensions on which no significant risk group differences were found. The strength of these findings is bolstered by the fact that, except for the narcissistic, passive-aggressive, and self-defeating dimensions, these HR–LR differences remained after statistically controlling for the participants' depressive symptom levels, based on their BDI scores. In addition, the risk group differences in the lifetime prevalence of episodic unipolar depressive disorders (major, minor, and HD) reported by Alloy et al. (2000) remained after statistically controlling for the effects of personality dysfunction. Therefore, although an association exists between negative cognitive style and personality disorder, personality dysfunction does not appear to be a sole mediator of the relation between cognitive vulnerability and depression.

Aside from *DSM* personality dysfunction, other personality characteristics have been linked to depression and deserve attention in regard to cognitive vulnerability for depression as well. For example, *sociotropy* and *autonomy* (Beck, 1983) represent two personality subtypes believed to confer vulnerability to depression when an individual experiences negative life events that are congruent with these personality traits. Sociotropy is believed to be a personality style characterized by concern about interpersonal relatedness and fear of rejection or abandonment. Individuals exhibiting this personality style are hypothesized to be prone to depression when they experience interpersonal stresses and losses, such as the break-up of a relationship or a fight with a friend. On the other hand, autonomy is believed to be a personality style characterized by concern for achievement, independence, and self-definition. Autonomous individuals are hypothesized to be at risk for depression when they experience failure to achieve goals they set for themselves, such as receiving a poor grade in school, or failing to get a promotion at work.

To date, there has been little published research on the relation between depressogenic cognitive styles and these two personality subtypes. In some analyses of the CVD project data, this relation was examined (Abramson, Alloy, & Hogan, 1997). HR participants showed greater sociotropy than did LR participants, even after controlling for their current level of depression. However, the opposite was found to be true with regard to autonomy. Specifically, HR individuals showed a trend toward less autonomy than LR individuals both before and after controlling for current depression levels. This suggests that HR individuals should be more prone to sociotropic, but not autonomous, depressions.

The aforementioned relations between cognitive vulnerability for depression and various personality dysfunction, disorders, and subtypes represent an important contribution to the continued evaluation and expansion of cognitive theories of depression. By incorporating an examination of personality and interpersonal functioning, these findings extend the growing body of research investigating the cognitive–behavioral–interpersonal configurations that confer risk for depression (e.g., Alloy, Fedderly, Kennedy-Moore, & Cohan, 1998; Gotlib & Hammen, 1992; Joiner, Alfano, & Metalsky, 1992; Panzarella et al., in press; Segrin & Abramson, 1994).

Developmental Antecedents of Cognitive Vulnerability to Depression

Evidence shows that negative cognitive styles do indeed confer vulnerability to future episodes of both depression and suicidality, so it is important to understand factors that may contribute to the development of such styles. Data from the CVD project allow an initial examination of several factors that may contribute to the development of these cognitive styles (see Alloy et al., 2004, for an in-depth review of the developmental findings from the CVD project). As part of the CVD project, we assessed the cognitive styles and lifetime history of psychopathology of 335 of our participants' parents (217 mothers, 118 fathers). In addition, participants and their parents were asked to report the parents' inferential feedback styles and parenting styles. Finally, participants' reports of childhood maltreatment were assessed.

Parental Psychopathology. Given previous research suggesting that children of depressed parents are at increased risk for the development of negative attributional styles (e.g., Garber & Flynn, 2001; Hammen, 1992) and episodes of depression (e.g., Downey & Coyne, 1990), data from the CVD project were used to examine the relation between participants' cognitive risk status and their parents' history of depression. Parental history of depression was assessed using the reports of our participants (i.e., family history RDC method; Andreason, Endicott, Spitzer, & Winokur, 1977), and from direct interviews of the parents themselves, using the expanded SADS–L.

Preliminary data from the CVD project suggest that there was a relation between participants' cognitive risk group status and their parents' histories of depression (Abramson et al., 2004). This relation, however, appears to be stronger for mothers' than for fathers' histories of depression. Specifically, HR participants, compared to LR participants, reported that their mothers were significantly more likely, and their fathers were marginally more likely, to have a past history of depression. In the direct interviews of the parents, mothers of HR participants were more likely to have had a past history of depression than were mothers of LR participants. There were no group differences, however, for fathers' histories of depression. These findings are unique in demonstrating a relation between parents' histories of depression and the cognitive styles of nondepressed individuals, and provide support for explorations of possible mediators of the association between parental depression and offspring's cognitive vulnerability to depression.

Modeling and Parental Inferential Feedback. Parents may influence the cognitive styles of their children through modeling their own negative cognitive style or by providing negative inferential feedback regarding the causes and consequences of negative events in their children's lives. However, studies have provided only limited support for a direct relation between parents' and their children's negative cognitive styles. For example, in the CVD project, the mothers of HR participants had more dysfunctional attitudes than did mothers of LR participants, even after controlling for the mothers' levels of depressive symptoms (Alloy et al., 2001). In contrast, there were no risk group differences in mothers' or fathers' inferential styles or in fathers' dysfunctional attitudes. In another study, however, third, fourth, and fifth graders' attributional styles were significantly related to those of their mothers, but not their fathers (Seligman et al., 1984). Finally, in a third study, no relation was found between sixth graders' attributional styles and those of their mothers (Garber & Flynn, 2001). Thus, although there is some evidence that children may model the cognitive styles of their parents, especially their mothers, future studies are needed to further examine this relation. Given the mixed results obtained thus far, future studies should examine potential moderating factors that may either strengthen or weaken the relation (e.g., amount of time spent with parent).

Studies have provided more consistent support for the hypothesis that negative parental inferential feedback may contribute to the development of a negative cognitive style in their children. For example, according to both participants' and their parents' reports and controlling for respondents' levels of depressive symptoms, both mothers and fathers of HR participants in the CVD project provided more stable, global attributional feedback than did mothers and fathers of LR participants (Alloy et al., 2001). Similarly, controlling for respondents' levels of depressive symptoms, mothers of HR participants also provided more negative consequence feedback for negative events in their child's life than did mothers of LR participants, according to both respondents' reports, as did fathers of HR participants according to the participants' reports. In addition, negative attributional and consequence feedback from mothers interacted with a history of high levels of childhood stressful life events to predict HR status (Crossfield, Alloy, Abramson, & Gibb, 2002). Moreover, the negative inferential feedback from parents predicted prospective onsets of depressive episodes in their children over the 2½-year follow-up period, mediated, in part or totally, by the children's cognitive risk status (Alloy et al., 2001).

These results have been supported in other studies. For example, sixth graders' attributional styles for positive and negative life events were correlated with their mothers' attributional styles for the same child-relevant events (Garber & Flynn, 2001). In addition, adolescents' attributional styles were significantly related to their fathers', but not mothers', attributional styles for the same child-relevant events (Turk & Bry, 1992). Thus, there is some evidence that parents may contribute to the development of negative cognitive styles in their children, not by the children modeling the attributions their parents make for negative events in the parents' lives, but by the attributional and consequence feedback the children receive from their parents for negative events in the children's own lives.

Parenting Styles. Studies have suggested that certain parenting styles may also contribute to the development of a negative cognitive style in children. For example, both HR participants in the CVD project and their fathers reported that the fathers exhibited less warmth and acceptance (and more rejection) than did fathers of LR participants (Alloy et al., 2001). There were no group differences, however, for fathers' levels of either psychological autonomy versus control or firm versus lax control (discipline), nor were there any group differences in the parenting styles of mothers. Fathers' acceptance scores also predicted prospective onsets of MD, MiD, and HD episodes in their children, but only the prediction of HD episodes was mediated by the children's cognitive risk status (Alloy et al., 2001). In a longitudinal study of sixth graders and their mothers, higher levels of maternal psychological control were associated with increasing negativity of their children's attributional styles over a 1-year follow-up, even after controlling for the mothers' histories of mood disorders (Garber & Flynn, 2001). In this study, neither parental acceptance versus rejection nor firm versus lax control were related to changes in the children's attributional styles. Finally, undergraduates with a negative cognitive style reported less maternal care when growing up than did undergraduates with a positive cognitive style (Whisman & Kwon, 1992). In this study, undergraduates' cognitive styles were not related to the degree of maternal overprotection reported during childhood.

Thus, although these studies suggest a relation between certain parenting styles and children's cognitive styles, they do not agree as to which parenting styles are the most detrimental. In addition, only one study (Alloy et al., 2001) from the CVD project has examined the parenting practices of fathers. Future studies, therefore, should seek to clarify the relation between parenting practices and children's negative cognitive styles and should seek to include fathers in this evaluation.

Childhood Maltreatment.   In extending the etiological chain of the hopelessness theory, Rose and Abramson (1992) proposed a developmental pathway by which negative life events, especially childhood maltreatment, may lead to the development of a negative cognitive style. Specifically, they suggested that when maltreatment occurs, individuals attempt to understand the cause, consequences, and meanings of the abuse so that future negative events may be avoided and hopefulness may be maintained. Thus, after the occurrence of maltreatment, children may initially make hopefulness-inducing attributions about its occurrence. For example, children may initially explain being beaten or verbally abused by their father by saying, "He was just in a bad mood today," which is an external, unstable, and specific explanation. With the repeated occurrence of maltreatment, however, these hopefulness-inducing attributions may be disconfirmed, leading children to begin making hopelessness-inducing attributions about its occurrence. For example, children may explain the maltreatment by thinking, "I'm a terrible person who deserves all the bad things that happen to me," which is an internal, stable, and global explanation that entails negative consequences and negative self-characteristics. Over time, these attributions may generalize to initially unrelated negative events. In this way, a relatively stable and global negative cognitive style may develop.

Researchers have only recently begun to evaluate the relation between childhood maltreatment and cognitive styles. These initial evaluations, however, have supported Rose and Abramson's hypotheses. For example, controlling for their levels of depressive symptoms, HR participants in the CVD project reported significantly higher levels of childhood emotional, but not physical or sexual, maltreatment than did LR participants (Gibb, Alloy, Abramson, Rose, Whitehouse, Donovan, et al., 2001). In addition, participants' cognitive risk status fully mediated the relation between reported levels of childhood emotional maltreatment and the occurrence of *DSM–III–R* and RDC nonendogenous MD during the first 2½ years of follow-up. Further, participants' cognitive risk status fully mediated, and their average levels of hopelessness partially mediated, the relation between reported levels of childhood emotional maltreatment and the occurrence of HD during the first 2½ years of follow-up. To address the possibility that the association of childhood emotional maltreatment with negative cognitive styles is actually due to genetic influences or a negative family environment in general, Gibb, Abramson, and Alloy (2004) also examined the relation between emotional maltreatment by nonrelatives (i.e., peer victimization) during development and negative cognitive styles. Gibb et al. (2004) found that even when parental maltreatment and parental history of psychopathology were controlled, peer victimization still was significantly associated with cognitive HR status. These findings are not easily explained by third variable accounts such as genetic influence or a general negative family context.

Similarly, examining the CVD project participants' average levels of suicidality (both questionnaire- and interview-assessed) across the first 2½ years of follow-up, participants' cognitive risk status and average levels of hopelessness partially mediated the relation between reported levels of childhood emotional maltreatment and average levels of suicidality (Gibb, Alloy, Abramson, Rose, Whitehouse, & Hogan, 2001). The results of a recent cross-sectional study were also supportive of Rose and Abramson's developmental model. Specifically, the results were consistent with the hypothesis that high levels of childhood emotional maltreatment lead to more negative inferences about that maltreatment, which then lead to the development of a negative inferential style, and this inferential style then leaves one vulnerable to hopelessness and the symptoms of hopelessness depression (Gibb, Alloy, Abramson, & Marx, 2003).

In addition to supporting Rose and Abramson's (1992) developmental model, these results also support their hypothesis that childhood emotional maltreatment may be more likely than either childhood physical or sexual maltreatment to contribute to the development of a negative cognitive style. Specifically, Rose and Abramson hypothesized that, with childhood emotional maltreatment, the depressogenic cognitions are directly supplied to the child by the abuser. With childhood physical and sexual maltreatment, however, children must supply their own negative cognitions. In this way, childhood physical and sexual maltreatment may allow greater opportunity for the child to make less depressogenic attributions and inferences for the occurrence of maltreatment. Although these studies provide preliminary evidence for a relation between childhood emotional maltreatment and negative cognitive styles, future longitudinal research is needed that assesses the degree to which emotional maltreatment contributes to increased negativity in cognitive styles over time.

Many important theoretical issues remain to be addressed with the CVD project data. Although analyses to date have indicated that individuals with negative cognitive styles are at higher risk for experiencing clinically significant depression, future analyses will need to be done to evaluate whether nondepressed individuals at high cognitive risk are more likely than low risk individuals to develop depression only when they experience stressful life events, or whether cognitive risk may confer vulnerability to depression even in the absence of negative life events. In the CVD project, negative life events were assessed repeatedly (every 6 weeks for the first 2½ years of follow-up) and dated to the day they occurred, which makes prospective evaluation of this cognitive vulnerability–stress hypothesis possible. Although preliminary investigations of the vulnerability–stress hypothesis have been conducted, a more thorough evaluation is necessary. In addition, it will be important to test if any predictive effect of the cognitive risk × stress interaction for future depressive episodes is mediated by the occurrence of hopelessness, as predicted by the hopelessness theory, and if it is specific to HD as opposed to other possible subtypes of depression. Other environmental and individual difference variables that may serve as protective factors against the development of hopelessness and depression will also need to be explored. For example, there is substantial evidence that social support can help buffer against the occurrence of depression when people experience stressful events (e.g., Cohen & Wills, 1985; Panzarella et al., in press). Future analyses of the CVD project data will allow an investigation of these potential protective factors.

There is much room for future research on cognitive vulnerabilities to depression outside of the CVD project as well. Most importantly, the CVD project combined both inferential styles and dysfunctional attitudes in defining negative cognitive style. Although this method of selecting participants provides the strongest possible test of the cognitive theories of depression, it does not allow examination of the unique contribution of inferential styles and dysfunctional attitudes in the prediction of depression. As such, the CVD project represents an important step in research examining cognitive vulnerability to depression. Future studies are needed, however, to more specifically test the predictions of Beck's theory and the hopelessness theory, separately (e.g., Haeffel et al., 2003). The role played by positive events should also be addressed in future studies. That is, do positive events provide a buffering effect, protecting against the occurrence of depression? Given the CVD project findings thus far, which have indicated a significant prospective relation between cognitive vulnerability and future depression, studies should continue to examine the therapeutic impact of modifying individuals' cognitive styles. For example, one study has suggested that cognitive behavioral therapists may reduce clients' depressive symptoms by reducing the negativity of clients' attributional styles (DeRubeis & Hollon, 1995). In addition, there is some evidence that training children to make less negative attributions about the negative events in their lives can help protect against future levels of depression (Gillham, Reivich, Jaycox, & Seligman, 1995; Jaycox, Reivich, Gillham, & Seligman, 1994). Given that negative cognitive styles may be especially likely to contribute vulnerability to depression when exacerbated by rumination, depressogenic cognitive styles may also be altered indirectly by training individuals in more effective methods of coping with stressful events, rather than directly trying to alter their cognitive style. Alternatively, it might be necessary to help cognitively vulnerable individuals decrease the stress in their environments.

Further, building positive cognitive styles in children by educating parents to model and provide feedback about more benign inferences for stressful events, as well as direct training in generating positive interpretations of stressful events in schools might help reduce the occurrence of negative cognitive style, and therefore, depression. Finally, parenting classes that teach parents less abusive ways of raising their children may also aid in the prevention of cognitive vulnerability to depression. All of these treatment and prevention models, based on the theorized existence of depressogenic cognitive styles, require further investigation if we are to more fully understand and utilize what we have learned from research on the cognitive theories of depression.

REFERENCES

Abramson, L. Y., & Alloy, L. B. (1990). Search for the "negative cognition" subtype of depression. In D. C. McCann & N. Endler (Eds.), *Depression: New directions in theory, research and practice* (pp. 77–109). Toronto: Wall & Thompson.

Abramson, L. Y., Alloy, L. B., Chiara, A., Tashman, N., Whitehouse, W. G., & Hogan, M. E. (2004). *The Temple–Wisconsin Cognitive Vulnerability to Depression Project: Axis I psychopathology in the parents of individuals at high and low cognitive risk for depression.* Manuscript in preparation. University of Wisconsin–Madison.

Abramson, L. Y., Alloy, L. B., Hankin, B. L., Haeffel, G. J., MacCoon, D. G., & Gibb, B. E. (2002). Cognitive vulnerability–stress models of depression in a self-regulatory and psychobiological context. In I. H. Gotlib & C. L. Hammen (Eds.), *Handbook of depression* (3rd ed., pp. 268–294). New York: Guilford.

Abramson, L. Y., Alloy, L. B., & Hogan, M. E. (1997). Cognitive/personality subtypes of depression: Theories in search of disorders. *Cognitive Therapy and Research, 21,* 247–265.

Abramson, L. Y., Alloy, L. B., Hogan, M. E., Whitehouse, W. G., Cornette, M., Akhavan, S., & Chiara, A. (1998). Suicidality and cognitive vulnerability to depression among college students. *Journal of Adolescence, 21,* 473–487.

Abramson, L. Y., Metalsky, G. I., & Alloy, L. B. (1989). Hopelessness depression: A theory-based subtype of depression. *Psychological Review, 96,* 358–372.

Akhavan, S. (2000). *Comorbidity of hopelessness depression with borderline and dependent personality disorders: Inferential, coping, and anger expression styles as risk factors.* Unpublished doctoral dissertation, Temple University.

Alloy, L. B., & Abramson, L. Y. (1999). The Temple–Wisconsin Cognitive Vulnerability to Depression (CVD) Project: Conceptual background, design and methods. *Journal of Cognitive Psychotherapy: An International Quarterly, 13,* 227–262.

Alloy, L. B., Abramson, L. Y., Gibb, B. E., Crossfield, A. G., Pieracci, A. M., Spasojevic, J., & Steinberg, J. A. (2004). Developmental antecedents of cognitive vulnerability to depression: Review of findings from the cognitive vulnerability to depression project. *Journal of Cognitive Psychotherapy: An International Quarterly, 18,* 115–133.

Alloy, L. B., Abramson, L. Y., Hogan, M. E., Whitehouse, W. G., Rose, D. T., Robinson, M. S., Kim, R. S., & Lapkin, J. B. (2000). The Temple–Wisconsin Cognitive Vulnerability to Depression Project: Lifetime history of Axis I psychopathology in individuals at high and low cognitive risk for depression. *Journal of Abnormal Psychology, 109,* 403–418.

Alloy, L. B., Abramson, L. Y., & Just, N. (1995, November). *Testing the cognitive vulnerability hypotheses of depression onset: Issues of research design.* Paper presented at the Association for the Advancement of Behavior Therapy Meeting, Washington, DC.

Alloy, L. B., Abramson, L. Y., Metalsky, G. I., & Hartlage, S. (1988). The hopelessness theory of depression: Attributional aspects. *British Journal of Clinical Psychology, 27,* 5–21.

Alloy, L. B., Abramson, L. Y., Murray, L. A., Whitehouse, W. G., & Hogan, M. E. (1997). Self-referent information processing in individuals at high and low cognitive risk for depression. *Cognition and Emotion, 11,* 539–568.

Alloy, L. B., Abramson, L. Y., Tashman, N. A., Steinberg, D. L., Hogan, M. E., Whitehouse, W. G., Crossfield, A. G., & Morocco, A. (2001). Developmental origins of cognitive vulnerability to depression: Parenting, cognitive, and inferential feedback styles of the parents of individuals at high and low cognitive risk for depression. *Cognitive Therapy and Research, 25,* 397–423.

Alloy, L. B., Abramson, L. Y., Whitehouse, W. G., Hogan, M. E., Panzarella, C., & Rose, D. T. (in press). Prospective incidence of first onsets and recurrences of depression in individuals at high and low cognitive risk for depression. *Journal of Abnormal Psychology.*

Alloy, L. B., & Clements, C. M. (1998). Hopelessness theory of depression: Tests of the symptom component. *Cognitive Therapy and Research, 22,* 303–335.

Alloy, L. B., Fedderly, S. S., Kennedy-Moore, E., & Cohan, C. L. (1998). Dysphoria and social interaction: An integration of behavioral confirmation and interpersonal perspectives. *Journal of Personality and Social Psychology, 74,* 1566–1579.

Alloy, L. B., Just, N., & Panzarella, C. (1997). Attributional style, daily life events, and hopelessness depression: Subtype validation by prospective variability and specificity of symptoms. *Cognitive Therapy and Research, 21,* 321–344.

Alloy, L. B., Lipman, A., & Abramson, L. Y. (1992). Attributional style as a vulnerability factor for depression: Validation by past history of mood disorders. *Cognitive Therapy and Research, 16,* 391–407.

American Psychiatric Association. (1987). *Diagnostic and statistical manual for mental disorders* (3rd rev. ed.). Washington, DC: Author.

American Psychiatric Association. (1994). *Diagnostic and statistical manual for mental disorders* (4th ed.). Washington, DC: Author.

Anderson, S. M. (1990). The inevitability of future suffering: The role of depressive predictive certainty in depression. *Social Cognition, 8,* 203–228.

Andreason, N., Endicott, J., Spitzer, R. L., & Winokur, G. (1977). The family history method using diagnostic criteria: Reliability and validity. *Archives of General Psychiatry, 34,* 1229–1235.

Barnett, P. A., & Gotlib, I. H. (1988). Psychosocial functioning and depression: Distinguishing among antecedents, concomitants and consequences. *Psychological Bulletin, 104,* 97–126.

Beck, A. T. (1967). *Depression: Clinical, experimental, and theoretical aspects.* New York: Harper & Row.

Beck, A. T. (1983). Cognitive therapy of depression: New perspectives. In P. J. Clayton & J. E. Barrett (Eds.), *Treatment of depression: Old controversies and new approaches* (pp. 265–284). New York: Raven.

Beck, A. T. (1987). Cognitive models of depression. *Journal of Cognitive Psychotherapy: An International Quarterly, 1,* 5–37.

Beck, A. T., Freeman, A., Davis, D. D., & Associates. (1990). *Cognitive therapy of personality disorders.* New York: Guilford.

Beck, A. T., Rush, A. J., Shaw, B. F., & Emery, G. (1979). *Cognitive therapy of depression.* New York: Guilford.

Berrebbi, D. S., Alloy, L. B., & Abramson, L. Y. (2004). *Stability in negative cognitive styles despite intervening episodes of depression.* Manuscript in preparation, Temple University.

Brown, G. W., & Harris, T. O. (1978). *Social origins of depression: A study of psychiatric disorder in women.* New York: The Free Press.

Cohen, S., & Wills, T. A. (1985). Stress, social support and the buffering hypothesis. *Psychological Bulletin, 98,* 310–357.

Cole, D. A., & Turner, J. E. (1993). Models of cognitive mediation and moderation in child depression. *Journal of Abnormal Psychology, 102,* 271–281.

Crossfield, A. G., Alloy, L. B., Abramson, L. Y., & Gibb, B. E. (2002). The development of depressogenic cognitive styles: The role of negative childhood life events and parental inferential feedback. *Journal of Cognitive Psychotherapy: An International Quarterly, 16,* 487–502.

Depue, R. A., Slater, J., Wolfstetter-Kausch, H., Klein, D., Goplerud, E., & Farr, D. (1981). A behavioral paradigm for identifying persons at risk for bipolar spectrum disorder: A conceptual framework and five validation studies (Monograph). *Journal of Abnormal Psychology, 90,* 381–437.

DeRubeis, R. J., & Hollon, S. D. (1995). Explanatory style in the treatment of depression. In G. M. Buchanan & M. E. P. Seligman (Eds.), *Explanatory style* (pp. 99–111). Hillsdale, NJ: Lawrence Erlbaum Associates.

Downey, G., & Coyne, J. C. (1990). Children of depressed parents: An integrative review. *Psychological Bulletin, 108,* 50–76.

Endicott, J., & Spitzer, R. A. (1978). A diagnostic interview: The Schedule for Affective Disorders and Schizophrenia. *Archives of General Psychiatry, 35,* 837–844.

Farmer, R., & Nelson-Gray, R. O. (1990). Personality disorders and depression: Hypothetical relations, empirical findings and methodological considerations. *Clinical Psychology Review, 10,* 453–476.

Finlay-Jones, R., & Brown, G. W. (1981). Types of stressful life event and the onset of anxiety and depressive disorders. *Psychological Medicine, 11,* 803–815.

Garber, J., & Flynn, C. (2001). Predictors of depressive cognitions in young adolescents. *Cognitive Therapy and Research, 25*, 353–376.

Gibb, B. E., Abramson, L. Y., & Alloy, L. B. (2004). Emotional maltreatment from parents, verbal peer victimization, and cognitive vulnerability to depression. *Cognitive Therapy and Research, 28*, 1–21.

Gibb, B. E., Alloy, L. B., Abramson, L. Y., & Marx, B. P. (2003). Childhood maltreatment and maltreatment-specific inferences: A test of Rose and Abramson's (1992) extension of the hopelessness theory. *Cognition and Emotion, 17*, 917–931.

Gibb, B. E., Alloy, L. B., Abramson, L. Y., Rose, D. T., Whitehouse, W. G., Donovan, P., Hogan, M. E., Cronholm, J., & Tierney, S. (2001). History of childhood maltreatment, depressogenic cognitive style, and episodes of depression in adulthood. *Cognitive Therapy and Research, 25*, 425–446.

Gibb, B. E., Alloy, L. B., Abramson, L. Y., Rose, D. T., Whitehouse, W. G., & Hogan, M. E. (2001). Childhood maltreatment and college students' current suicidal ideation: A test of the hopelessness theory. *Suicide and Life Threatening Behavior, 31*, 405–415.

Gillham, J. E., Reivich, K. J., Jaycox, L. H., & Seligman, M. E. P. (1995). Prevention of depressive symptoms in schoolchildren: Two-year follow-up. *Psychological Science, 6*, 343–351.

Gotlib, I. H., & Hammen, C. L. (1992). A marital/family discord model of depression: Implications for therapeutic intervention. In N. S. Jacobson & A. S. Gurman (Eds.), *Clinical handbook of couple therapy* (pp. 411–436). New York: Guilford.

Gotlib, I. H., Lewinsohn, P. M., Seeley, J. R., Rohde, P., & Redner, J. E. (1993). Negative cognitions and attributional style in depressed adolescents: An examination of stability and specificity. *Journal of Abnormal Psychology, 102*, 607–615.

Haeffel, G. J., Abramson, L. Y., Voelz, Z. R., Metalsky, G. I., Halberstadt, L., Dykman, B. M., Donovan, P., Hogan, M. E., Hankin, B. L., & Alloy, L. B. (2003). Cognitive vulnerability to depression and lifetime history of Axis I psychopathology: A comparison of negative cognitive styles (CSQ) and dysfunctional attitudes (DAS). *Journal of Cognitive Psychotherapy: An International Quarterly, 17*, 3–22.

Hammen, C. (1992). The family–environment context of depression: A perspective on children's risk. In D. Cicchetti & S. Toth (Eds.), *Rochester symposium of developmental psychopathology* (Vol. 4, pp. 145–153). Rochester, NY: University of Rochester Press.

Hankin, B. L., Abramson, L. Y., & Siler, M. (2001). A prospective test of the hopelessness theory of depression in adolescence. *Cognitive Therapy and Research, 25*, 607–632.

Ingram, R. E., Miranda, J., & Segal, Z. V. (1998). *Cognitive vulnerability to depression.* New York: Guilford.

Jaycox, L. H., Reivich, K. J., Gillham, J., & Seligman, M. E. P. (1994). Prevention of depressive symptoms in school children. *Behaviour Research and Therapy, 32*, 801–816.

Joiner, T. E., Alfano, M. S., & Metalsky, G. I. (1992). When depression breeds contempt: Reassurance-seeking, self-esteem, and rejection of depressed college students by their roommates. *Journal of Abnormal Psychology, 101*, 165–173.

Joiner, T. E., Jr., & Rudd, M. D. (1996). Toward a categorization of depression-related psychological constructs. *Cognitive Therapy and Research, 20*, 51–68.

Joiner, T. E., Steer, R. A., Abramson, L. Y., Alloy, L. B., Metalsky, G. I., & Schmidt, N. B. (2001). Hopelessness depression as a distinct dimension of depressive symptoms among clinical and nonclinical samples. *Behaviour Research and Therapy, 39*, 523–536.

Joiner, T. E., & Wagner, K. D. (1995). Attribution style and depression in children and adolescents: A meta-analytic review. *Clinical Psychology Review, 15*, 777–798.

Just, N., Abramson, L. Y., & Alloy, L. B. (2001). Remitted depression studies as tests of the cognitive vulnerability hypotheses of depression onset: A critique and conceptual analysis. *Clinical Psychology Review, 21*, 63–83.

Just, N., & Alloy, L. B. (1997). The response styles theory of depression: Tests and an extension of the theory. *Journal of Abnormal Psychology, 106*, 221–229.

Lewinsohn, P. M., Steinmertz, J., Larson, D., & Franklin, J. (1981). Depression related cognitions: Antecedents or consequences? *Journal of Abnormal Psychology, 90,* 213–219.

Loranger, A. W. (1988). *Personality Disorder Examination (PDE) manual.* Yonkers, NY: DV Communications.

Metalsky, G. I., Halberstadt, L. J., & Abramson, L. Y. (1987). Vulnerability to depressive mood reactions: Toward a more powerful test of the diathesis–stress and causal mediation components of the reformulated theory of depression. *Journal of Personality and Social Psychology, 52,* 386–393.

Metalsky, G. I., & Joiner, T. E. (1992). Vulnerability to depressive symptomatology: A Prospective test of the diathesis–stress and causal mediation components of the hopelessness theory of depression. *Journal of Personality and Social Psychology, 63,* 667–675.

Metalsky, G. I., & Joiner, T. E., Jr. (1997). The Hopelessness Depression Symptom Questionnaire. *Cognitive Therapy and Research, 21,* 359–384.

Metalsky, G. I., Joiner, T. E., Hardin, T. S., & Abramson, L. Y. (1993). Depressive reactions to failure in a naturalistic setting: A test of the hopelessness and self-esteem theories of depression. *Journal of Abnormal Psychology, 102,* 101–109.

Monroe, S. M., & Hadjiyannakis, K. (2002). The social environment and depression: Focusing on severe life stress. In I. H. Gotlib & C. L. Hammen (Eds.), *Handbook of depression* (3rd ed., pp. 314–340). New York: Guilford.

Morrow, J., & Nolen-Hoeksema, S. (1990). Effects of responses to depression on the remediation of depressive affect. *Journal of Personality and Social Psychology, 69,* 176–190.

Nolen-Hoeksema, S. (1991). Responses to depression and their effects on the duration of the depressive episode. *Journal of Abnormal Psychology, 100,* 20–28.

Nolen-Hoeksema, S. (2000). Ruminative responses predict depressive disorders. *Journal of Abnormal Psychology, 109,* 504–511.

Nolen-Hoeksema, S., Girgus, J. S., & Seligman, M. E. P. (1986). Learned helplessness in children: A longitudinal study of depression, achievement, and explanatory style. *Journal of Personality and Social Psychology, 51,* 435–442.

Nolen-Hoeksema, S., Girgus, J. S., & Seligman, M. E. P. (1992). Predictors and consequences of childhood depressive symptoms: A five-year longitudinal study. *Journal of Abnormal Psychology, 101,* 405–422.

Nolen-Hoeksema, S., & Morrow, J. (1991). A prospective study of depression and posttraumatic stress symptoms after a natural disaster: The 1989 Loma Prieta Earthquake. *Journal of Personality and Social Psychology, 61,* 115–121.

Nolen-Hoeksema, S., Morrow, J., & Fredrickson, B. L. (1993). Response style and the duration of episodes of depressed mood. *Journal of Abnormal Psychology, 102,* 20–28.

Nolen-Hoeksema, S., Parker, L. E., & Larson, J. (1994). Ruminative coping with depressed mood following loss. *Journal of Personality and Social Psychology, 67,* 92–104.

Panak, W. F., & Garber, J. (1992). Role of aggression, rejection, and attributions in the prediction of depression in children. *Development and Psychopathology, 4,* 145–165.

Panzarella, C., Alloy, L. B., & Whitehouse, W. G. (in press). Expanded hopelessness theory of depression: On the mechanisms by which social support protects against depression. *Cognitive Threapy and Research.*

Persons, J. B., & Miranda, J. (1992). Cognitive theories of vulnerability to depression: Reconciling negative evidence. *Cognitive Therapy and Research, 16,* 485–502.

Peterson, C. R., Semmel, A., von Baeyer, C., Abramson, L. Y., Metalsky, G. I., & Seligman, M. E. P. (1982). The Attributional Style Questionnaire. *Cognitive Therapy and Research, 6,* 287–300.

Raniere, D. F. (2000). *Long-term stability of inferences about major stressful life-events: Comparing retrospective reports among individuals at high versus low cognitive risk for depression.* Unpublished doctoral dissertation, Temple University.

Robinson, M. S. (1997). *The role of negative inferential style and stress-reactive rumination on negative inferences in the etiology of depression: Empirical investigation and clinical implications.* Unpublished doctoral dissertation, Temple University.

Robinson, M. S., & Alloy, L. B. (2003). Negative cognitive styles and stress-reactive rumination interact to predict depression: A prospective study. *Cognitive Therapy and Research, 27*, 275–291.

Robinson, N. S., Garber, J., & Hilsman, R. (1995). Cognitions and stress: Direct and moderating effects on depressive versus externalizing symptoms during the junior high transition. *Journal of Abnormal Psychology, 104*, 453–463.

Rose, D. T., & Abramson, L. Y. (1992). Developmental predictors of depressive cognitive style: Research and theory. In D. Cicchetti & S. L. Toth (Eds.), *Rochester symposium on developmental psychopathology* (Vol. 4, pp. 323–349). Hillsdale, NJ: Lawrence Erlbaum Associates.

Rose, D. T., Abramson, L. Y., Hodulik, C., Halberstadt, L. J., & Leff, G. (1994). Heterogeneity of cognitive style among inpatient depressives. *Journal of Abnormal Psychology, 103*, 419–429.

Safford, S. M., & Alloy, L. B. (1999, March). *Negative cognitive style and negative life events in predicting depression.* Poster presented at American Psychopathological Association 89th annual meeting, New York.

Segal, Z. V. (1988). Appraisal of the self-schema construct in cognitive models of depression. *Psychological Bulletin, 103*, 147–162.

Segal, Z. V., & Ingram, R. E. (1994). Mood priming and construct activation in tests of cognitive vulnerability to unipolar depression. *Clinical Psychology Review, 14*, 663–695.

Segrin, C., & Abramson, L. Y. (1994). Negative reactions to depressive behaviors: A communication theories analysis. *Journal of Abnormal Psychology, 103*, 655–668.

Seligman, M. E. P., Peterson, C., Kaslow, N. J., Tannenbaum, R. L., Alloy, L. B., & Abramson, L. Y. (1984). Attributional style and depressive symptoms among children. *Journal of Abnormal Psychology, 93*, 235–238.

Smith, J., Grandin, L., Alloy, L. B., & Abramson, L. Y. (2004). *Cognitive vulnerability to depression and Axis II personality dysfunction.* Manuscript submitted for publication.

Spangler, D. L., Simons, A. D., Monroe, S. M., & Thase, M. E. (1997). Comparison of cognitive models of depression: Relationships between cognitive constructs and cognitive diathesis–stress match. *Journal of Abnormal Psychology, 106*, 395–403.

Spasojevic, J., & Alloy, L. B. (2001). Rumination as a common mechanism relating depressive risk factors to depression. *Emotion, 1*, 25–37.

Spitzer, R. L., Endicott, J., & Robins, E. (1978). Research diagnostic criteria: Rationale and reliability. *Archives of General Psychiatry, 35*, 773–782.

Steinberg, J. A., Oelrich, C., Alloy, L. B., & Abramson, L. Y. (2004). *Negative self-referent information processing as a moderator vs. mediator of negative cognitive styles in predicting prospective onsets of depression.* Manuscript in preparation, Temple University.

Tiggemann, M., Winefield, A. H., Winefield, H. R., & Goldney, R. D. (1991). The prediction of psychological distress from attributional style: A test of the hopelessness model of depression. *Australian Journal of Psychology, 43*, 125–127.

Turk, E., & Bry, B. H. (1992). Adolescents' and parents' explanatory styles and parents' causal explanations about their adolescents. *Cognitive Therapy and Research, 16*, 349–357.

Weissman, A., & Beck, A. T. (1978, November). *Development and validation of the Dysfunctional Attitude Scale: A preliminary investigation.* Paper presented at the meeting of the American Educational Research Association, Toronto, Ontario, Canada.

Whisman, M. A., & Kwon, P. (1992). Parental representations, cognitive distortions, and mild depression. *Cognitive Therapy and Research, 16*, 557–568.

3

Cognitive Vulnerability to Depression

Rick E. Ingram
University of Kansas

Jeanne Miranda
University of California, Los Angeles

Zindel Segal
Centre for Addiction and Mental Health

An argument has been made that nothing brings mental health professionals closer to understanding the essential features of disorders than does the construct of vulnerability (Ingram & Price, 2001). Nowhere is this assertion probably more true than in the case of depression, where the study of vulnerability has begun to emerge as a focal point in efforts to understand and prevent this disorder. This chapter discusses theory and research that has examined the essential features of vulnerability to depression. A number of conceptual paradigms (e.g., biological, genetic) have offered important insights into the nature of vulnerability to depression. However, because cognitive factors have been widely recognized in the psychological-science community to play an important role in risk for depression, the focus is on cognitive approaches to vulnerability.

Several assumptions about vulnerability are addressed, and then cognitive theories of depression, and the statements they make about vulnerability factors, are examined. The research relevant to these theories is reviewed, focusing first on research conducted with adults and then the more limited data available on vulnerable children. Following this review, several ideas are suggested about the nature of cognitive vulnerability that emerge from extant theories and data. Before beginning, however, note that space limitations preclude an exhaustive review of all of the information relevant to theory and research on cognitive vulnerability to depression. Nevertheless, although the review is selective, each of the major topics is considered in terms of how it pertains to depression and cognitive vulnerability. Readers interested in a more detailed account of the various topics and issues should consult Ingram, Miranda, and Segal (1998) and Gotlib and Hammen (2002).

CONCEPTUAL ASSUMPTIONS UNDERLYING THEORY AND RESEARCH ON COGNITIVE VULNERABILITY TO DEPRESSION

Before starting the exploration of cognitive vulnerability to depression, it is important to briefly examine several assumptions that underlie much of the theory and research in this area. These assumptions reflect the diathesis–stress nature of depression, the cognitive diathesis proposed in depression theories, and ideas about definitions of vulnerability.

Diathesis–Stress

Most cognitive models of depression, and by extension cognitive vulnerability models of depression, are explicitly diathesis–stress models; these models argue that depression is the result of the interaction between cognitive factors and environmental stressors. The diathesis–stress approach specifies that, under ordinary conditions, people who are vulnerable to the onset of depression are indistinguishable from nonvulnerable people (Segal & Ingram, 1994). According to this idea, only when confronted with certain stressors do cognitive differences between vulnerable and nonvulnerable people emerge, which then turn into depression for those who are vulnerable (Ingram & Luxton, in press; Monroe & Hadjiyannakis, 2002; Monroe & Simons, 1991; Segal & Shaw, 1986). More specifically, most cognitive models propose that when stressful life events are encountered by vulnerable people, these events precipitate a pattern of negative, biased, self-referent information processing that initiates the first cycle in the downward spin of depression (Segal & Shaw, 1986). Alternatively, individuals who do not possess this diathesis react with an appropriate level of depressive affect to the event, but do not become depressed.

The Cognitive Diathesis in Diathesis–Stress Models

The cognitive diathesis proposed by most cognitive models can be traced to the depression theory proposed by Beck (1963, 1967). Beck was the first to argue that depression is the result of maladaptive cognitive structures; in particular, that schemas about the self are causally linked to the disorder and are triggered by stressful life events. Although definitions vary somewhat, many investigators conceptualize self-schemas as organized representations of an individual's prior experiences (Segal, 1988). Cognitive structures such as schemas are not randomly distributed throughout the memory system, but are instead connected to each other in varying degrees of association. Functionally, the self-schema significantly influences information processing by selecting what information is extracted from both internal and external sources, and by affecting the encoding as well as the retrieval of information (Alba & Hasher, 1983; Kihlstrom & Cantor, 1984). Although not shared by all cognitive theories of depression, cognitive structures such as schemas represent the guiding conceptual principle that underlies most contemporary accounts of depression.

Definitions of Vulnerability

There are few explicit definitions of vulnerability available in the literature (Ingram et al., 1998; Ingram & Price, 2001). However, theory and research on vulnerability suggest a number of features essential to the construct of vulnerability and can therefore be used to arrive at a suitable definition of vulnerability. The most fundamental of these features is that vulnerability is conceptualized as a trait rather than as the kind of state that characterizes the appearance of depression. That is, even as episodes of depression emerge and then disappear, vulnerability remains constant. It is important to note in this regard that even though vulnerability is seen as a trait, this does not mean it is necessarily permanent or unalterable. Although psychological vulnerability may be resistant to change, corrective experiences can occur that attenuate vulnerability (e.g., therapy). Vulnerability is also viewed as *endogenous* to the person (in contrast to risk that is a function of external forces),[1] as well as typically being viewed as *dormant* unless it is activated in some fashion. Related to this notion of dormancy, *stress* can also be viewed as a central aspect of vulnerability in that cognitive diatheses cannot precipitate depression without the occurrence of stressful life events.

COGNITIVE THEORIES OF VULNERABILITY

Although few cognitive theories of depression focus extensively on vulnerability, all make statements about the causes of depression, and it is in the discussion of such causes that these theories arrive at a conceptualization of vulnerability. It is important to note in this regard these theories

---

[1]External forces are conceptualized in terms of risk factors (e.g., poverty) rather than vulnerability because they do not specify the mechanisms of onset or maintenance; the term *vulnerability* refers to these mechanisms.

are usually aimed at understanding depression in adulthood, but to the extent that they focus on vulnerability, these models typically propose that events in childhood create cognitive vulnerability. Even though some only briefly allude to this vulnerability (e.g., Ingram, 1984), others provide more detailed descriptions of the origins of cognitive vulnerability (e.g., Abramson, Metalsky, & Alloy, 1989; Beck, 1967). In addition, some models are not explicitly models of depression, but the cognitive variables they describe are relevant to understanding the development of cognitive vulnerability factors to depression (e.g., Bowlby, 1980). The theories that speak to cognitive vulnerability are examined, first by briefly describing the basic elements of these theories, and then through a look at the statements they make about the development of cognitive vulnerability.

Cognitive Schema Models

As previously noted, Beck (1967) proposed the first cognitive theory of depression. Beck argued that dysfunctional cognitions, such as cognitive errors, are important causal elements for depression. However, this theory goes beyond cognitive errors and suggests that "deeper" cognitive structures are also involved in precipitating depression. Specifically, Beck contended that there are three "layers" of cognition involved in the causes of depression. First, automatic thoughts are the recurring, intrusive, and negative thoughts that occur in depressed individuals. Second, underlying these automatic thoughts are irrational cognitions or beliefs, sometimes referred to as "conditionals." These beliefs tend to take the form of "if–then" beliefs that are negative in nature. For example, a depressive conditional belief might be, "If I don't get the job I applied for, then I am stupid." Third, automatic thoughts and irrational beliefs are a function of a deeper depressive self-schema that organizes thoughts, beliefs, and information processing in a negative way. A number of theories other than Beck's have been proposed, and although they differ in some respects, all tend to rely on similar theoretical notions (e.g., Ingram, 1984; Ingram et al., 1998; Teasdale, 1983; Teasdale & Barnard, 1993).

Although most cognitive schema theories of depression suggest the operation of a more or less generalized negative self-schema, some investigators have specified a specific problematic organization of these cognitive structures. For example, in more recent statements on the nature of depressive self-schemas, Beck (1987) refined his theory to include two categories of problematic schema content (see also Robins, 1990; Robins & Block, 1988; Robins & Luten, 1991). The first is interpersonal in nature, and is referred to as *sociotropy/dependency*; individuals with this concept embedded in their cognitive schemas value positive interchange with others and focus on acceptance, support, and guidance from others. The second type of cognitive content is concerned with achievement and is called *autonomy/self-criticism*; these individuals rely on independence, mobility, and achievement, and are prone to be self-critical. According to this formulation, the experience of stressors congruent with these themes should activate these dysfunctional cognitive structures and precipitate depression. For example, disruptions in interpersonal relationships should be especially problematic for the person with the sociotropic schema whereas problems in achievement situations (e.g., work) should activate depressive experiences for the person with the autonomous schema type.

Origins of Vulnerability in Cognitive Schema Models. Theories that focus on cognitive schemas in depression generally suggest these schemas develop in response to stressful or traumatic events in childhood and adolescence (Ingram et al., 1998). In adulthood, these schemas sensitize individuals to respond in a cognitively and emotionally dysfunctional fashion to events similar to those experienced in childhood. For example, Beck (1967) suggested that "in childhood and adolescence, the depression-prone individual becomes sensitized to certain types of life situations. The traumatic situations initially responsible for embedding or reinforcing the negative attitudes that comprise the depressive constellation are the prototypes of the specific stresses that may later activate these constellations. When a person is subjected to situations reminiscent of the original traumatic experiences, he may then become depressed" (p. 278). Beck's theory thus locates the nexus of vulnerability, even for adults, in childhood experiences. Other theories (e.g., Goodman & Gotlib, 1999; Ingram et al., 1998) make similar statements.

Hopelessness Depression

The hopelessness theory of depression represents a conceptual progression that started with the original learned helplessness theory (e.g., Seligman, 1975). This progression began in 1978 when learned helplessness theory was reformulated to focus on individuals' tendencies to make certain kinds of attributions about the causes of events (Abramson, Seligman, & Teasdale, 1978). In particular, the tendency to make unstable, specific, and external attributions for positive events, and to make stable, global, and internal attributions for negative events, was proposed to lead to depression. Most recently, Abramson et al. (1989) refined this theoretical approach, which they referred to as the hopelessness theory of depression. In addition to dysfunctional attributional tendencies, Abramson et al. (1989) argued that the cause of hopelessness depression is the expectation that highly desired outcomes will not occur, or that highly aversive outcomes will occur, coupled with the perception that no responses are possible that will be able to change the likelihood of these outcomes.

Origins of Vulnerability in the Hopelessness Model.   Rose and Abramson (1992) and Gibb, Alloy, Abramson, and Marx (2003) suggested several possible developmental factors that may underlie hopelessness theory. Specifically, they argued that children who experience negative events such as maltreatment attempt to find the causes, consequences, and meaning of these events. They further noted that young children evidence a tendency to make internal attributions for all events, including negative events; thus these children tend to see themselves as the cause of maltreatment. In some situations, the variables involved in this process precipitate the development of the negative attributional style that produces risk for depression. For example, the occurrence of negative events that are internalized affects the child's self-concept and, in so doing, may lead to broad tendencies to internalize negative events. These attributional tendencies alone, however, are insufficient to lead to the hopelessness attributional style. Rather, to the extent that negative events are repetitive and occur in the context of relationships with significant others (e.g., parents), these events will undermine the need for the child to maintain a positive self-image as well as optimism about future positive events. Additionally, the persistence of these events will produce a pattern of attributions for negative events that, over time, will become both stable and global. Attributional patterns thus become more traitlike, and in this way provide the foundation for hopelessness in the face of stressors in the future—a process that produces hopelessness depression.

Attachment Theory

As proposed by Bowlby (1969, 1973, 1980), attachment theory addresses processes that shape the capacity of people to form meaningful emotional bonds with others throughout their lives.[2] Although attachment begins in infancy, and is thus thought to be primarily a childhood process, the effects of attachment do not end in childhood; several investigators have argued that, once developed, attachment patterns persist into adulthood and affect a multitude of relationships (Ainsworth, 1989; Bartholomew & Horowitz, 1991; Doane & Diamond, 1994; Ricks, 1985). Indeed, Bowlby summed up this lifelong process most succinctly by suggesting that attachment is a process that stretches from "cradle to grave."

---

[2]The terms *bonding* and *attachment* are used interchangeably, even though some authors (e.g., Parker, 1979) have argued that they are not the same. For the purposes of this chapter, however, they are similar enough to be thought of as reflecting the same construct.

The quality of contact with caretakers is a key determinant of the individual's attachment patterns (Ainsworth, Blehar, Waters, & Wall, 1978). In particular, consistently affectionate, nurturant, and protective interactions with parents promote the development of the child's ability to form normal behavioral, cognitive, and emotional bonds with others throughout life. However, attachment does not always function normally; deviations from secure attachment result when bonding processes are disrupted in some fashion. Moreover, such dysfunctional attachment patterns in children and adolescents have been suggested to be related to peer rejection, problematic self-control, social competence deficits, alcohol abuse, conduct disorders (see P. M. Cole & Zahn-Waxler, 1992; Doane & Diamond, 1994), and risk for depression (Bemporad & Romano, 1992; Cummings & Cicchetti, 1990).

Cognitive Vulnerability According to Attachment Theory. The risk that appears to originate from dysfunctional attachment or bonding patterns may stem from cognitive variables (Ingram et al., 1998). In particular, attachment theory has long emphasized the concept of internal working models. Quite similar to schema models, these are thought to reflect the cognitive representation of relationships that have been generalized through interactions with key figures early in the individual's life. According to most attachment theorists, once developed these working models continue to influence the cognitions and feelings that individuals experience about relationships with important others. Insecure attachment will be reflected in the organization and functioning of the individual's working models, leading to distorted information about interpersonal interactions and thus to an increased risk for maladaptive relations with others (see Bowlby, 1988). Given the importance of interpersonal relationships for providing support and buffering against stress, dysfunctional relationships that are caused by maladaptive information processing provide the basis for vulnerability to depression.

COGNITIVE VULNERABILITY RESEARCH

Although by no means an exhaustive list, the models reviewed represent the major cognitive approaches to the conceptualization of depression and depression risk. Next consider the research that is relevant to the depression risk proposals of these models. Even though these models diverge in some theoretical respects, they also converge on a number of important constructs (e.g., how maladaptive information processing can lead to depression risk), as well as on the notion that the developmental genesis of depression risk resides in the effects of interactions with significant others early in life. Accordingly, although each approach has stimulated a somewhat different research tradition, and tested somewhat different ideas about vulnerability, this research tends to concentrate on assessing the link between cognition and vulnerability to depression, and how this link might be related to important developmental experiences and interactions between parents and children.

Priming Studies

A central premise of some cognitive approaches to depression is that vulnerable individuals possess cognitive risk factors that are largely inactive until individuals encounter adversity in a domain that is central to their sense of self-worth. For example, in Beck's model, stress in the person's environment is postulated to activate the negative self-schema, particularly stress matching the individuals' core doubts and concerns about self-worth (Segal, Shaw, Vella, & Katz, 1992). Even though a number of studies have assessed cognitive functioning during a depressive episode, because this cognitive functioning could be a consequence of depression, these studies are usually uninformative about cognitive processes that are thought to be linked to the onset of a depressive episode (Barnett & Gotlib, 1988). Additionally, research examining cognitive functioning in currently nondepressed but vulnerable individuals has generally failed to show that they think in depressotypic ways, but this too is also uninformative because it fails to take into account the diathesis–stress nature of most cognitive theories (Ingram et al., 1998).

   In contrast, "priming" studies explicitly focus on diathesis–stress perspectives that are central to many cognitive theories of depression (Hollon, 1992), and thus assess the outcomes associated with the activation of negative self-referent cognitive structures in response to stresslike encounters. These studies typically rely on inducing a negative mood state in nondepressed but vulnerable individuals, with the hope of modeling in the laboratory the effect that stress has on most people—that is, the production of negative mood. In theory, this brief negative mood state should activate the kind of cognitions that serve as vulnerability factors for the more severe mood state that is a depressive episode. More generally, these studies seek to model the processes whereby the normal sad mood states that are occasionally experienced by everyone energize the mechanisms the lead to a downward spiral into depression for some people (i.e., those who are vulnerable). In more specific terms, vulnerability is conceptualized as the availability of relatively well-developed and well-elaborated cognitive structures that are linked to negative affective structures (Ingram, 1984; Ingram et al., 1998). Once brought about by any variety of life events, the structures responsible for the experience of sadness provide access to the extensive and elaborate processing of depressive information. This process serves to generate a downward extension of normal depressed mood into the more significant and debilitating experience of depression by those who possess these networks. Thus, once this intricate system of dysfunctional themes is activated by the type of negative mood that is thought to follow the experience of stress, a pattern of negative self-referent information processing is precipitated that escalates into depression for vulnerable people (Segal & Shaw, 1986). Priming studies are intended to model this process.

Some priming failures have been reported in the literature. For example, Brosse, Craighead, and Craighead (1999) found that increased endorsement of dysfunctional attitudes following a negative mood induction was unrelated to depression history. Dykman (1997) also documented that shifts in dysfunctional attitudes following a mood induction were unrelated to depression history. Similarly, Solomon, Haaga, Kirk, and Friedman (1998) failed to find differences in irrational beliefs between never depressed and recovered depressed persons following priming by negative sociotropic and autonomous event scenarios.

Despite some failures, there is enough evidence of priming effects to support a consensus that vulnerable individuals do possess dormant but reactive cognitive schemas of the type that should be linked to cognitive vulnerability to depression (Gotlib & Krasnoperova, 1998; Ingram et al., 1998; Scher, Segal, & Ingram, in press; Segal & Ingram, 1994). For instance, using a variety of cognitive measures that reflect dysfunctional cognition, studies by Teasdale and Dent (1987), Dent and Teasdale (1988), Miranda, Persons, and Byers (1990), Miranda, Gross, Persons, and Hahn (1998), Hedlund and Rude (1995), Ingram, Bernet, and McLaughlin (1994), Ingram and Ritter (2000), Taylor and Ingram (1999), and Segal, Gemar, and Williams (1999) all supported the activation of what appear to be cognitive diatheses. Some research has described evidence of cognitive diatheses in children as young as 8 years old (i.e., Taylor & Ingram, 1999).

The previous studies supported the activation of dysfunctional self-schemas, but Segal et al. (1999) in particular provided evidence that these schemas not only can be activated, but that they appear to be associated with vulnerability to the experience of depression. In this study, depressed patients who had recovered after being treated with either cognitive behavioral therapy (CBT) or pharamacotherapy (PT) completed ratings of dysfunctional attitudes before and after a priming procedure (i.e., a negative mood induction). Following priming, PT patients showed a significant increase in dysfunctional cognitions, a finding that is consistent with other priming data (see Segal & Ingram, 1994). CBT patients, on the other hand, showed no change in DAS scores. Several years after initial testing, a follow-up study reassessed patients and found that their cognitive reactions to the mood induction predicted relapse, even after controlling for the effects of previous depression history. Thus, these data suggest a link between cognitive reactivity and risk for later depressive relapse, a key element of schema theories of depression.

Behavioral High Risk Research

Another approach to empirically assessing cognitive vulnerability uses a behavioral high risk paradigm, which employs a theoretically defined risk factor and selects people who, on the basis of the risk factor, are assumed to be vulnerable to depression. Although a number of studies have used this paradigm, two well-known high risk approaches have provided data on cognitive vulnerability: the Temple–Wisconsin Cognitive Vulnerability to Depression Project and the depressogenic personality/life stress congruency approach.

The Temple–Wisconsin Cognitive Vulnerability to Depression Project. One of the more comprehensive studies undertaken to assess vulnerability is the Temple–Wisconsin project (Alloy & Abramson, 1999, see also Abramson et al., 2002). This two-site longitudinal study examines the etiological proposals of both the hopelessness model and cognitive schema theory as represented by Beck's (1967) model. This study assesses a group of individuals who, upon entry into college, were identified as possessing negative inferential styles or negative self-schemas, and compares their outcomes with individuals who do not show these cognitive characteristics.

Data reported from this project thus far have suggested a number of cognitive factors that may be linked to vulnerability. Most critically, those identified as being at high cognitive risk are more likely to experience depression at some point in the future (Abramson et al., 1999). Results have also suggested that, compared to the low risk group, high risk subjects process negative self-referent information more fully than positive self-referent information (Alloy, Abramson, Murray, Whitehouse, & Hogan, 1997). Regarding the origins of vulnerability, Alloy et al. (2001) also reported that the mothers of cognitively high risk individuals exhibit more negative cognition than do the mothers of low risk individuals, the fathers of high risk students are less emotionally accepting, and both the mothers and fathers of high risk students are more likely to make more stable and global attributions for the stressful events that their children experience. Gibb et al. (2001) also found more reports of emotional maltreatment in high risk individuals in the Temple–Wisconsin data. Overall, data from the Temple–Wisconsin project indicate that cognitive factors can predict the eventual onset of depression, they are related to dysfunctional information processing, are associated with parents' cognitive processing, and to some degree may be the result of emotional maltreatment.

Congruency Between Personality and Life Stress and Vulnerability to Depression. A different conceptual and operational definition of high risk stems from research examining the match between the occurrence of key life events and specific sensitivities. Recall that sociotropy/dependency and autonomy/self-criticism describe cognitive styles that leave people vulnerable to depression when congruent stressful life events occur. Although most of this research is cross-sectional, evidence in support of the congruency hypothesis has begun to accumulate (e.g., Robins, 1990; Segal et al., 1992). For instance, in reviewing findings from 24 studies, Nietzel and Harris (1990) concluded that the match between cognitive style and congruent life stress places is associated with depression more so than is the nonmatching of events of similar severity. They also found that some types of matches were especially problematic; for example, the combination of elevated sociotropy/dependency interacting with negative social events led to greater depression than did the autonomy/self-criticism matching or the other two mismatches. Coyne and Whiffen (1995) acknowledged the greater predictive power of personality by life stress matches over mismatches, but because they did not believe this model is complex enough to accommodate fluctuations in the course of people's live, they were more skeptical about the relevance of this model to the study of depression vulnerability. This skepticism not withstanding, the empirical findings are clearly supportive of cognitive models of depression that locate vulnerability in the activation of individuals' meaning and need structures, and how these structures match up with life events (see Zuroff, Mongrain, & Santor, 2004).

Parent–Child Interactions in the Production of Cognitive Vulnerability. Different kinds of parent–child interactions may be associated with the development of cognitive vulnerability to depression. This section discusses research that has assessed some of these interactions, in particular, data that have been reported on attachment/bonding and cognitive vulnerability to depression, and data examining the link between cognitive vulnerability and abuse.

Parent–Child Bonding and Attachment

As already noted, attachment and the cognition that is linked to attachment and depression is considered an important outcome of parent–child interactions. Moreover, the idea that problematic parent–child interactions can produce vulnerability to depression is a theme that tends to occur across cognitive models. Several studies have assessed this theme. For example, a number of the studies examining the impact of parental interactions on depression and cognition have assessed the recall of certain kinds of interactions as they pertain to possible cognitive vulnerability. Two types of interactions that have been of particular interest to theorists and researchers are parental care and parental overprotection. Parker (1979, 1983) suggested that low levels of parental care (defined as either neglect or by overt rejection) lead to future cognitive vulnerability by disrupting the child's self-esteem. In contrast to low levels of expressed care, overprotectiveness is thought to operate on vulnerability because the parent is so anxious or intrusive that a genuine caring relationship cannot be established with the child.

Studies that examine the cognitive component of the link between interactions such as these and depression, however, are much less common than those assessing the link between parent–child interactions and the development of depression per se.[3] McCranie and Bass (1984) reported that among women nursing students, an overcontrolling mother was associated with greater dependency needs, whereas for students who reported both a mother and a father who were overcontrolling, a greater tendency toward self-criticism was found. Likewise, in a study among medical students, Brewin, Firth-Cozens, Furnham, and McManus (1992) reported that higher levels of self-criticism were related to reports of inadequate parenting. This was especially true for individuals who consistently reported high levels of self-criticism. Similar results have been found by Blatt, Wein, Chevron, and Quinlan (1979). Because both self-criticism and dependency are thought to be possible cognitive vulnerability factors, and have been shown in other studies to be associated with depressive states (Blatt & Zuroff, 1992), these data may be relevant for understanding the development of the cognitive diatheses for depression.

From a somewhat different perspective, studies by Whisman and Kwon (1992), Roberts, Gotlib, and Kassel (1996) and Whisman and McGarvey (1995) generally examined current attachment levels in adults, and found that insecure attachment is related to higher levels of depressive symptoms (similar to data from a number of other studies examining the link between attachment/bonding and depression). More importantly from a cognitive vulnerability perspective, however, they also found that this relation was mediated by depressotypic attitudes and dysfunctional

---

[3]A number of studies have assessed the relation between attachment/bonding and depression, and have typically found that poor attachment/bonding is in fact related to the development of depression as well as to anxiety (for reviews see Blatt & Homann, 1992; Burbach & Borduin, 1986; and Gerlsma, Emmelkamp, & Arrindell, 1990). Because the focus of this chapter is on cognitive vulnerability, the focus here is primarily on those studies that have examined the link between attachment, depression, and cognition.

attributions of the type that have been proposed by various depression theories to be central to the development of depression. These studies thus provide empirical evidence that disturbed parent–child interactions may not only create risk factors for depression, but that these risk factors are cognitive in nature.

Other studies have suggested that disruptions in the parent–child bonding process may be associated with cognitive vulnerability to depression. For instance, Manian, Strauman, and Denney (1998) found that self-discrepancy patterns of the type thought to be related to emotional regulation are associated with recollections of parenting warmth and rejection—dimensions quite similar to the caring scale of the PBI. Such data imply that parental rejection may be a key factor in not only the development of depression, but in the origin of cognitive vulnerability to this depression. Likewise, Parker (1979) found recollections of diminished maternal care to be associated with the kind of cognitive deficits frequently seen in depression. Echoing this finding, Ingram, Overbey, and Fortier (2000) indicated that recollections of maternal care were associated with deficits in positive cognition and excesses in negative cognition. Dysfunctional cognition of this type has been specified by depression theories to represent a key causal agent in the onset and maintenance of the disorder.

In another study assessing the possible childhood antecedents of cognitive vulnerability to depression, Ingram and Ritter (2000) found that college students, who were thought to be vulnerable because they had previously experienced an episode of depression, displayed more negative errors on an information-processing task when they had been primed by a sad mood than did unprimed vulnerable people or primed nonvulnerable subjects. In addition, prior ratings of maternal care were negatively associated with errors on the negative stimulus aspects of the task, suggesting that lower levels of care were associated with the processing of more negative information when vulnerable individuals were in a negative mood. This study, along with those previously reviewed, clearly points in the direction of early interactional patterns leading to the kinds of cognitive patterns linked to depression. More specifically, these data suggest that a perceived lack of caring by mothers in particular may set the stage for the development of a cognitive self-schema that is activated in response to a sad mood and that eventually leads to depression.[4]

Early Abuse and Maltreatment Experiences. A related but different kind of parent–child interaction has been examined in studies that assess

---

[4]Such interpretations do not suggest that fathers are unimportant in these possible vulnerability functions, but rather that these data simply tend to be less likely to detect a role for fathers.

abuse experiences. Although different in focus, just as research has shown consistent relations between perceptions of the quality of parental care and later depression, data have also suggested a consistent relation between reports of abuse, particularly sexual abuse, and depression (for reviews, see Browne & Finkelhor, 1986; Cutler & Nolen-Hoeksema, 1991; and Kendall-Tackett, Williams, & Finkelhor, 1993). In one of the few studies that investigated cognitive variables within the context of abuse and depression, Kuyken and Brewin (1995) assessed memory retrieval in depressed patients, some of whom had experienced sexual and/or physical abuse as children. They found that depressed women who had been sexually (but not physically) abused showed an inability to recall specific memories in response to both positive and negative cues. According to their study, such abuse may lead to the avoidance of key memories and disruptions in working memory, which may then play a role in mediating the relation between abuse and depression.

Rose, Abramson, Hodulik, Halberstadt, and Leff (1994) also examined the mediational effect of cognitive variables on the relation between sexual abuse and depression, albeit from a very different perspective. In this study, one subgroup of depressed individuals who had experienced childhood sexual abuse was also characterized by negative cognitive styles. It was speculated that these adverse early experiences led to the development of negative cognitive processing patterns linked to vulnerability to depression. This speculation was further supported by Rose and Abramson (1995), who indicated that degree of childhood maltreatment was correlated with degree of dysfunctional cognition. Taken together, the data reported by Kuyken and Brewin (1995), Rose et al. (1994), and Rose and Abramson (1995) suggest that a history of early adverse experiences (e.g., sexual abuse) may produce the early cognitive patterns that lead to the later development of depression.

Summary of Research on Cognitive Vulnerability to Depression

The extant data clearly suggest that negative self-related cognitions, whether conceptualized from a cognitive schema standpoint or an attributional standpoint, serve as cognitive vulnerability factors within the context of a diathesis–stress relation. Priming data show that these cognitive factors exist in vulnerable individuals, and they can be activated by the effects of stresslike experiences, such as the occurrence of negative mood. Moreover, some of these data, along with data on attributional styles, show that dysfunctional cognitive factors are associated with the onset of depression in response to stressful events. High risk research has also shown that the match between the type of event and the particular content of the negative cognitions is an important factor in determining whether depressive reactions will occur.

The data also reveal that disrupted interactions with parents pose a risk factor for later depression as a function of the development of cognitive vulnerability mechanisms. Such disruptions may take the form of poor parenting, as in overcontrol and a lack of care, or may be more malevolent, as in the sexual or emotional abuse of children and adolescents. Although theoretical perspectives suggest that the link between these parental behaviors and later depression in adulthood is cognitive in nature, the empirical data on the cognitive effects of these disturbed interactions are relatively sparse. Nevertheless, the extant data do support the idea that cognitive variables form mediational pathways between troublesome parent–child/adolescent interactions and depression. Of course, these data are not the only types that bear on the issue of cognitive vulnerability to depression and the origins of cognitive vulnerability. Most of the studies reviewed thus far have examined these factors in adults—most of them young adults. A body of data also exists on such factors in children and adolescents.

COGNITIVE VULNERABILITY FACTORS IN HIGH RISK CHILDREN

A number of studies have assessed cognitive functioning in depressed children (see Garber & Flynn, 2001b). Although important, these data are relatively uninformative about vulnerability factors inasmuch as cognitive patterns that occur during depression, and may therefore appear to serve as a vulnerability factor, may instead be a consequence of the disorder (Barnett & Gotlib, 1988). However, one way to examine the origins and development of cognitive vulnerability for depression is to examine cognitive functioning in children who are not depressed, but who are at risk for depression. One group of high risk children are those whose mothers are depressed (Goodman & Gotlib, 1999; Hammen, 1991a).

Only a limited number of studies have examined cognitive functioning in high risk children. In one study that did so, the negative attributional styles of children with mood-disordered mothers were assessed. Findings indicated that the children of depressed mothers reported more negatively toned self-attributions than did children of nondepressed mothers (Radke-Yarrow, Belmont, Nottelmann, & Bottomly, 1990). Rake-Yarrow et al. also found some correspondence between mother and child statements; for example, a mother who endorsed the statement "I hate myself" was likely to have a child who endorsed the statement "I am bad."

A particularly thorough study was reported by Jaenicke et al. (1987) as part of a larger project conducted by Hammen (1991a). In this study, the offspring of unipolar, bipolar, nonpsychiatric medical patients, and normal mothers were examined using a self-referent incidental recall task (e.g., Rogers, Kuiper, & Kirker, 1977). In this task, the incidental recall of personally relevant adjectives can be used to make inferences about schemas and information processing that are operative in depression (Ingram & Kendall, 1986). This task has been used most frequently in the assessment of adults, but was modified for use with children by Hammen and Zupan (1984). Recall results suggested a lack of positive information recall for the children of both unipolar and bipolar mothers. On other tasks, children in the unipolar and bipolar groups also reported a less positive self-concept and evidenced a more negative attributional style.

In another study assessing possible cognitive vulnerability mechanisms in the children of depressed mothers, Taylor and Ingram (1999) examined information-processing indices of negative self-schemas in both high risk (children whose mothers were depressed) and low risk children (children whose mothers were not depressed). Prior to completing a self-referent encoding and recall task, half of the children in the Taylor and Ingram (1999) study participated in a priming (mood induction) task. When recall patterns were examined, negative mood enhanced the recall of negative personally relevant stimuli for only high risk children, suggesting the emergence of negative cognitive schemas in these children, but not in low risk children. Thus, these data purport that depressed mothers may transmit negative cognitive characteristics to their children, which form the basis of a negative self-schema that is activated in response to negative mood producing events.

Garber and Flynn (2001a) assessed perceptions of self-worth, attributional style, and hopelessness in the children of depressed mothers. They reported that maternal depression was related to all three of these negative cognitions, and beyond maternal depression, low maternal care was associated with limited child self-worth. Children's attributional style also was found to mirror maternal attributions for child-related events; that is, children made the same types of attributions for child-related events as did their mothers.

In a longitudinal study of the perceptions of control in children, Rudolph, Kurlakowsky, and Conley (2001) found that both stress and family were associated with deficits in the perception of control, and in more helplessness. To the extent that these perceptions and a sense of helplessness contribute to vulnerability to depression, the results reported by Rudolph et al. (2001) suggest that, although parenting may be important in producing vulnerability, other factors also play a role. In fact, data from D. A. Cole, Jacquez, and Maschman (2001) and Williams, Connolly, and

Segal (2001) also evidence that other individuals (e.g., teachers and romantic partners) may play a role in creating cognitive vulnerability in children and adolescents.

In sum, data from studies examining the cognitive characteristics of children who are at risk for depression support the idea that these children have negative cognitive structures available, and that depressed parents may transmit these negative cognitive characteristics to their children. The data also indicate, however, that even though parents are extremely important, other interpersonal relationships may also contribute to this cognitive vulnerability creation. Clearly, children at risk for depression appear to have negative self-schemas that, when accessed, are linked to the appearance of self-devaluing and pessimistic thoughts, as well as to dysfunctional information processing. Theory and data thus make a strong case that negative events in childhood are essential elements in the formation of cognitive structures that place children at risk, and that eventually predispose adults to the experience of depression (Goodman & Gotlib, 1999).

THE NATURE OF COGNITIVE VULNERABILITY TO DEPRESSION: SUMMARY AND SOME DIRECTIONS FOR THE FUTURE

This chapter has reviewed some of the major theories of depression and examined the statements these theories make about cognitive vulnerability. It has also examined the data that has sought to empirically address the risk variables featured in these theories. These theories and the data that follow from them do not chart a single course through the multitude of constructs that have been proposed; rather, theories and research conceptualize and examine these factors from a variety of different perspectives. Despite this diversity, some themes that run through these theories and studies provide important clues about the nature of cognitive vulnerability and the origins of this vulnerability process. Next consider some of these themes, as well as some theoretical speculations on the nature of cognitive vulnerability to depression.

The Role of Interpersonal Events

It may seem surprising for a chapter on cognitive vulnerability to highlight interpersonal events, but they are nevertheless crucial for understanding cognitive vulnerability as well as the factors that create it. Indeed, the apparent antipathy between cognitive and interpersonal models of depression is not only unnecessary, but also quite arbitrary (Gotlib &

Hammen, 1992; Joiner & Coyne, 2002). Although a variety of interpersonal events are important in creating cognitive vulnerability, current theory and data have suggested that attachment processes play a critical role in this process. We thus address some of the implications of the idea that attachment processes play this critical role.

Attachment and Bonding in the Creation of Cognitive Vulnerability.
The fact that attachment processes occur throughout a number of different species, including humans, suggests that it has considerable evolutionary significance. Bowlby (1988) was quite clear on this point: "It is . . . more than likely that a human being's powerful propensity to make these deep and long-term relationships is the result of a strong gene-determined bias to do so, a bias that has been selected during the course of evolution" (p. 81). The motivation to bond is thus hardwired in our past. Although there are a number of functions that attachment and bonding serve, the ongoing maintenance of affective bonds plays a critical role in our most basic emotional needs—the maintenance of proximity to individuals of our own kind.

It is thus not an evolutionary accident that interpersonal loss is one of the most powerful precipitants of depression (Ingram et al., 1998). Indeed, humans are biologically wired to not only seek out interactions with others, but to seek out intimate interactions with at least some people. This social behavior reflects a biologically driven process that eventuates in reproductive success (Gilbert, 1992) and has thus been selected for by evolutionary processes because it helps to perpetuate our species. Indeed, at the other end of the continuum, when social-contact seeking is absent it is considered a reflection of psychopathology of another type (e.g., schizoid personality disorder).

A variety of negative effects may occur when events happen in childhood that adversely affect attachment processes; childhood is obviously a time of enormous learning and thus the occurrence of negative events can have a profound effect on the child's developing cognitive and affective neural connections (Ingram et al., 1998; Goodman & Gotlib, 1999). Because occasional negative events are a routine part of growing up, it is to the extent that negative events occur in abundance, occur in the context of multiple and likely interacting domains (e.g., a very dysfunctional family, divorce, high levels of poverty, problematic peer relationships), are chronic or extremely traumatic, or are depriving of the child's emotional needs, that cognitive and affective development will be proportionally impacted. Moreover, the long-term effects of negative events are likely to be particularly virulent when they involve key attachment figures. For instance, lack of caring or involvement (evidenced in the extreme by abandonment) most likely leaves a vulnerability to depression. This lack of caring can be reflected by neglect in some cases, or in others, extreme criticism or abuse. In fact, although other factors certainly play some role, data have begun to suggest that lack of care may be the single most important factor in producing vulnerability to depression (Ingram et al., 1998).

Possible Mechanisms of the Development of Depressive Self-Schemas

What are the mechanisms by which interpersonal experiences such as a lack of care might lead to depressive cognitive structures? Within the context of having a depressed mother, Goodman and Gotlib (1999) named a variety of factors that may be linked to the development of negative cognitive structures, such as modeling negative cognition and interactions, and exposure to depressive behaviors and affect. Similarly, D. A. Cole et al. (2001) pointed out the relevance of the "looking glass" hypothesis for the development of depressive cognitive structures. Originally proposed by Cooley (1902) and by Mead (1934), the looking glass hypothesis suggests that the view of oneself is constructed by the perceptions of others of the person, and the communication of these perceptions. In the child who is developing a schema of the self, negative experiences like a lack of care and rejection by attachment figures are likely to generate personal themes of derogation and unworthiness that become deeply encoded in self-structures. Also deeply encoded are concepts linked to the experience of disrupted attachment such as representations about the behavior of significant others. In the terminology of attachment theory, these experiences should not only determine the schemas, or working models, of oneself, but should also determine how one is inclined to see others, as well as the expectations of how to interact with others.

Attachment disruptions are almost certainly characterized by the experience of negative affect. It is thus important to note that during critical maturation periods, cognitive structures are not the only neural networks that are developing. The affective structures with which we are all born (see LeDoux, 1996, 2000) are also in the process of becoming more differentiated and developing associations to other structures (see Jordan & Cole, 1996). As these cognitive and affective structures collaterally develop, connections between them almost certainly develop in such a way that negative cognitive self-structures become closely linked to negative affective structures. Negative affect is thus associated with unfavorable conceptions of the self. Hence, the depressive self-schema does not only represent a negative view of the self, but also a connection to negative affective structures.

If attachment disruptions are brief and secure attachment interactions are reestablished, then negative cognitive representations are likely to be limited and more weakly associated with negative affective networks. Alternatively, if the attachment process is more problematic, then such connections between negative self-representations and negative affect should become more extensive and more strongly linked. Thus, if negative emotion-producing events related to the self are numerous, particularly traumatic, or chronic, they will have a correspondingly profound effect on the development of, and connections between, representations of the self and others, and on the experience of negative affective states. The soon-to-be vulnerable to depression person thus develops a schema of the self as unlikable and unlovable that is strongly tied to the experience of negative affect.

Depressogenesis of Cognitive Mechanisms

All individuals encounter stress and negative emotions in their lives, but not all experience depression as a result of this stress and emotion. However, when individuals who have negative cognitive structures that are connected to negative affective structures encounter these experiences, not only will they experience negative emotions, but these negative emotions will also activate a variety of maladaptive cognitions about the self; the experience of negative affect thus brings the negative self-schema "on-line." Life stress, or negative events, that are cognitively interpreted in terms of one's own inadequacy and inferiority thus turn a "normal" negative affective state into depression (Teasdale, 1988). We are reminded in this regard of Freud's differentiation between mourning and melancholia: In mourning the person's response to a loss is "*this* is terrible," whereas in melancholia the person's response to this loss is "*I* am terrible." Therefore, the vulnerability function, or depressogenesis of the cognitive mechanisms outlined, lies in the transition from normal negative affective states to a depressive psychopathological state via the connection between negative cognitive self-structures and negative affective structures.

Maintenance of Depression

Thus far, comments about cognitive vulnerability and the causes of depression have been aimed largely at the onset of the depressed state. Onset, however, is not the only aspect of causality (Ingram et al., 1998); depressed people tend to stay depressed for a period of time, and thus the factors that maintain this state may be as, or even more important than, onset. After all, if people encountered the onset of depression only to have it lift a day or two later, then depression would not constitute the disabling disorder that it is. Next consider the implications for maintenance of the cognitive factors that have been discussed.

External Information Processing: The Tyrannical Self-Schema. The cognitive maintenance process is reminiscent of ideas presented in an article by Greenwald (1980) entitled "The Totalitarian Ego: Fabrication and Revision of Personal History." Greenwald reviewed numerous studies suggesting that, through information-processing biases such as selective attention, people have a tendency to revise their personal history in order to psychologically protect themselves; they "rewrite" their experiences to make themselves feel better. Greenwald labeled this behavior totalitarian because of the psychological similarity to totalitarian societies that maintain control through the manipulation of information; for example, history books are rewritten to serve certain views. But another aspect of totalitarian societies might be more metaphorically germane for depressed people; totalitarian societies maintain control not only through rewriting history, but also through oppression and tyranny. It is in this sense that depressed people might be seen as operating under the constraints of a totalitarian ego (or perhaps a "tyrannical" self-schema). Such a schema does not serve to psychologically protect individuals, but rather "oppresses" them through information processing that provides full access to self-degrading, negative, and pessimistic data. Structuring the self, the future, and the worldview in a negative fashion (e.g., Beck's negative cognitive triad) is one manner in which depression is maintained.

Top-Down/Bottom-Up Information Processing. The maintenance of depression may also be seen in the context of an overreliance on top-down information processing. It has been recognized for some time that information processing can stem from the top-down, indicating the influence of cognitive structures on the data to be processed, or alternatively, from the bottom-up, which suggests that information processing is directed from the data available (e.g., Norman, 1986). Healthy individuals most likely employ a combination or balance of top-down and bottom-up information processing. That is, healthy people employ schemas to help structure and order information processing, but they are also responsive to the data that are available, which in turn influences the operation and content of schemas (see Neisser, 1967). Depressed individuals, on the other hand, are more likely to disregard the information available. Such "cognitive intransigence" (Ingram, 1990) is particularly problematic when the cognitive structures are so dysfunctional in nature. Therefore, one way to view the cognitive maintenance of depression (and vulnerability to depression) is not only via the operation and content of cognitive self-structures, but in terms of deviations from the normal balance between top-down and bottom-up processing; depression maintenance may be the result of an overabundance of top-down processing to the relative exclusion of bottom-up processing.

Final Pathways: The Cognitive-Interpersonal Link
in Depression and Vulnerability

In the cognitive vulnerability processes described, interpersonal events play several key roles. For instance, during key developmental periods, distressful interpersonal events involving key attachment figures activate innate negative affective structures, lead to the development of negative cognitive self-structures, and correspondingly begin the process of developing connections between these cognitive and affective structures. In addition, once these vulnerability structures are in place, distressful interpersonal events serve as the triggering agents for the activation of depressive cognitive processes.

Although it has been acknowledged that interpersonal events play a pivotal role as potent triggers for the activation of proximal vulnerability, there has been no comment on the broader relation between cognitive and interpersonal functioning in depression vulnerability. Although there are any number of psychological models of vulnerability to depression, including interpersonal models, we propose that cognitive factors serve as the final common pathway to depression, at least for depression that is primarily psychologically mediated as opposed to that which is primarily biologically mediated (e.g., bipolar depression) (see also Ingram et al., 1998). That is, although numerous psychological factors are related to the onset and maintenance of depression, we contend that these all operate via cognitive processes. Like Akiskal's (1979; Akiskal & McKinney, 1973, 1975) examination of depression from a neuroanatomical level of analysis (the diencephalon as the final neuroanatomical pathway), by final common pathway we suggest that cognitive factors mediate all other psychological vulnerability processes, including interpersonal processes.

To help illustrate the idea that cognitive processes serve as the pathway through which factors like interpersonal events are linked to depression, consider the hypotheses and data that have been advanced about stress-generation and depression (Hammen, 1991b). In some—perhaps many—cases, stressful interpersonal events do not simply happen to people independently of their actions. All social behavior is cognitively mediated to the extent that it must be processed and interpreted if even at very subconscious levels. Therefore, by interpreting social information, and determining behavioral responses, cognitive structures such as working models provide the template for how other's actions are viewed. Individuals thus process and interpret social information and respond "accordingly." In the case of depression vulnerability, others' behaviors, verbalizations, and nonverbal cues are processed and interpreted through the filter of the depressogenic vulnerability schema. Benign interactions have the potential to be viewed as critical, leading to an "appropriate response." If the vulnerable individual responds to a perceived critical remark in kind, then interpersonal difficulties ensue as a cycle of social rejection is engendered. Hence, interpersonal stress is generated or caused by cognitive factors.

Of course, some people are in fact criticized, or do experience stressful events that are not of their own making. For vulnerable or currently depressed people, such criticisms or events, when interpreted via negative cognitive structures, will lead to exacerbated negative responses. Whereas the person with a healthy self-concept who is criticized by being called a "loser" will probably respond with some negative affect (but will be unlikely to enter a dysfunctional interpersonal cycle), the person who has incorporated "loserness" into schemas or working models will respond both cognitively and behaviorally in a very different way to such a comment. Similarly, whereas stressful events create negative emotions for even the healthiest of people, for the vulnerable person these stressful events are interpreted through a meaning system that distorts the impact of the event, and creates negative affect that fuels further dysfunctional cognitions. Therefore, the person who has been sensitized to losses because of the abandonment by a key attachment figure will interpret these losses through the lens of a negative cognitive structure that will create more stress, more negative affect, and lead to more biological disregulation than will the person who experiences a loss but who has a relatively healthy self-concept and functional self-schema.

The final common pathway hypothesis suggests that the interpretation of stressful events, and interactions with others, are dependent on the cognitive processing functions of depressogenic cognitive structures. The idea that cognition serves as the central mediating process is not new, and goes back at least to Beck's (1967) speculations on the nature of depression. In a discussion of stress generation in depression, Hammen (1991b) summed up this perspective nicely: "Negative cognitions about themselves and events may alter their responses to circumstances or may contribute to an inability to cope with emergent situations and may also determine reactions to personally meaningful events [i.e., stress-generation]. In a sense, therefore, depression causes future depression through the mediation of stressors and cognitions about the self and circumstances" (p. 559). Hence, cognition is the psychological bond that holds the rest of the vulnerability process together. This is the essence of the final pathway hypothesis.

This chapter has reviewed several of the major cognitive theories of depression, noted the statements they make about the nature of vulnerability, and examined their ideas about the origins of this cognitive vulnerability. It also has looked at the empirical data relevant to these theories.

These data have assessed possible vulnerability factors in both adults and children, although the amount of data on children lags behind that which has been reported for adults. Although not completely uniform, the bulk of these data suggest that cognitive factors do play an important role in both the onset and maintenance of the depressed state. Moreover, the data also show that these cognitive factors develop in childhood, and are most likely the result of disrupted interaction patterns with key attachment figures such as parents (although individuals other than parents may also contribute to vulnerability). Similar types of interaction patterns may carry on throughout the vulnerable individual's life, and thus constitute an important aspect of the depression process. As important as these processes are, however, we propose that cognitive variables serve as the final common pathway to depression. That is, to have meaning to the person, interpersonal interactions or putatively stressful events must be processed through the lens of cognitive schemas, that in the case of depression-proneness are quite negative in nature; in this manner, "normal" negative events turn into depression. This idea is not new, but its time has come.

REFERENCES

Abramson, L. Y., Alloy, L. B., Hogan, M. E., Whitehouse, W. G., Donovan, P., Rose, D., Panzarella, C., & Raniere, D. (1999). Cognitive vulnerability to depression: Theory and evidence. *Journal of Cognitive Psychotherapy, 13*, 5–20.

Abramson, L. Y., Alloy, L. B., Hogan, M. E., Whitehouse, W. G., Donovan, P., Rose, D. T., Panzarella, C., & Raniere, D. (2002). Cognitive vulnerability to depression: Theory and evidence. In R. L. Leahy & E. T. Dowd (Eds.), *Clinical advances in cognitive psychotherapy: Theory and application* (pp. 75–92). New York: Springer.

Abramson, L. Y., Metalsky, G. I., & Alloy, L. B. (1989). Hopelessness depression: A theory-based subtype of depression. *Psychological Review, 96*, 358–372.

Abramson, L. Y., Seligman, M. E. P., & Teasdale, J. (1978). Learned helplessness in humans: Critique and reformulation. *Journal of Abnormal Psychology, 87*, 49–74.

Akiskal, H. S. (1979). A biobehavioral approach to depression. In R. A. Depue (Ed.), *The psychobiology of depressive disorders* (pp. 409–433). New York: Academic Press.

Akiskal, H. S., & McKinney, W. T. (1973). Depressive disorders: Toward a unified hypothesis. *Science, 182*, 20–29.

Akiskal, H. S., & McKinney, W. T. (1975). Overview of recent research in depression: Integration of ten conceptual models into a comprehensive clinical frame. *Archives of General Psychiatry, 32*, 285–305.

Alba, J. W., & Hasher, L. (1983). Is memory schematic? *Psychological Bulletin, 93*, 207–231.

Alloy, L. B., & Abramson, L. Y. (1999). The Temple–Wisconsin Cognitive Vulnerability to Depression Project: Conceptual background, design, and methods. *Journal of Cognitive Psychotherapy, 13*, 227–262.

Alloy, L. B., Abramson, L. Y., Murray, L. A., Whitehouse, W. G., & Hogan, M E. (1997). Self-referent information processing in individuals at high and low risk for depression. *Cognition and Emotion, 11*, 539–568.

Alloy, L. B., Abramson, L. Y., Tashman, N. A., Steinberg, D. L., Hogan, M. E., Whitehouse, W. G., Crossfield, A. G., & Morocco, A. (2001). Developmental origins of cognitive vulnerability to depression: Parenting, cognitive, and inferential feedback styles on the parents of individuals at high and low cognitive risk for depression. *Cognitive Therapy and Research, 25,* 397–424.

Ainsworth, M. D. S. (1989). Attachments beyond infancy. *American Psychologist, 44,* 709–716.

Ainsworth, M. D. S., Blehar, M. C., Waters, E., & Wall, S. (1978). *Patterns of attachment: A psychological study of the strange situation.* Hillsdale, NJ: Lawrence Erlbaum Associates.

Bartholomew, K., & Horowitz, L. M. (1991). Attachment styles among young adults: A test of a four-category model. *Journal of Personality and Social Psychology, 61,* 226–244.

Barnett, P. A., & Gotlib, I. H. (1988). Psychosocial functioning in depression: Distinguishing among antecedents, concomitants, and consequences. *Psychological Bulletin, 104,* 97–126.

Beck, A. T. (1963). Thinking and depression: Vol. 1. Idiosyncratic content and cognitive. *Archives of General Psychiatry, 9,* 324–333.

Beck, A. T. (1967). *Depression: Causes and treatment.* Philadelphia: University of Pennsylvania Press.

Beck, A. T. (1987). Cognitive models of depression. *Journal of Cognitive Psychotherapy, 1,* 5–37.

Bemporad, J. R., & Romano, S. J. (1992). Childhood maltreatment and adult depression: A review of research. In D. Cicchetti & S. L. Toth (Eds.), *Developmental perspectives on depression* (pp. 351–376). Rochester, NY: University of Rochester Press.

Blatt, S. J., & Homann, E. (1992). Parent–child interaction in the etiology of dependent and self-critical depression. *Clinical Psychology Review, 12,* 47–91.

Blatt, S. J., Wein, S. J., Chevron, E., & Quinlan, D. M. (1979). Parental representations and depression in normal young adults. *Journal of Abnormal Psychology, 88,* 388–397.

Blatt, S. J., & Zuroff, D. C. (1992). Interpersonal relatedness and self-definition: Two prototypes for depression. *Clinical Psychology Review, 12,* 527–562.

Bowlby, J. (1969). *Attachment and loss: Vol. 1. Attachment.* New York: Basic Books.

Bowlby, J. (1973). *Attachment and loss: Vol. 2. Separation, anxiety, and anger.* New York: Basic Books.

Bowlby, J. (1980). *Attachment and loss: Vol. 3. Loss: Sadness and depression.* New York: Basic Books.

Bowlby, J. (1988). *A secure base: Parent–child attachment and healthy human development.* New York: Basic Books.

Brewin, C. R., Firth-Cozens, J., Furnham, A., & McManus, C. (1992). Self-criticism in adulthood and recalled childhood experience. *Journal of Abnormal Psychology, 101,* 561–566.

Brosse, A. L., Craighead, L. W., & Craighead, W. E. (1999). Testing the mood-state hypothesis among previously depressed and never-depressed individuals. *Behavior Therapy, 30,* 97–115.

Browne, A., & Finkelhor, D. (1986). Impact of child sexual abuse: A review of the research. *Psychological Bulletin, 99,* 66–77.

Burbach, D. J., & Borduin, C. M. (1986). Parent–child relations and the etiology of depression. *Clinical Psychology Review, 6,* 133–153.

Cole, D. A., Jacquez, F. M., & Maschman, T. L. (2001). Social origins of depressive cognitions: A longitudinal study of self-perceived competence in children. *Cognitive Therapy and Research, 25,* 377–396.

Cole, P. M., & Zahn-Waxler, C. (1992). Emotional dysregulation in disruptive behavior disorders. In D. Cicchetti & S. L. Toth (Eds.), *Developmental perspectives on depression* (pp. 173–209). Rochester, NY: University of Rochester Press.

Cooley, C. H. (1902). *Human nature and the social order.* New York: Scribner's.

Coyne, J. C., & Whiffen, V. E. (1995). Issues in personality as diathesis for depression: The case of sociotropy dependency and autonomy self criticism. *Psychological Bulletin, 118,* 358–378.

Cummings, E. M., & Cicchetti, D. (1990). Toward a transactional model of relations between attachment and depression. In M. Greenberg & D. Cicchetti (Eds.), *Attachment in the preschool years: Theory research, and intervention* (pp. 339–372). Chicago: University of Chicago Press.

Cutler, S. E., & Nolen-Hoeksema, S. (1991). Accounting for sex differences in depression through female victimization: Childhood sexual abuse. *Sex Roles, 24*, 425–438.

Dent, J., & Teasdale, J. D. (1988). Negative cognition and the persistence of depression. *Journal of Abnormal Psychology, 97*, 29–34.

Doane, J. A., & Diamond, D. (1994). *Affect and attachment in the family: A family based treatment of major psychiatric disorder*. New York: Basic Books.

Dykman, B. M. (1997). A test of whether negative emotional priming facilitates access to latent dysfunctional attitudes. *Cognition and Emotion, 11*, 197–222.

Garber, J., & Flynn, C. (2001a). Predictors of depressive cognitions in young adolescents. *Cognitive Therapy and Research, 25*, 353–376.

Garber, J., & Flynn, C. (2001b). Vulnerability to depression in childhood and adolescence. In R. E. Ingram & J. M. Price (Eds.), *Vulnerability to psychopathology: Risk across the lifespan* (pp. 175–225). New York: Guilford.

Gerlsma, C., Emmelkamp, P. M., & Arrindell, W. A. (1990). Anxiety, depression, and perception of early parenting: A meta-analysis. *Clinical Psychology Review, 10*, 251–277.

Gibb, B. E., Alloy, L. B., Abramson, L. Y., & Marx, B. P. (2003). Childhood maltreatment and maltreatment-specific inferences: A test of Rose and Abramson's (1992) extension of the hopelessness theory. *Cognition and Emotion, 17*, 917–931.

Gibb, B. E., Alloy, L. B. Abramson, L. Y., Rose, D. T., Whitehouse, W. G., Donovan, P., Hogan, M. E. Cronholm, J., & Tierney, S. (2001). History of childhood maltreatment, negative cognitive styles, and episodes of depression in adulthood. *Cognitive Therapy and Research, 25*, 425–446.

Gilbert, P. (1992). *Depression: The evolution of powerlessness*. New York: Guilford.

Goodman, S. H., & Gotlib, I. H. (1999). Risk for psychopathology in the children of depressed mothers: A developmental model for understanding mechanisms of transmission. *Psychological Review, 106*, 458–490.

Gotlib, I. H., & Hammen, C. L. (1992). *Psychological aspects of depression: Toward a cognitive-interpersonal integration*. Chichester, England: Wiley.

Gotlib, I. H., & Hammen, C. L. (Eds.). (2002). *Handbook of depression* (3rd ed.). New York: Guilford.

Gotlib, I. H., & Krasnoperova, E. (1998). Biased information processing as a vulnerability factor for depression. *Behavior Therapy, 29*, 603–617.

Greenwald, A. (1980). The totalitarian ego: Fabrication and revision of personal history. *American Psychologist, 35*, 603–618.

Hammen, C. (1991a). *Depression runs in families: The social context of risk and resilience in children of depressed mothers*. New York: Springer-Verlag.

Hammen, C. (1991b). The generation of stress in the course of unipolar depression. *Journal of Abnormal Psychology, 100*, 555–561.

Hammen, C., & Zupan, B. A. (1984). Self-schemas and the processing of personal information in children. *Journal of Experimental Child Psychology, 37*, 598–608.

Hedlund, S., & Rude, S. S. (1995). Evidence of latent depressive schemas in formerly depressed individuals. *Journal of Abnormal Psychology, 104*, 517–525.

Hollon, S. D. (1992). Cognitive models of depression from a psychobiological perspective. *Psychological Inquiry, 3*, 250–253.

Ingram, R. E. (1984). Toward an information processing analysis of depression. *Cognitive Therapy and Research, 8*, 443–477.

Ingram, R. E. (1990). Self-focused attention in clinical disorders: Review and a conceptual model. *Psychological Bulletin, 107*, 156–176.

Ingram, R. E., Bernet, C. Z., & McLaughlin, S. C. (1994). Attentional allocation processes in individuals at risk for depression. *Cognitive Therapy and Research, 18,* 317–332.

Ingram, R. E., & Kendall, P. C. (1986). Cognitive clinical psychology: Implications of an information processing perspective. In R. E. Ingram (Ed.), *Information processing approaches to clinical psychology* (pp. 4–21). Orlando: Academic Press.

Ingram, R. E., & Luxton, D. (in press). Vulnerability-stress models. In B. L. Hankin & J. R. Z. Abela (Eds.), *Development of psychopathology: A vulnerability–stress perspective.* New York: Sage.

Ingram, R. E., Miranda, J., & Segal, Z. V. (1998). *Cognitive vulnerability to depression.* New York: Guilford.

Ingram, R. E., Overbey, T., & Fortier, M. (2001). Individual differences in dysfunctional automatic thinking and parental bonding: Specificity of maternal care. *Personality and Individual Differences, 30,* 401–412.

Ingram, R. E., & Price, J. M. (2001). The role of vulnerability in understanding psychopathology. In R. E. Ingram & J. M. Price (Eds.), *Vulnerability to psychopathology: Risk across the lifespan* (pp. 3–19). New York: Guilford.

Ingram, R. E., & Ritter, J. (2000). Vulnerability to depression: Cognitive reactivity and parental bonding in high-risk individuals. *Journal of Abnormal Psychology, 109,* 588–596.

Jaenicke, C., Hammen, C. L., Zupan, B., Hiroto, D., Gordon, D., Adrain, C., & Burge, D. (1987). Cognitive vulnerability in children at risk for depression. *Journal of Abnormal Child Psychology, 15,* 559–572.

Joiner, T., & Coyne, C. (2002). *The interactional nature of depression.* Washington, DC: American Psychological Association.

Jordan, A., & Cole, D. A. (1996). Relation of depressive symptoms to the structure of self-knowledge in childhood. *Journal of Abnormal Psychology, 105,* 530–540.

Kendall-Tackett, K. A., Williams, L. M., & Finkelhor, D. (1993). Impact of sexual abuse on children: A review and synthesis of recent empirical studies. *Psychological Bulletin, 113,* 164–180.

Kihlstrom, J. F., & Cantor, N. (1984). Mental representations of the self. In L. Berkowitz (Ed.), *Advances in experimental social psychology* (Vol. 15, pp. 360–399). New York: Academic Press.

Kuyken, W., & Brewin, C. R. (1995). Autobiographical memory functioning in depression and reports of early abuse. *Journal of Abnormal Psychology, 104,* 585–591.

LeDoux, J. E. (1996). *The emotional brain: The mysterious underpinnings of emotional life.* New York: Simon & Schuster.

LeDoux, J. E. (2000). Emotion circuits in the brain. *Annual Review of Neuroscience, 23,* 155–184.

Manian, N., Strauman, T., & Denney, N. (1998). Temperament, recalled parenting styles, and self-regulation: Testing the developmental postulates of self-discrepancy theory. *Journal of Personality and Social Psychology, 75,* 1321–1332.

McCranie, E. W., & Bass, J. D. (1984). Childhood family antecedents of dependency and self-criticism: Implications for depression. *Journal of Abnormal Psychology, 93,* 3–8.

Mead, G. H. (1934). *Mind, self, and society.* Chicago: University of Chicago Press.

Miranda, J., Gross, J., Persons, J., & Hahn, J. (1998). Mood matters: Negative mood induction activates dysfunctional attitudes in women vulnerable to depression. *Cognitive Therapy and Research, 22,* 363–376.

Miranda, J., Persons, J. B., & Byers, C. (1990). Endorsement of dysfunctional beliefs depends on current mood state. *Journal of Abnormal Psychology, 99,* 237–241.

Monroe, S. M., & Hadjiyannakis, K. (2002). The social environment in depression: Focusing on severe life stress. In I. H. Gotlib & C. L. Hammen (Eds.), *Handbook of depression* (3rd ed., pp. 314–340). New York: Guilford.

Monroe, S. M., & Simons, A. D. (1991). Diathesis–stress theories in the context of life stress research: Implications for the depressive disorders. *Psychological Bulletin, 110,* 406–425.

Neisser, U. (1967). *Cognitive psychology*. New York: Appleton.

Nietzel, M. T., & Harris, M. J. (1990). Relationship of dependency and achievement/autonomy to depression. *Clinical Psychology Review, 10,* 279–297.

Norman, D. A. (1986). Toward a theory of memory and attention. *Psychological Review, 75,* 522–536.

Parker, G. (1979). Parental characteristics in relation to depressive disorders. *British Journal of Psychiatry, 134,* 138–147.

Parker, G. (1983). Parental "affectionless control" as an antecedent to adult depression: A risk factor delineated. *Archives of General Psychiatry, 40,* 956–960.

Radke-Yarrow, M., Belmont, B., Nottelmann, E. D., & Bottomly, L. (1990). Young children's self-conceptions: Origins in the natural discourse of depressed mothers and their children. In D. Cicchetti & M. Beeghly (Eds.), *The self in transition: Infancy to childhood. The John D. and Catherine T. MacArthur foundation series on mental health and development* (pp. 345–361). Chicago: University of Chicago Press.

Ricks, M. (1985). The social transmission of parental: Attachment across generations. In I. Bretherton & E. Waters (Eds.), Growing points in attachment theory and research. *Monographs of the Society for Research in Child Development, 50*(1–2, Serial No. 209), 445–466.

Roberts, J. E., Gotlib, I. H., & Kassel, J. D. (1996). Adult attachment security and symptoms of depression: The mediating roles of dysfunctional attitudes and low self-esteem. *Journal of Personality and Social Psychology, 70,* 310–320.

Robins, C. J. (1990). Congruence of personality and life events in depression. *Journal of Abnormal Psychology, 99,* 393–397.

Robins, C. J., & Block, P. (1988). Personal vulnerability, life events, and depressive symptoms: A test of a specific interactional model. *Journal of Personality and Social Psychology, 54,* 847–852.

Robins, C. J., & Luten, A. G. (1991). Sociotropy and autonomy: Differential patterns of clinical presentation in unipolar depression. *Journal of Abnormal Psychology, 100,* 74–77.

Rogers, T. B., Kuiper, N. A., & Kirker, W. S. (1977). Self-reference and the encoding of personal information. *Journal of Personality and Social Psychology, 35,* 677–688.

Rose, D. T., & Abramson, L. Y. (1992). Developmental predictors of depressive cognitive style: Research and theory. In D. Cicchetti & S. L. Toth (Eds.), *Developmental perspectives on depression* (pp. 323–350). Rochester, NY: University of Rochester Press.

Rose, D. T., & Abramson, L. Y. (1995). *Developmental maltreatment and cognitive vulnerability to hopelessness depression.* Paper presented at the meeting of the Association for the Advancement of Behavior Therapy, Washington, DC.

Rose, D. T., Abramson, L. Y., Hodulik, C. J., Halberstadt, L., & Leff, G. (1994). Heterogeneity of cognitive style among depressed inpatients. *Journal of Abnormal Psychology, 103,* 419–429.

Rudolph, K. D., Kurlakowsky, K. D., & Conley, C. S. (2001). Developmental and social-contextual origins of depressive control-related beliefs and behavior. *Cognitive Therapy and Research, 25,* 447–476.

Scher, C. D. Segal, Z., & Ingram, R. E. (in press). Beck's theory of depression: Origins, empirical status, and future directions for cognitive vulnerability. In R. L. Leahy (Ed.), *New advances in cognitive therapy*. New York: Guilford.

Segal, Z. V. (1988). Appraisal of the self-schema construct in cognitive models of depression. *Psychological Bulletin, 103,* 147–162.

Segal, Z. V., Gemar, M., & Williams, S. (1999). Differential cognitive response to a mood challenge following successful cognitive therapy or pharmacotherapy for unipolar depression. *Journal of Abnormal Psychology, 108,* 3–10.

Segal, Z. V., & Ingram, R. E. (1994). Mood priming and construct activation in tests of cognitive vulnerability to unipolar depression. *Clinical Psychology Review, 14,* 663–695.

Segal, Z. V., & Shaw, B. F. (1986). Cognition in depression: A reappraisal of Coyne & Gotlib's critique. *Cognitive Therapy and Research, 10,* 671–694.

Segal, Z. V., Shaw, B. F., Vella, D. D., & Katz, R. (1992). Cognitive and life stress predictors of relapse in remitted unipolar depressed patients: Test of the congruency hypothesis. *Journal of Abnormal Psychology, 101,* 26–36.

Seligman, M. E. P. (1975). *Helplessness: On depression, development, and death.* San Francisco: Freeman.

Solomon, A., Haaga, D. A. F., Kirk, L., & Friedman, D. G. (1998). Priming irrational beliefs in recovered-depressed people. *Journal of Abnormal Psychology, 107,* 440–449.

Taylor, L., & Ingram, R. E. (1999). Cognitive reactivity and depressotypic information processing in the children of depressed mothers. *Journal of Abnormal Psychology, 108,* 202–210.

Teasdale, J. D. (1983). Negative thinking in depression: Cause, effect, or reciprocal relationship? *Advances in Behaviour Therapy and Research, 5,* 3–25.

Teasdale, J. D. (1988). Cognitive vulnerability to persistent depression. *Cognition and Emotion, 2,* 247–274.

Teasdale, J. D., & Barnard, P. J. (1993). *Affect, cognition, and change.* Hillsdale, NJ: Lawrence Erlbaum Associates.

Teasdale, J. D., & Dent, J. (1987). Cognitive vulnerability to depression: An investigation of two hypotheses. *British Journal of Clinical Psychology, 26,* 113–126.

Whisman, M. A., & Kwon, P. (1992). Parental representations, cognitive distortions, and mild depression. *Cognitive Therapy and Research, 16,* 557–568.

Whisman, M. A., & McGarvey, A. L. (1995). Attachment, depressotypic cognitions, and dysphoria. *Cognitive Therapy and Research, 19,* 633–650.

Williams, S., Connolly, J., & Segal, Z. V. (2001). Intimacy in relationships and cognitive vulnerability to depression in adolescent girls. *Cognitive Therapy and Research, 25,* 477–496.

Zuroff, D. C., Mongrain, M., & Santor, D. A. (2004). Conceptualizing and measuring personality vulnerability to depression: Comment on Coyne and Wiffen. *Psychological Bulletin, 130,* 489–511.

4

Cognitive Vulnerability to Bipolar Spectrum Disorders

Lauren B. Alloy
Temple University

Noreen A. Reilly-Harrington
Harvard Medical School

David M. Fresco
Case Western Reserve University

Ellen Flannery-Schroeder
University of Rhode Island

Until recently, the basis of the research and theories covering bipolar disorder has been almost exclusively biological in nature. Despite the pioneering work of Kraepelin (1921) suggesting that environmental factors play a part in precipitating manic and depressive episodes, conceptions of bipolar disorder as a genetically based biological illness have dominated over the past century—and rightfully so. The data from family, twin, and adoption studies suggesting that bipolar disorder carries a strong genetic predisposition (Goodwin & Jamison, 1990; Nurnberger & Gershon, 1992) and from pharmacotherapy trials indicating the effectiveness of lithium and anticonvulsive drugs in controlling the cycling of bipolar disorder (e.g., Keck & McElroy, 1996) are rather convincing (Miklowitz & Alloy, 1999).

However, there has been a growing interest in the role of psychosocial processes in the onset, course, and treatment of bipolar spectrum disorders. This resurgence of interest in psychological and environmental processes in bipolar disorder is largely attributable to four factors. First, although genetic and biochemical processes are undeniably important in the etiology, course, and treatment of bipolar disorder, they cannot fully account for differences in the expression of the disorder or the timing and frequency of symptoms (O'Connell, 1986). Second, there has been an increased recognition of the limitations of prophylactic lithium usage. In fact, in a 1990 workshop report, the National Institute of Mental Health called for a further exploration of the impact of psychosocial factors on the course of bipolar disorder as well as the development of psychosocial treatments as an adjunct to pharmacotherapy (Prien & Potter, 1990). Third, there is growing evidence that stressful life events and negative family interactions influence the course of bipolar disorder (Johnson & Roberts, 1995; Miklowitz, Goldstein, & Nuechterlein, 1995). Finally, the huge success of cognitive models (e.g., Abramson, Metalsky, & Alloy, 1989; Beck, 1967, 1987) in understanding the etiology, course, and treatment of unipolar depression has led to the extension of these models to bipolar spectrum disorders with promising initial results (e.g., Alloy, Abramson, Walshaw, & Neeren, in press; Alloy, Reilly-Harrington, Fresco, Whitehouse, & Zechmeister, 1999; Hammen, Ellicott, & Gitlin, 1992; Reilly-Harrington, Alloy, Fresco, & Whitehouse, 1999).

Consequently, this chapter reviews recent theory and empirical research on the role of cognitive styles and life events as vulnerability factors for the onset and course of bipolar spectrum disorders. It begins by describing the nature of the bipolar spectrum. Then it presents the cognitive vulnerability–stress models of unipolar depression and the logic of their extension to bipolar spectrum disorders. Next, it discusses the methodological challenges posed by the group of bipolar disorders for vulnerability research. It covers the extant studies of life events and cognitive styles associated with bipolar disorders and predictive of bipolar symptoms and episodes. Finally, it looks at the implications of the current findings for the continued development of cognitive behavioral adjunctive treatments for bipolar disorders. The exploration of cognitive vulnerability–stress approaches to bipolar disorders is only at its beginning. Hopefully, spurred on by the current review, future investigators will conduct further, more sophisticated studies of the impact of cognition and stress on the onset and course of bipolar spectrum disorders.

THE BIPOLAR SPECTRUM

Although Kraepelin (1921) grouped most major forms of depression under the general rubric of "manic-depressive illness," it was not until Leonhard's (1957) work that patients with both depressive and manic episodes, whom Leonhard termed "bipolar," were distinguished from those exhibiting only recurrent depressions. Since 1957, more than 100 studies have examined the family history, natural course, clinical symptoms, personality factors, biology, and pharmacological treatments associated with the bipolar–unipolar distinction (e.g., Depue & Monroe, 1978; Goodwin &

Jamison, 1990; Johnson & Kizer, 2002). Within the bipolar category, a group of disorders appear to form a continuum or spectrum from the milder, subsyndromal form of manic depression, known as "Cyclothymia," to full-blown manic depression, known as Bipolar I Disorder. Indeed, the *Diagnostic and Statistical Manual of Mental Disorders* (4th ed., *DSM–IV*; American Psychiatric Association, 1994) identified four types of bipolar disorders: Bipolar I Disorder, Bipolar II Disorder, Cyclothymic Disorder, and Bipolar Disorder Not Otherwise Specified (NOS).

According to *DSM–IV*, Bipolar I Disorder is defined by at least one episode of mania. Symptoms of mania include euphoria and/or irritability, high energy/activity, rapid speech and increased talkativeness, racing thoughts, high self-confidence/grandiosity, decreased sleep, distractability, and impulsive, reckless behaviors with a high propensity for negative consequences. Individuals with Bipolar I Disorder may have had prior depressive episodes and most will have subsequent manic or depressive episodes. They may also experience hypomanic episodes and mixed depressive/manic episodes. The lifetime prevalence of Bipolar I Disorder is approximately 1.2% (Smith & Weissman, 1992), with community samples yielding prevalence estimates ranging from 0.4% to 1.6% (Weissman, Bruce, Leaf, Florio, & Holzer, 1990). Completed suicide occurs in 10% to 15% of individuals with Bipolar I Disorder (*DSM–IV*; APA, 1994). Unlike unipolar depression, Bipolar I Disorder is equally common in men and women (Weissman et al., 1988) and has a mean age of onset of around 24 years, with many onsets in adolescence and even childhood (Geller & DelBello, 2003; Goodwin & Jamison, 1990). Bipolar I Disorder is associated with episodic antisocial behavior, divorce, and school or occupational failure (*DSM–IV*; APA, 1994; Hammen, Gitlin, & Altshuler, 2000). With regard to familial pattern, first-degree biological relatives of individuals with Bipolar I Disorder have elevated rates of Bipolar I (4%–24%), Bipolar II (1%–5%), and Major Depressive (4%–24%) Disorders (Goodwin & Jamison, 1990).

Bipolar II Disorder differs from Bipolar I in that individuals exhibit one or more hypomanic, instead of full-blown manic, episodes accompanied by the presence of one or more major depressive episodes. Bipolar II Disorder is more common in women than in men and its lifetime prevalence is estimated at approximately 0.5% (Weissman et al., 1988). As in Bipolar I Disorder, completed suicide occurs in from 10% to 15% of cases, and the associated psychosocial impairment is also similar. *DSM–IV* (APA, 1994) reports a familial pattern for Bipolar II, with first-degree biological relatives exhibiting elevated rates of Bipolar II, Bipolar I, and Major Depressive Disorders.

Cyclothymic Disorder is characterized by recurrent and intermittent mood episodes in which the individual oscillates, or "cycles," between periods of depression and hypomania, with or without normal, euthymic periods in between. However, unlike major depression and mania, both types of mood episodes are of subsyndromal intensity and duration (2–3 days, on average; Alloy & Abramson, 2000). Historically, there has been controversy about whether Cyclothymia is best conceptualized as a temperament, a personality disorder, or a subsyndromal mood disorder (Alloy & Abramson, 2000). Friends and family often describe cyclothymic individuals as "moody," "high-strung," "hyperactive," and "explosive" (Akiskal, Djenderedjian, Rosenthal, & Khani, 1977), and they are often perceived as exhibiting features of personality disorder rather than mood disorder at first clinical presentation.

However, Kraepelin (1921) believed that Cyclothymia is on a continuum with full-blown Bipolar I Disorder and, indeed, may be a precursor to it. Five lines of evidence support this continuum model and suggest that Cyclothymia is an integral part of the bipolar spectrum (Alloy & Abramson, 2000). First, the behavior of cyclothymics is qualitatively similar to that of individuals with Bipolar I and II Disorders (Akiskal et al., 1977; Akiskal, Khani, & Scott-Strauss, 1979; Depue et al., 1981). Second, similar to Bipolar I and II patients, cyclothymics show high rates of comorbidity of anxiety, alcohol and substance use, eating, and attention deficit hyperactivity disorders (Alloy, Flannery-Schroeder, Safford, Floyd, & Abramson, 1999; Brady & Lydiard, 1992; Pergui, Toni, & Akiskal, 1999). Third, equivalent rates of bipolar disorder have been found in the first- and second-degree relatives of cyclothymic and Bipolar I individuals (Akiskal et al., 1977; Depue et al., 1981; Dunner, Russek, Russek, & Fieve, 1982), and increased rates of Cyclothymia are found in the offspring of Bipolar I patients (Klein, Depue, & Slater, 1985). In addition, among monozygotic twins, when one twin was diagnosed with manic depression, the co-twin, if not also manic depressive, was frequently cyclothymic (Bertelsen, Harvald, & Hauge, 1977). These findings suggest that Cyclothymia shares a common genetic predisposition with bipolar disorder. Fourth, like Bipolar I patients, cyclothymics often experience an induction of hypomanic episodes when treated with tricyclic antidepressants (Akiskal et al., 1977) and often improve on lithium prophylaxis (Akiskal et al., 1979). Finally, up to 80% of bipolar patients exhibit cyclothymia premorbidly (Goodwin & Jamison, 1990); cyclothymics are at increased risk of developing full-blown bipolar disorder in the future (Akiskal et al., 1977).

In *DSM–IV*, Bipolar Disorder NOS includes individuals with bipolar features that do not meet criteria for Bipolar I, Bipolar II, or Cyclothymic Disorders. Such cases include recurrent hypomanic episodes without intercurrent depressive symptoms or rapid alternation between manic/hypomanic symptoms and depressive symptoms that do not meet minimal duration criteria for a manic, hypomanic, or depressive episode.

THE COGNITIVE VULNERABILITY–STRESS MODELS
OF UNIPOLAR DEPRESSION

Given that people vary in their responses to stressful life events, the cognitive theories of unipolar depression have sought to explain why some individuals are vulnerable to depression when confronted with stressful events, whereas others do not become depressed at all or suffer only mild, short-lived dysphoria. From the cognitive perspective, the meaning or interpretation people give to their life experiences influences their vulnerability to depression. According to the hopelessness theory of depression (Abramson et al., 1989; Alloy, Abramson, Metalsky, & Hartlage, 1988), individuals who tend to attribute negative life events to stable (enduring) and global (general) causes infer that further negative consequences will follow from a current negative event, and infer that the occurrence of a negative event in their lives means that they are deficient or unworthy are hypothesized to be more likely to experience an onset of depression or a worsening of current depression when confronted with stressors than are individuals who do not exhibit these negative inferential styles. Individuals who exhibit any of these three negative inferential styles should be more likely to make negative attributions and inferences about actual negative events they encounter, thereby incrementing the likelihood of becoming hopeless, the proximal cause of the symptoms of depression. However, in the absence of negative events, individuals who exhibit the hypothesized depressogenic inferential styles should be no more likely to develop depression than persons without these styles.

In Beck's (1967) model of depression, negative self-schemata organized around themes of failure, inadequacy, loss, and worthlessness serve as vulnerabilities for the onset and exacerbation of depression that are activated by the occurrence of stressful events relevant to the content of the self-schemata. Such negative self-schemata are often represented as a set of dysfunctional attitudes in which the individuals believe that their happiness and self-worth depend on being perfect or on others' approval. Consistent with cognitive science operationalizations of the schema construct (e.g., Alba & Hasher, 1983; Taylor & Crocker, 1981), Beck (1967) hypothesized that depressive self-schemata influence the perception, interpretation, and recall of personally relevant experiences, thereby leading to a negatively biased construal of one's personal world. When activated by the occurrence of negative events, depressive self-schemata lead to the onset or exacerbation of depressive symptoms through their effect on preferential encoding and retrieval of negative self-referent information. In Beck's (1987) model, individual differences in the value people place on various life experiences serve as additional vulnerabilities for depression. People who are high in sociotropy place great importance on intimacy, social relationships, and acceptance from others and are vulnerable to depression when they experience interpersonal disappointments or losses, whereas those high in autonomy value achievement, freedom, and independence and are at risk for depression when they encounter failures or events that impinge on their personal choice.

The vulnerability hypotheses of the cognitive theories of unipolar depression have received considerable empirical support (see Abramson et al., 1999, 2002; Alloy, Abramson, Whitehouse, et al., 1999; Alloy, Abramson, Safford, & Gibb, chap. 2, this vol. for reviews). The logic of these models may be extended to bipolar spectrum disorders. The same cognitive processes that contribute vulnerability to unipolar depressive episodes in response to negative life events may also confer risk to the depressive episodes experienced by bipolar individuals following negative events.

Based on the logic behind cognitive theories of unipolar depression, two predictions can be made concerning vulnerability to manic and hypomanic episodes. On the one hand, based on the hopelessness theory, individuals who characteristically exhibit positive inferential styles for positive life events (stable, global attributions for positive events, positive consequences and positive self-implications of positive events) should react to the occurrence of positive events by becoming hopeful and, in turn, developing euphoria and hypomanic/manic symptoms. Similarly, Beck (1976) suggested that manic individuals are characterized by a set of positive self-schemata, consisting of unrealistically positive attitudes about the self, world, and future. Beck hypothesized that when these individuals experience positive events, their positive schemata are activated and promote the development of manic symptoms. Alternatively, given that negative life events have been found to trigger manic episodes as well as depressive episodes in bipolar individuals (Johnson & Roberts, 1995; see later section, "Life Events and Bipolar Spectrum Disorders"), it may be that bipolar individuals' cognitive styles for interpreting negative events, rather than their styles for construing positive events, are more important in influencing their vulnerability to manic and hypomanic episodes. A review of the role of cognitive styles as vulnerability factors for bipolar disorders shows that there is evidence for both of these alternatives. There is also discussion of the conditions under which cognitive styles for interpreting negative events may promote vulnerability to manic/ hypomanic episodes versus depressive episodes at different times in the same individual.

METHODOLOGICAL CHALLENGES
OF VULNERABILITY RESEARCH
IN BIPOLAR SPECTRUM DISORDERS

From a conceptual and research design perspective, a putative vulnerability factor for a disorder must be demonstrated to meet two criteria (Alloy, Abramson, Raniere, & Dyller, 1999; Ingram, Miranda, & Segal, 1998): It must temporally precede the initial onset of the disorder or, in the case of a vulnerability factor for the course of a disorder, precede episodes or symptom exacerbations of the disorder; and it must exhibit some degree of stability independent of the symptoms of the disorder (but see Just, Abramson, & Alloy, 2001, for the argument that a vulnerability factor does not need to be immutable). Given these criteria, some research designs are more appropriate than others for testing vulnerability hypotheses (Alloy, Abramson, Raniere, et al., 1999). For example, cross-sectional studies that compare a group with the disorder of interest to a normal control group (and possibly, a group with a different disorder) on several characteristics can generate hypotheses about potential vulnerabilities, but are wholly inadequate for establishing temporal precedence or stability independent of symptoms of the disorder. Designs that compare individuals who have remitted from an episode of the disorder of interest to a normal control group on the potential vulnerability factors or that longitudinally compare individuals with the disorder in their symptomatic versus remitted states are an improvement because they can demonstrate independence of the potential vulnerabilities from the symptoms of the disorder. However, such "remitted disorder designs" cannot distinguish between the alternative possibilities that the characteristics are risk factors for the disorder or consequences ("scars") of the disorder (Just et al., 2001; Lewinsohn, Steinmetz, Larson, & Franklin, 1981). Thus, ideally, a prospective, longitudinal design is needed in which the potential vulnerability factor is assessed prior to the onset of the disorder. Such prospective designs can establish both the vulnerability factor's temporal precedence and independence from symptoms (Alloy, Abramson, Raniere, et al., 1999; Alloy, Abramson, Whitehouse, et al., 1999).

Unfortunately, few studies examining the role of life events as proximal triggers or cognitive styles as distal vulnerabilities for bipolar spectrum disorders have used the preferred prospective designs. Thus, the review here makes note of those studies that do. Indeed, as a group, the bipolar spectrum disorders present especially difficult methodological challenges for conducting tests of vulnerability hypotheses. First, they are highly recurrent with significant interepisode symptomatology and functional impairment. As a consequence, it is very difficult to assess proximal life events or distal cognitive styles at a time when the individual is asymptomatic in order to establish independence of these potential vulnerabilities from symptoms of mania/hypomania or depression. One has to be concerned with the possibility that residual symptoms may bias the assessment of life events or cognitions. Second, bipolar disorders have their initial onset at an early age (mean onset of 14 years old for Cyclothymia; Akiskal et al., 1977, 1979). Thus, to truly establish temporal precedence for initial onset of bipolar disorder, one would have to assess life events or cognitive styles in childhood or early adolescence. No study to date has done this. Third, as a consequence of many mood swings and interepisodic symptoms, many bipolar individuals lead chaotic lives. This, in turn, increases the likelihood that they actually contribute to the occurrence of stressors in their lives through poor judgment, poor coping skills, and other symptoms (Alloy, Abramson, Raniere, et al., 1999; Hammen, 1991; Johnson & Roberts, 1995). To deal with this problem, some investigators of life events and bipolar disorders have included only those events that are independent of the participants' behavior, and we note these studies in our review. Given these methodological challenges for vulnerability research, much work remains to be done in investigating the role of cognitive styles and life events as vulnerabilities for bipolar spectrum disorders.

LIFE EVENTS AND BIPOLAR SPECTRUM DISORDERS

A growing body of evidence suggests that life events may have an impact on the onset and course of bipolar spectrum disorders (Johnson & Kizer, 2002; Johnson & Roberts, 1995). For the most part, these studies have found that bipolar individuals experienced increased stressful events prior to onset or subsequent episodes of their disorder. Moreover, most have found that the manic/hypomanic, as well as the depressive, episodes of bipolar individuals were preceded by negative life events (Johnson & Roberts, 1995). However, several methodological limitations make interpretation of many of these studies difficult. First, many studies used retrospective rather than prospective designs. Retrospective designs have the problems that recall of events may decrease over time and become biased by the individuals' attempts to explain the cause of their disorder to themselves (Brown, 1974, 1989). Second, many studies do not distinguish between the depressive and manic/hypomanic episodes of bipolar individuals; thus, it is unclear whether stressful events contribute to the onset of mania and depression. Third, several do not include a control group. Fourth, some use admission to the hospital or the start of a treatment regimen as the time of episode onset, which does not necessarily correspond well with the actual date of episode onset. Finally, many studies have failed to differentiate between events that are independent of or dependent on people's behavior, a distinction of considerable importance given the chaotic lifestyles of those with bipolar disorders. We review the more limited retrospective studies first, followed by the stronger prospective studies.

Retrospective Studies

Several retrospective studies relied on review of medical charts to assess life events in patients with bipolar disorder. Based on retrospective chart review, Leff, Fischer, and Bertelson (1976) found that 35% of bipolar inpatients reported a stressful event rated as independent of their behavior in the month prior to onset of episode. Clancy, Crowe, Winokur, and Morrison (1973) also used retrospective chart review and found that 39% of unipolar, 27% of bipolar, and 11% of schizophrenic patients had a stressful event in the 3 months prior to onset of their disorder. No significant differences were found for types of precipitating stressful events for bipolar versus unipolar patients. Ambelas (1979, 1987) conducted two retrospective chart review studies. In the 1979 study, 28% of 67 hypomanic or manic inpatients versus 6% of 60 surgical control patients had experienced an independent stressful event during the 4 weeks prior to hospital admission. In almost all the cases reported, the stressful event precipitating mania or hypomania was a loss or threat event. In his study of 90 bipolar manic inpatients, Ambelas (1987) found that compared with 8% of an age-matched surgical control group, 66% of first episode bipolar patients and 20% of repeat admission bipolar patients reported a severe independent event in the 4 weeks before admission.

An improvement over retrospective chart reviews is represented by retrospective studies that actually conducted interviews with or administered questionnaires to bipolar individuals regarding their past experiences of life events. Only some of these studies assessed the independence of the events from bipolar individuals' behavior and differentiated manic from depressive episodes. Glassner, Haldipur, and Dessauersmith (1979) retrospectively interviewed 25 bipolar patients and their relatives about the patients' life events preceding their first and most recent episodes of disorder. They found that 75% of first episode and 56% of subsequent episode patients reported a stressful event prior to onset. Utilizing the same methodology with 46 bipolar patients and their relatives, Glassner and Haldipur (1983) reported that 64% of late onset (onset after age 20) versus 23% of early onset bipolar patients reported a stressful event preceding their initial episode. Bidzinska (1984) reported that acute and chronic stress preceded the onset of illness in 90% of bipolar and 89.4% of unipolar patients in Warsaw, with no differences between men and women in either group. However, bipolar patients reported more work-related stressors than did unipolar patients. In a study of 79 bipolar patients attending a lithium clinic that did distinguish between manic and depressive episodes, Dunner, Patrick, and Fieve (1979) retrospectively assessed stressful events occurring in a 3-month period prior to the initial or later episodes of depression or mania. About one half of the patients recalled a stressful event in the 3 months before their initial episode and an increase in work and interpersonal difficulties was associated with onset of a manic versus a depressed episode.

Most of the retrospective studies that examined relatively independent stressful events also found that bipolar individuals experienced increased stress prior to episode onsets. Kennedy, Thompson, Stancer, Roy, and Persad (1983) found that compared to control participants or to the period following admission to the hospital, manic patients experienced twice as many stressful events during the 4-month period prior to hospital admission. Life events having significant objective, negative, and traumatic impact were distinctly more common prior to admission, independent of the affective illness. Among bipolar patients in a lithium clinic, Aronson and Shukla (1987) found a significant increase in relapse 2 weeks after a major hurricane, a severe independent life event. Although there were no differences between relapsers and nonrelapsers in age, duration of illness, or lithium level, relapsers had less symptom stability before the hurricane than did nonrelapsers. Joffe, MacDonald, and Kutcher (1989) matched 14 recently relapsed manics to more stable bipolar patients and also found significantly more uncontrollable and unexpected life events among the relapsers prior to onset. Similarly, Davenport and Adland (1982) reported a 50% onset rate of mood disorder episodes among 40 bipolar men during or immediately following their wives' pregnancies.

In a sample of remitted depressed bipolar and unipolar patients retrospectively assessed over a long 1-year interval, Perris (1984) found that bipolar patients reported an average of 2.5 independent events and unipolar patients reported an average of 1.9 independent events in the year prior to episode onset. Using both a retrospective and prospective design, Sclare and Creed (1990) reported that manic patients experienced more independent events prior to onset than after recovery. In a study of manic, psychotically depressed, and schizophrenic patients and nonpsychiatric controls, Bebbington et al. (1993) reported that the psychotically depressed patients experienced more severe, independent life events in the 6 months prior to onset of psychosis than did both manic and schizophrenic patients. However, the manic patients also reported more severe, independent events prior to relapse than did the nonpsychiatric controls. In contrast, Chung, Langeluddecke, and Tennant (1986) found that the rate of independent threatening events in the 26 weeks prior to onset for 14 manic patients did not differ significantly from that of controls (even though the rate was twice as high in the manics). Finally, in a retrospective study of childhood stressful events, Grandin, Alloy, and Abramson (2004) pointed out that compared to demographically matched normal controls, bipolar spectrum (Bipolar II, Cyclothymic, Bipolar NOS) participants experienced more childhood stressors that were independent of their behavior prior to the age of onset of their bipolar symptomatology.

Prospective Studies

Stronger evidence for the role of stressful life events as proximal triggers of affective episodes in individuals with bipolar disorders comes from the more methodologically adequate prospective studies. Hall, Dunner, Zeller, and Fieve (1977) assessed 38 bipolar patients prospectively at monthly intervals for a total of 10 months. Although overall numbers of life events did not differ for patients who relapsed versus those who did not, hypomanic relapsers had greater numbers of employment-related events than did nonrelapsers. In another report from this study, Hall (1984) noted that a higher number of severe loss events, as well as work-related events, also were reported prior to manic relapse in this sample. Limitations of this study included the failure to control for medication or illness duration, as well as the lack of structured diagnostic interviews to determine relapse.

In a study of 62 bipolar patients followed for 2 years, with interviews designed to assess life events and mental state conducted every 3 months, Hunt, Bruce-Jones, and Silverstone (1992) revealed that 19% of 52 relapses were preceded by a severe event in the previous month, compared to a background rate of 5% of patients experiencing a severe event each month at other times. Manic and depressive relapses did not differ on the rate of prior life events. In contrast, using similar methods, McPherson, Herbison, and Romans (1993) found no difference in the number of moderately severe, independent events in the month preceding relapse as compared with control periods. The McPherson et al. study was limited by a high dropout rate and the absence of a required well period prior to study entrance. Johnson and Roberts (1995) reported that all studies requiring a well period or full recovery prior to study entrance have obtained a positive association between life stress and relapse.

In a prospective study of 61 bipolar outpatients followed over a 2-year period with systematic interviewing procedures to assess life events, symptoms, levels of medication maintenance, and observance of treatment regimen, Ellicott, Hammen, Gitlin, Brown, and Jamison (1990) obtained a significant association between life events and relapse of the disorder. Indeed, bipolar outpatients with high stress showed a four-and-one-half-fold greater relapse rate than those with lower stress and these findings were not accounted for by differences in levels of medication or adherence. Using similar methodology in a subsample of 52 bipolar outpatients, Hammen and Gitlin (1997) again found that patients with relapses during the 2-year follow-up period had more severe events and more total stress during the preceding 6 months, and more total stress during the preceding 3 months, than those with no episodes. In addition, inconsistent with Post's (1992) "stress sensitization" hypothesis that stressors play a larger role in precipitating initial episodes than later episodes of mood disorder, Hammen and Gitlin reported that patients with more prior episodes were more likely to have episodes preceded by major life events and relapsed more quickly than patients with fewer prior episodes.

Johnson and Miller (1997) examined negative life events as a predictor of time to recovery from an episode of bipolar disorder. They studied 67 individuals recruited during hospitalization for bipolar disorder and conducted monthly structured interview assessments of stressful life events. Bipolar patients who experienced a severe, independent event during the index episode took three times as long to recover from the episode as those who did not experience a severe, independent event and this effect was not mediated by medication compliance.

Several investigators have considered biological mechanisms through which stressful life events may influence the onset and course of bipolar spectrum disorders. For example, some theorists (e.g., Ehlers, Frank, & Kupfer, 1988; Healy & Williams, 1988) have suggested that life events affect the course of mood disorders through their destabilizing effects on critical circadian rhythms. Consistent with this view, Malkoff-Schwartz et al. (1998) explained that bipolar patients in a manic episode had significantly more pre-onset life events characterized by social rhythm disruptions (e.g., change in the sleep–wake cycle) than did depressed bipolars.

In summary, although relatively few in number, the methodologically sound prospective studies suggest that the occurrence of stressful life events may contribute proximal risk to the onset of mood episodes in individuals with bipolar disorders. Given the more extensive literature on the role of stress as a precipitant of episodes of unipolar depression, it is not surprising that negative events may trigger bipolar depressive episodes. However, our review, as well as Johnson and Roberts' (1995) review, indicates that negative events may also contribute risk for manic/hypomanic episodes. Given that almost none of the studies on stress and bipolar disorder have investigated positive life events, future research on life events and bipolar disorder should examine whether positive events also play a role in the course of bipolar spectrum disorders. Such positive events as achievements and gains could activate bipolar individuals' engagement in goal striving, which in turn might lead to hypomanic/manic symptoms such as high activity and energy levels, racing thoughts, increased self-confidence, and risky behaviors (Harmon-Jones et al., 2002). In the next section, we review the evidence on the role of cognitive styles as distal vulnerabilities for bipolar spectrum disorders that increase the likelihood of depressive and manic/hypomanic episodes in response to stressful life events. In so doing, we address the applicability of the cognitive vulnerability–stress models of unipolar depression (Hopelessness and Beck's theories) to bipolar spectrum disorders.

COGNITIVE STYLES AND BIPOLAR SPECTRUM DISORDERS

Investigators have largely ignored the role of cognitive processes in bipolar spectrum conditions, mainly focusing on the cognitive factors involved in unipolar depression. Consequently, little is known about the cognitive styles characteristic of individuals with bipolar disorders or whether such cognitive styles increase bipolar individuals' vulnerability to depressive and manic/hypomanic episodes in combination with life events. However, in the last decade, there has been increasing interest in the role of cognitive styles as vulnerabilities for episodes of bipolar disorder. Thus, this section reviews the extant cross-sectional research on the cognitive patterns associated with bipolar spectrum disorders and the stability of such patterns as well as longitudinal research on the manner in which cognitive styles may contribute vulnerability to bipolar episodes in response to life events.

Cognitive Styles Associated with Bipolar Spectrum Disorders

Relatively few studies have directly examined the cognitive styles or information processing of individuals with bipolar mood disorders. Based on the grandiosity that is a common symptom of mania and hypomania, one might expect bipolar individuals (who experience manic or hypomanic episodes) to exhibit cognitive patterns more positive than those of unipolar depressive individuals. On the other hand, based on psychodynamic formulations suggesting that the grandiosity of manic or hypomanic periods is a "defense" or counterreaction to underlying depressive tendencies (Freeman, 1971), bipolar individuals would be expected to exhibit cognitive styles as negative as those of unipolar depressives. In a more modern version of the psychodynamic hypothesis, Neale (1988) suggested that grandiose ideas have the function of keeping distressing cognitions out of awareness and are precipitated by underlying low self-regard. Similarly, based on an extension of the cognitive theories of unipolar depression to bipolar spectrum disorders, it might also be expected that the cognitive patterns of bipolar individuals would be negative. In fact, the studies conducted to date imply that the observed positivity or negativity of bipolar individuals' cognitive patterns depends to some degree both on whether they are in a depressed or manic/hypomanic episode or a euthymic state at the time of the assessment and on whether the assessment of the cognitive patterns is based on explicit or implicit tasks. That is, most studies indicate that persons with bipolar disorders show cognitive styles and self-referent information processing as negative as those of unipolar depressives, but sometimes present themselves in a positive fashion on more explicit cognitive tasks.

Those studies examining the cognitive styles and information processing of currently depressed bipolar individuals have generally found their cognitive patterns to be as negative as those of unipolar depressives. For example, Hollon, Kendall, and Lumry (1986) noted that both depressed unipolar and bipolar patients showed similarly negative automatic thoughts and dysfunctional attitudes characteristic of depression (see also C. V. Hill, Oei, & M. A. Hill, 1989). In a comparison of 57 depressed unipolar women, 9 depressed bipolar women, and 24 nonpsychiatric control women on the self-criticism and dependency scales of the Depressive Experiences Questionnaire (Blatt, D'Afflitti, & Quinlan, 1976), Rosenfarb, Becker, Khan, and Mintz (1998) found that both depressed unipolar and bipolar women were more self-critical than controls. On the other hand, whereas depressed unipolar women were also more dependent than controls, depressed bipolar women did not differ from controls on dependency. In a comparison of the subset of their sample (31 unipolar, 7 bipolar) currently in a depressed episode with 23 normal controls and the currently nondepressed mood disordered participants, Reilly-Harrington et al. (1999) offered that both currently depressed bipolar and unipolar participants exhibited more internal, stable, global attributional styles for negative events, more external, unstable, specific attributional styles for positive events, and more negative self-referent information processing for depression-relevant content than did nondepressed participants.

Three studies have examined the cognitive patterns of currently manic or hypomanic individuals and obtained results consistent with the importance of distinguishing between explicit and implicit assessments of cognitions. Bentall and Thompson (1990) compared students who scored high versus low on a hypomania scale on an emotional Stroop test in which the participants named the ink colors of depression-related and euphoria-related words written in different colored inks. Consistent with prior findings on the emotional Stroop task with unipolar depressed patients (Ingram et al., 1998), Bentall and Thompson found that hypomanic students took longer to color name the depression-related words, but not the euphoria-related words. These findings were replicated by French, Richards, and Scholfield (1996), even after controlling for the effects of anxiety on Stroop task performance. Lyon, Startup, and Bentall (1999) administered Bentall and Thompson's (1990) emotional Stroop test, Winters and Neale's (1985) pragmatic inference task that assesses attributions for hypothetical scenarios in an implicit manner, an explicit attribution questionnaire, and a self-referent incidental recall task designed to assess Beck's concept of self-schema to 15 bipolar manic patients, 15 bipolar depressed patients, and 15 normal controls. Consistent with the hypothesis that bipolar depressed individuals possess negative cognitive styles like those of unipolar depressives, Lyon et al. explained that bipolar depressed patients attributed negative events more than positive events to internal, stable, and global causes on both the attribution questionnaire and the pragmatic inference task, exhibited slowed color-naming for depression-related words on the Stroop task, and endorsed as self-descriptive and recalled more negative trait adjectives on the incidental recall task. Although, like the normal controls, the bipolar manic patients showed a self-serving bias on the explicit attribution questionnaire, taking credit for positive events more than negative events, and endorsed more positive than negative words, on the more implicit tasks, the manic patients exhibited negative cognitive styles or information processing like those of depressed individuals. Specifically, manic patients attributed negative events internally rather than externally on the pragmatic inference task, showed slower color naming for depression-related rather than euphoria-related words on the Stroop task, and recalled more negative than positive words on the self-referent incidental recall task.

Stability of Cognitive Styles Associated With Bipolar Spectrum Disorders

The handful of studies examining the stability of the cognitive patterns of bipolar individuals have employed one of two research designs: cross-sectional studies of bipolar individuals who are currently euthymic and have remitted from a depressive or hypomanic/manic episode or longitudinal studies of bipolar individuals across depressed, hypomanic, and euthymic periods. Most studies have used the remitted design and thus are not optimal for examining the stability of cognitive styles across different phases of the bipolar disorder.

Four studies have obtained support for negative cognitive styles and information processing in remitted bipolar individuals. For example, Winters and Neale (1985) assessed groups of remitted bipolar and unipolar patients and normal controls on a battery of self-report measures of self-esteem, social desirability, and self-deception as well as on an implicit pragmatic inference task designed to measure causal attributions for hypothetical scenarios. They found that although the remitted bipolar patients showed higher self-esteem, social desirability, and self-deception than the remitted unipolar patients and normal controls on the self-report measures, they generated causal inferences as negative as those of the remitted unipolar patients on the more implicit pragmatic inference task. Among their subsample of 17 remitted unipolar depressed women, 11 remitted bipolar women, and 24 nonpsychiatric control women, Rosenfarb et al. (1998) found that both the remitted unipolar and bipolar women were more self-critical than the controls. The remitted unipolar women did not differ from the controls on dependency, whereas the remitted bipolar women were actually less dependent than the controls. Thus, only self-criticism was exhibited by both currently depressed and remitted unipolar and bipolar women. Scott, Stanton, Garland, and Ferrier (2000) found that 41 remitted bipolar inpatients exhibited more dysfunctional attitudes, greater sociotropy, greater overgeneral recall on an autobiographical memory task, and fewer solutions on a social problem-solving task than did 20 normal controls. Finally, as part of their Longitudinal Investigation of Bipolar Spectrum Disorders (LIBS) Project, Alloy, Abramson, and colleagues (Alloy, Abramson, Walshaw, et al., 2004; Alloy, Abramson, Grandin, et al., 2004) compared the cognitive styles and self-schema processing of 206 euthymic bipolar spectrum (Bipolar II, Cyclothymia, Bipolar NOS) and 214 demographically matched normal participants. The bipolar group exhibited more negative inferential styles, dysfunctional attitudes (particularly, perfectionism), sociotropy (particularly, concern about disapproval), autonomy (particularly, mobility/freedom from control), self-criticism, self-consciousness (particularly, private self-consciousness), and ruminative response styles than did the normal control group (see Table 4.1). The two groups did not differ on dependency or attachment. In addition, bipolar participants showed greater processing of negative depression-relevant content and less processing of positive, depression-relevant content on the Self-Referent Information Processing Task Battery (Alloy, Abramson, Murray, Whitehouse, & Hogan, 1997) compared to the normal controls. Thus, these studies suggest that euthymic bipolar individuals exhibit negative cognitive patterns characterized especially by concerns with performance evaluation, perfectionism, autonomy, self-criticism, and rumination, rather than by dependency or attachment concerns, as is often true of unipolar depressed individuals.

Three other studies of remitted bipolar individuals did not obtain much evidence of negative cognitive processes in the remitted state. According to Tracy, Bauwens, Martin, Pardoen, and Mendlewicz (1992), remitted unipolar patients made more stable attributions for negative events than remitted bipolar patients and controls, with no other differences among the three groups. In the same sample, Pardoen, Bauwens, Tracy, Martin, and Mendlewicz (1993) reported that remitted unipolar patients had lower self-esteem than remitted bipolar patients and controls, who did not differ from each other. Similarly, Reilly-Harrington et al. (1999) did not obtain differences in attributional style for negative or positive events, dysfunctional attitudes, or most of their measures of self-referent information processing among 66 remitted unipolar, 37 remitted bipolar, and 23 normal control undergraduates. They did find, however, that remitted bipolar individuals were more likely to endorse as self-

TABLE 4.1
Means and Standard Deviations for Cognitive Styles
in Bipolars and Normal Controls

Measure	Bipolar II	Cyclothymic/ Bipolar NOS	Normal Control
CSQ–Neg	206.20$_a$ (41.4)	195.92$_a$ (47.7)	169.32$_b$ (37.4)
CSQ–Pos	240.59$_a$ (41.0)	251.55$_b$ (35.5)	248.89$_b$ (33.6)
DAS–PE	3.34$_a$ (0.1)	2.79$_b$ (0.1)	2.28$_c$ (0.1)
DAS–AO	3.94$_a$ (0.1)	3.79$_{ab}$ (0.1)	3.66$_{bc}$ (0.1)
SAS–S–CD	26.29$_a$ (0.6)	25.38$_a$ (0.9)	22.36$_b$ (0.5)
SAS–S–AS	42.70$_a$ (0.6)	42.59$_a$ (1.1)	42.03$_a$ (0.5)
SAS–S–PO	23.58$_a$ (0.4)	23.50$_{ab}$ (0.7)	22.02$_{bc}$ (0.4)
SAS–A–IA	45.95$_a$ (0.5)	47.03$_{ab}$ (0.8)	44.58$_{ac}$ (0.4)
SAS–A–MF	40.66$_a$ (0.5)	41.36$_a$ (0.8)	36.14$_b$ (0.4)
SAS–A–SP	16.94$_a$ (0.3)	17.92$_a$ (0.5)	14.48$_b$ (0.3)
DEQ–Dep	−0.46$_a$ (0.1)	−0.60$_a$ (0.1)	−0.62$_a$ (0.1)
DEQ–SC	0.34$_a$ (0.1)	0.09$_a$ (0.1)	−0.96$_b$ (0.1)
SCS–Pri	27.37$_a$ (0.4)	26.21$_a$ (0.7)	22.82$_b$ (0.4)
SCS–Pub	19.06$_a$ (0.4)	18.72$_a$ (0.7)	16.70$_b$ (0.3)
SCS–SA	12.17$_a$ (0.5)	12.69$_a$ (0.8)	10.22$_b$ (0.4)
RSQ–Rum	52.47$_a$ (0.8)	51.33$_a$ (1.3)	36.39$_b$ (0.7)
RSQ–Dis	26.04$_a$ (0.4)	26.96$_a$ (0.7)	27.24$_a$ (0.4)

Note: CSQ = Cognitive Style Questionnaire; Neg = Negative Events Composite; Pos = Positive Events Composite; DAS = Dysfunctional Attitudes Scale; PE = Performance Evaluation; AO = Approval by Others; SAS = Sociotropy Autonomy Scales; S = Sociotropy; CD = Concern about Disapproval; AS = Attachment/Separation; PO = Pleasing Others; A = Autonomy; IA = Individualistic Achievement; MF = Mobility/Freedom from Control; SP = Solitary Pleasures; DEQ = Depressive Experiences Questionnaire; Dep = Dependency; SC – Self Criticism; SCS = Self-Consciousness Scale; Pri = Private; Pub = Public; SA = Social Anxiety; RSQ = Response Styles Questionnaire; Rum = Rumination; Dis = Distraction. Means with differing subscripts in each row differ by at least $p < .05$. From *Depressive Cognitive Styles and Bipolar Spectrum Disorders: A Unique Behavioral Approach System (BAS) Profile?* by L. B. Alloy, L. Y. Abramson, P. D. Walshaw, et al., 2004.

descriptive depression-relevant than nondepression-relevant adjectives and predicted that they would be more likely to behave in depression-relevant than nondepression-relevant ways in the future than did remitted unipolar and control participants, and these differences were not attributable to any effects of treatment.

Two studies used a longitudinal design to investigate the stability of cognitive styles across the naturally occurring mood swings of individuals with bipolar mood disorders. Eich, Macaulay, and Lam (1997) noted that recall of autobiographical memories was more negative in the depressed than the manic state in a group of 10 rapid cycling bipolar patients. Alloy, Reilly-Harrington, et al. (1999) assessed attributional styles and dysfunctional attitudes, as well as state cognitions about the self, in 13 cyclothymic, 8 dysthymic, 10 hypomanic, and 12 normal control under-graduates on three separate occasions as the different mood states charac-teristic of their disorder naturally occurred. At Time 1, all groups were as-sessed in a normal mood state. At Time 2, cyclothymics and dysthymics were in a depressed period, hypomanics were in a hypomanic period, and normals were in a normal mood state. At Time 3, dysthymics were in an-other depressed period, cyclothymics and hypomanics were in a hypo-manic period, and normals were in a normal mood state. The interval be-tween each of the sessions averaged 4.7 weeks, with a range of from 1 to 9 weeks.

Alloy, Reilly-Harrington, et al. (1999) reported analyses on partici-pants' depression and hypomanic symptom scores that indicated that, as intended, they had been successful in assessing participants in the differ-ent mood states appropriate to their diagnoses at each time point (see Ta-ble 4.2). Consistent with the hypothesis that attributional styles and dys-functional attitudes would be stable across participants' mood swings, Alloy et al. found that the group × time interaction was not significant, al-though there was a main effect of group (see Table 4.2). As shown in Table 4.2, across mood states, cyclothymics' and dysthymics' dysfunctional atti-tudes and attributional styles for negative events did not differ from each other and both groups had more negative cognitive styles than hypo-manics and normal controls, whose scores also did not differ from each other. In contrast, the more statelike cognitions about the self did differ as a function of current mood state. Whereas the four groups did not differ on self-perceptions at Times 1 or 3, at Time 2, when cyclothymics and dysthymics were in a depressed state and hypomanics were in a hypo-manic state, dysthymics' and cyclothymics' thoughts about the self did not differ from each other, but were more negative than those of hypo-manics and normal controls. Also, cyclothymics' self-referent thoughts were more negative when they were depressed (Time 2) than when they were either hypomanic (Time 3) or in a normal mood (Time 1).

The Alloy, Reilly-Harrington, et al. (1999) findings are intriguing in several respects. First, in contrast to cyclothymics, hypomanic participants, who have no depressive episodes as part of their phenomenology, showed much more positive attitudes and attributional styles, similar to those of normal controls. This suggests that the cognitive styles of unipolar mania/hypomania may be quite different and more positive in character than ma-nia/hypomania in the context of a history of depression. Further studies are needed that examine other cognitive processes and information-processing biases in bipolar versus unipolar manic/hypomanic groups to determine whether unipolar manic/hypomanic individuals exhibit more positive cognitions in general than do individuals who experience mania or hypo-mania in the context of a history of depressive episodes. Second, the cog-

TABLE 4.2
Means and Standard Deviations for Study
Measures as a Function of Mood State

Measure	Time/Mood	Cyclothymics	Dysthymics	Hypomanics	Normals
BDI	Time 1/Nor	10.1_{ax} (6.1)	13.6_{ax} (8.8)	5.6_{bx} (6.3)	4.1_{bx} (3.8)
	Time 2/Dep	20.5_{ay} (13.0)	22.8_{ay} (11.2)	2.3_{bx} (2.3)	2.0_{bx} (3.1)
	Time 3/Hyp	6.0_{ax} (5.7)	19.1_{by} (12.6)	3.7_{ax} (4.0)	3.2_{ax} (4.4)
HMI	Time 1/Nor	18.8_{ax} (9.0)	14.9_{ax} (6.5)	19.5_{ax} (9.8)	17.9_{ax} (5.6)
	Time 2/Dep	15.7_{ax} (9.9)	14.7_{ax} (5.8)	28.1_{by} (13.5)	14.0_{ax} (5.5)
	Time 3/Hyp	23.9_{ay} (8.4)	16.5_{bx} (8.9)	27.7_{ay} (16.9)	10.8_{cy} (4.4)
DAS	Time 1/Nor	137.9_{ax} (26.4)	153.9_{ax} (32.9)	110.3_{bx} (30.3)	112.5_{bx} (23.3)
	Time 2/Dep	139.1_{ax} (17.9)	166.9_{ax} (30.1)	110.6_{bx} (32.1)	105.5_{bx} (27.3)
	Time 3/Hyp	134.7_{ax} (18.6)	163.1_{ax} (36.3)	109.4_{bx} (30.8)	101.9_{bx} (25.7)
ASQ–NC	Time 1/Nor	13.7_{ax} (2.6)	16.9_{ax} (4.3)	12.1_{bx} (2.8)	12.0_{bx} (2.1)
	Time 2/Dep	14.8_{ax} (2.2)	15.0_{ax} (2.9)	11.8_{bx} (3.4)	12.0_{bx} (2.3)
	Time 3/Hyp	13.5_{ax} (3.5)	15.8_{ax} (3.3)	11.4_{bx} (3.5)	12.6_{bx} (1.7)
ASQ–PC	Time 1/Nor	17.2_{ax} (2.5)	16.5_{ax} (4.1)	16.1_{ax} (2.2)	16.4_{ax} (2.0)
	Time 2/Dep	16.6_{ax} (3.2)	15.0_{ax} (4.3)	17.1_{ax} (2.1)	16.2_{ax} (2.0)
	Time 3/Hyp	17.8_{ax} (3.1)	14.4_{ax} (3.7)	16.9_{ax} (2.3)	15.2_{ax} (2.3)
SPQ	Time 1/Nor	390.1_{ax} (56.2)	332.7_{ax} (77.1)	396.8_{ax} (44.1)	418.0_{ax} (65.5)
	Time 2/Dep	330.4_{ay} (64.0)	294.4_{ax} (74.2)	426.6_{bx} (72.8)	416.2_{bx} (70.5)
	Time 3/Hyp	400.4_{ax} (44.1)	317.5_{ax} (66.8)	420.5_{ax} (79.6)	426.7_{ax} (72.9)

Note: BDI = Beck Depression Inventory; HMI = Halberstadt Mania Inventory; DAS = Dysfunctional Attitudes Scale; ASQ = Attributional Style Questionnaire; NC = Negative Composite; PC = Positive Composite; SPQ = Self Perception Questionnaire; Nor = Normal; Dep = Depressed; Hyp = Hypomanic. The mood states refer to those of the cyclothymic participants; dysthymics were in a depressed state at both Times 2 and 3; hypomanics were in a hypomanic state at both Times 2 and 3; normals were in a normal state at all 3 times. Means with differing subscripts in each row (letters a–d) or each column (letters x–z) differ at $p < .05$. Adapted from "Cognitive Styles and Life Events in Subsyndromal Unipolar and Bipolar Mood Disorders: Stability and Prospective Prediction of Depressive and Hypomanic Mood Swings," by L. B. Alloy, N. Reilly-Harrington, D. M. Fresco, W. G. Whitehouse, J. S. Zechmeister, 1999, *Journal of Cognitive Psychotherapy: An International Quarterly, 13,* p. 30. Adapted with permission from Springer Publishing Co.

nitive vulnerabilities (negative attributional styles and dysfunctional attitudes) featured in the cognitive theories of unipolar depression showed considerable stability across large changes in naturally occurring mood states. This is in contrast to the results of at least some studies of remitted bipolar and unipolar patients described earlier. Alloy et al. speculated that participants' cognitive styles showed stability across mood swings in their study because they had a sample of untreated individuals. In most of the prior remitted depression studies involving treated samples, cognitive styles may have improved as a treatment by-product rather than as a naturally occurring result of symptom remission without intervention. Finally, whereas cyclothymics exhibited similar distal negative cognitive styles (attributional styles, dysfunctional attitudes) across mood states, their proximal cognitions (self perceptions) varied as a function of current mood state and were more positive in a hypomanic than in a depressive period. This suggests that whereas bipolar individuals may exhibit negative cognitive styles that are relatively stable, they may also possess more latent positive self-schemata that are only activated in positive mood states (see also Eich et al., 1997). Future studies need to examine this proposal directly.

Cognitive Vulnerability–Stress Prediction of Bipolar Mood Episodes

Do the negative cognitive styles or self-referent information processing featured as vulnerabilities in the cognitive theories of unipolar depression also act as vulnerability factors for bipolar spectrum disorders in response to life events? That is, do negative cognitive styles increase the likelihood that bipolar individuals become depressed or hypomanic/manic when confronted with positive or negative life events? Five studies have examined the cognitive vulnerability–stress hypothesis for bipolar disorders.

Hammen, Ellicott, Gitlin, and Jamison (1989) tested Beck's (1987) event congruence, vulnerability–stress hypothesis in 22 unipolar and 25 bipolar patients. Specifically, the patients were categorized into sociotropic and autonomous subtypes and then followed for 6 months with independent assessments of symptoms and life events. Based on Beck's (1987) theory, it was predicted that patients who experienced a preponderance of negative life events that were congruent with their personality style (interpersonal events for sociotropic patients and achievement events for autonomous patients) would be more likely to experience an onset or exacerbation of symptoms. Hammen et al. obtained support for the event congruence hypothesis only in the unipolar patients. However, there were trends consistent with the hypothesis for the bipolar patients as well and Hammen et al. suggested that a longer period of follow-up might be needed to obtain the effect in bipolar patients. Indeed, in a later study, Hammen et al. (1992) followed a larger sample of 49 remitted bipolar patients for an average of 18 months. Although onset of symptoms was not associated with a preponderance of negative events that matched the bipolar patients' personality type, subsequent symptom severity was significantly related to the interaction of sociotropy and negative interpersonal events, consistent with Beck's (1987) hypothesis. Similarly, in analyses using the first 6 months of follow-up data in the LIBS Project, Francis-Raniere, Alloy, and Abramson (2004) revealed that among bipolar participants, after controlling for initial depressive symptoms and total negative life events experienced, the interaction of autonomous cognitive styles with congruent, autonomy-relevant negative events, and the interaction of sociotropic cognitive styles with congruent, sociotropy-relevant negative events, each predicted increases in depressive symptoms over the 6 months. In addition, after controlling for initial hypomanic symptoms and total positive events experienced, the autonomous styles × autonomy-relevant positive events and sociotropic styles × sociotropy-relevant positive events interactions each predicted increases in hypomanic symptoms over the 6 months.

Two studies tested the cognitive vulnerability–stress hypotheses of both the Beck (1967) and hopelessness (Abramson et al., 1989) theories in samples including bipolar individuals. Alloy, Reilly-Harrington, et al. (1999) examined whether attributional styles and/or dysfunctional attitudes assessed at Time 1 in a normal mood state interacted with subsequent positive and negative life events to predict prospective increases in depressive and hypomanic symptoms among their sample of undergraduates with untreated subsyndromal unipolar and bipolar mood disorders. Consistent with the hopelessness theory, an internal, stable, global attributional style for negative events at Time 1 interacted with subsequent negative life events to predict increases in depressive symptoms at Times 2 and 3 (see Fig. 4.1 for prediction to Time 2). In addition, an internal, stable, global attributional style for positive events at Time 1 interacted with subsequent positive life events to predict increases in hypomanic symptoms at Time 2 (see Fig. 4.2). Dysfunctional attitudes at Time 1 did not interact with positive or negative life events to predict changes in either depressive or hypomanic symptoms at Times 2 or 3.

In a longitudinal design, Reilly-Harrington et al. (1999) also examined whether the interaction of Time 1 attributional styles, dysfunctional attitudes, and negative self-referent information processing (as assessed by a battery of tasks) and intervening negative life events predicted increases in 97 unipolar (most of them remitted) and 49 bipolar (most of them remitted) individuals' clinician-rated depressive and manic symptomatology at Time 2, a month later. Consistent with both hopelessness and Beck's theories, negative attributional style, dysfunctional attitudes, and negative self-referent information processing each interacted significantly with subsequent negative life events to predict increases in depressive symptoms (see Table 4.3) and, within the bipolar group, manic symptoms (see Table 4.4) at Time 2. As predicted, only individuals with negative cognitive styles or information processing at Time 1 who reported a high number of negative life events experienced increases in depressive and manic symptoms at Time 2. Moreover, these findings were maintained when the data of the few unipolar and bipolar students who had received treatment were removed from the analyses.

In summary, the results of the few vulnerability–stress studies to date are promising in supporting the applicability of the cognitive theories of unipolar depression to bipolar spectrum disorders. As such, they suggest

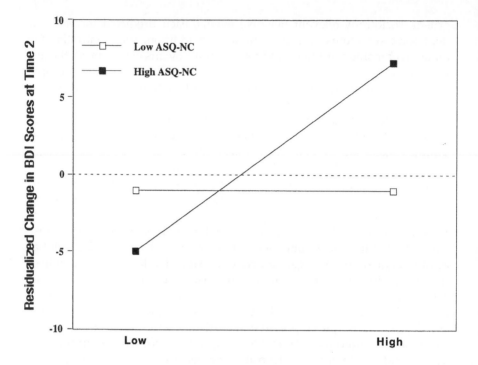

Proportion of Negative Events

FIG. 4.1.   Residualized change in Beck Depression Inventory (BDI) scores at Time 2 as a function of attributional style for negative events and the proportion of negative life events (total negative events/total events) experienced. High ASQ–NC refers to a more internal, stable, global attributional style for negative events and Low ASQ–NC is a less internal, stable, global attributional style for negative events. Adapted from "Cognitive Styles and Life Events in Subsyndromal Unipolar and Bipolar Mood Disorders: Stability and Prospective Prediction of Depressive and Hypomanic Mood Swings," by L. B. Alloy, N. Reilly-Harrington, D. M. Fresco, W. G. Whitehouse, and J. S. Zechmeister, 1999, *Journal of Cognitive Psychotherapy: An International Quarterly, 13*, p. 33. Adapted with permission from Springer Publishing Co.

that similar cognitive and psychosocial processes may contribute vulnerability to both unipolar and bipolar forms of mood disorder. Two issues raised by the findings of the vulnerability–stress studies to date remain to be resolved in future research. First, although two studies (Hammen et al., 1992; Reilly-Harrington et al., 1999) found that negative life events in interaction with negative cognitive styles predicted both depressive and manic symptoms among bipolar individuals, two other studies (Alloy, Reilly-Harrington, et al., 1999; Francis-Raniere et al., 2004) indicated that positive life events predicted increases in hypomanic symptoms in combi-

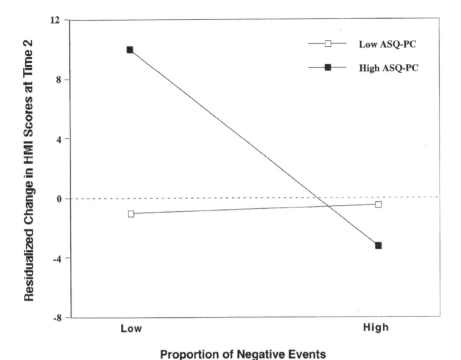

FIG. 4.2. Residualized change in Halberstadt Mania Inventory (HMI) scores at Time 2 as a function of attributional style for positive events and the proportion of negative life events (total negative events/total events) experienced. High ASQ–PC refers to a more internal, stable, global attributional style for positive events and Low ASQ–PC is a less internal, stable, global attributional style for positive events. Adapted from "Cognitive Styles and Life Events in Subsyndromal Unipolar and Bipolar Mood Disorders: Stability and Prospective Prediction of Depressive and Hypomanic Mood Swings," by L. B. Alloy, N. Reilly-Harrington, D. M. Fresco, W. G. Whitehouse, and J. S. Zechmeister, 1999, *Journal of Cognitive Psychotherapy: An International Quarterly, 13*, p. 35. Adapted with permission from Springer Publishing Co.

nation with positive cognitive styles. Thus, more work is needed to understand the conditions under which positive versus negative events and positive versus negative cognitive styles provide vulnerability to mania/hypomania. Second, given that some of the studies reviewed here found that negative life events interact with negative cognitive styles and information processing to predict increases in both depressive and manic symptoms, what determines which type of episode a bipolar individual will experience at any particular time? Reilly-Harrington et al. (1999) speculated that the particular kind of stressful event may be key, with manic/hypomanic episodes more likely to follow stressors that disrupt the sleep–wake cycle (i.e., social rhythm disruptors; Malkoff-Schwartz et al.,

TABLE 4.3
Hierarchical Multiple Regression Analyses to Predict Change in
Clinician-Rated (SADS) Depression in Bipolar and Unipolar Participants

Step	Predictor	Beta In	pr	t	df	Total R^2	R^2 Change
1	ASQ–NC	2.60	.22	2.37*	109	.05	.05
2	NEGEV	0.15	.10	1.05	108	.06	.01
3	ASQ–NC × NEGEV	0.60	.21	2.24*	107	.10	.04
1	DAS	0.05	.24	2.48*	101	.06	.06
2	NEGEV	0.25	.16	1.62	100	.08	.02
3	DAS × NEGEV	0.02	.33	3.46***	99	.18	.10
1	SRIP–NC	2.89	.25	2.63**	100	.06	.06
2	NEGEV	0.16	.11	1.13	99	.08	.02
3	SRIP–NC × NEGEV	0.95	.36	3.77***	98	.20	.12

Note: ASQ–NC = Time 1 Attributional Style Questionnaire composite for negative events; NEGEV = Time 2 Life Experiences Survey total number of negative events; DAS = Time 1 Dysfunctional Attitudes Scale; SRIP–NC = Time 1 Self-referent Information Processing Task Battery composite for negative depression-relevant stimuli. Adapted from "Cognitive Styles and Life Events Interact to Predict Bipolar and Unipolar Symptomatology," by N. A. Reilly-Harrington, L. B. Alloy, D. M. Fresco, and W. G. Whitehouse, 1999, *Journal of Abnormal Psychology, 108*, p. 574. Copyright © 1999 by the American Psychological Association. Adapted with permission.
*$p < .05$. **$p < .01$. ***$p < .001$.

TABLE 4.4
Hierarchical Multiple Regression Analyses to Predict Change in
Clinician-Rated (SADS) Mania in Bipolar Participants

Step	Predictor	Beta In	pr	t	df	Total R^2	R^2 Change
1	ASQ–NC	0.23	.03	0.19	36	.00	.00
2	NEGEV	0.27	.24	1.45	35	.06	.06
3	ASQ–NC × NEGEV	0.62	.33	2.01*	34	.16	.10
1	DAS	0.03	.28	1.68+	33	.08	.08
2	NEGEV	0.24	.22	1.28	32	.13	.05
3	DAS × NEGEV	0.01	.43	2.67**	31	.29	.16
1	SRIP–NC	1.27	.22	1.30	34	.05	.05
2	NEGEV	0.21	.20	1.17	33	.09	.04
3	SRIP–NC × NEGEV	0.38	.30	1.78+	32	.17	.08

Note: ASQ–NC = Time 1 Attributional Style Questionnaire composite for negative events; NEGEV = Time 2 Life Experiences Survey total number of negative events; DAS = Time 1 Dysfunctional Attitudes Scale; SRIP–NC = Time 1 Self-referent Information Processing Task Battery composite for negative depression-relevant stimuli. Adapted from "Cognitive Styles and Life Events Interact to Predict Bipolar and Unipolar Symptomatology," by N. A. Reilly-Harrington, L. B. Alloy, D. M. Fresco, and W. G. Whitehouse, 1999, *Journal of Abnormal Psychology, 108*, p. 575. Copyright © 1999 by the American Psychological Association. Adapted with permission.
+$p < .10$. *$p < .05$. **$p < .01$. ***$p < .001$.

1998) and depressive episodes more likely to follow loss events (e.g., Brown & Harris, 1978). Alternatively, the perceived controllability of stressful life events may be important. In accord with Wortman and Brehm's (1975) reactance model, when bipolar individuals experience negative life events they perceive to be completely uncontrollable, depression may ensue; whereas when they experience stressors that appear to be surmountable, they may react with increased energy and goal directedness and hypomania may result. Clearly, future work involving assessments of both objective characteristics and subjective interpretations of the nature of the stressful events that trigger depressive and manic/ hypomanic episodes is needed to test both of these intriguing hypotheses.

Treatment Implications

Although pharmacotherapy has been the mainstay of treatment for bipolar disorder, the findings discussed in this chapter lend support for the use of adjunctive psychotherapy. In particular, cognitive behavioral therapy (CBT) for bipolar disorder is directed at modifying maladaptive cognitive styles and improving the management of psychosocial stressors. Numerous studies document the efficacy of CBT for unipolar depression (Dobson, 1989), even in severe and medication-resistant cases (Fava, Savron, Grandi, & Rafanelli, 1997). However, CBT has only recently been recognized as an adjunctive treatment for bipolar disorder. Although lifelong pharmacotherapy is generally indicated for bipolar patients, negative beliefs about medication and medication-related side effects, such as cognitive dysfunction or weight gain, may interfere with adherence to pharmacotherapy (Gitlin, Cochran, & Jamison, 1989; Jamison & Akiskal, 1983). Jamison and Akiskal (1983) surveyed 22 patients and found that 50% regarded psychotherapy as very important in medication compliance.

Preliminary studies suggest that CBT may help to reduce relapse, improve medication compliance, and improve quality of life (Newman, Leahy, Beck, Reilly-Harrington, & Gyulai, 2002; Otto, Reilly-Harrington, Kogan, Henin, & Knauz, 1999). The earliest controlled trial of CBT for bipolar disorder randomized 28 bipolar patients on lithium treatment to a 6-week adjunctive individual therapy protocol or to standard pharmacotherapy alone (Cochran, 1984). Patients in the therapy condition received an intervention based on Beck's CBT aimed at altering the behaviors and cognitions that interfered with medication compliance. The intervention improved compliance with the lithium regime both at posttreatment and 3-month follow-up. In addition, patients in the intervention were less likely to discontinue lithium, to be hospitalized during the follow-up period, and to have episodes precipitated by medication noncompliance. Similarly, a recent controlled trial of CB group treatment as an adjunct to standard pharmacotherapy for bipolar disorder (Hirshfeld et al., 1998) reported that patients who completed the adjunctive CB group treatment had longer periods of euthymia and fewer new episodes than controls treated with standard pharmacotherapy alone.

Cognitive behavioral therapy for bipolar disorder is a structured, active treatment aimed at solving current problems and modifying dysfunctional thinking and behavior. In the depressive phase of bipolar disorder, patients may view situations in a negatively distorted way. Alternatively, the thinking of hypomanic patients may be positively or negatively biased and associated with risky or impulsive behavior. The techniques of CBT teach patients to recognize and test out such "cognitive errors" utilizing cognitive restructuring and written dysfunctional thought records. Behavioral strategies, such as a "two-person feedback rule," are used to interfere with impulsive, risky decision making. Given the high rates of suicide in this population, strategies for coping with suicidal ideation and behaviors are also heavily emphasized. A focus on psychoeducation ensures that patients understand the symptoms of bipolar disorder, the role of pharmacotherapy, and the importance of regular sleep patterns. Behavioral strategies include daily mood monitoring and regulation of sleep, activity, and medication regimens. They may also be incorporated for dealing with medication-related side effects, such as weight gain. Problem solving focuses on dealing more effectively with stressful life events and interpersonal conflicts.

Strategies are also geared toward the recognition and prevention of new episodes. Patients are encouraged to challenge nostalgic feelings about past hypomanic episodes and to weigh the costs and benefits of future manic episodes. They are also taught to watch out for early warning signs of relapse and to recognize personal triggers of mood episodes. Patients are encouraged to formulate a support system comprised of family members, friends, and so on, who will participate with them in their treatment contract. In this contract, the patient identifies early warning signs of hypomania and depression and specifies a plan for preventing and coping with future episodes. Patients often give support system members specific directives, such as contacting their doctor, removing credit cards, or encouraging sleep when noticing hypomanic symptoms (Otto et al., 1999).

Cognitive behavioral therapy for bipolar disorder (Otto et al., 1999) is one of three psychosocial treatments currently under study in the large-scale, multisite National Institute of Mental Health sponsored Systematic Treatment Enhancement Program for Bipolar Disorder (STEP–BD). Two other specialized psychotherapies that have shown promise for the treatment of bipolar disorder—Family Focused Treatment (Miklowitz & Goldstein, 1997) and Interpersonal and Social Rhythm Therapy (Frank, Kupfer, Ehlers, & Monk, 1994)—are also being studied. In this sample of 5,000 patients, data is being collected on cognitive styles and life events and may help to further elucidate the role of these factors as distal vulnerabilities and proximal triggers, respectively, in the course of bipolar disorders.

———————

This review suggested that the cognitive vulnerability–stress models of unipolar depression may also be applicable to understanding vulnerability processes in bipolar spectrum disorders. It appears that both stressful life events and negative cognitive styles and information processing contribute to risk for depressive and manic/hypomanic episodes in bipolar disorders. However, several issues remain to be clarified in future research. Although the review indicated that negative life events may trigger manic/hypomanic episodes, do some kinds of positive life events also precipitate mania/hypomania? And, do negative events trigger manic or hypomanic reactions in unipolar manic individuals as well as in bipolar individuals? Finally, under what conditions do bipolar individuals exhibit positive versus negative cognitive styles and information-processing biases, and what are the mechanisms that determine whether a depressive or manic/hypomanic episode occurs at any particular time? When these issues are resolved, the cognitive vulnerability–stress perspective will provide a more powerful model for understanding psychological vulnerability processes in bipolar disorders.

REFERENCES

Abramson, L. Y., Alloy, L. B., Hankin, B. L., Haeffel, G. J., MacCoon, D. G., & Gibb, B. E. (2002). Cognitive vulnerability–stress models of depression in a self-regulatory and psychobiological context. In I. H. Gotlib & C. L. Hammen (Eds.), *Handbook of depression* (pp. 268–294). New York: Guilford.

Abramson, L. Y., Alloy, L. B., Hogan, M. E., Whitehouse, W. G., Donovan, P., Rose, D. T., Panzarella, C., & Raniere, D. (1999). Cognitive vulnerability to depression: Theory and evidence. *Journal of Cognitive Psychotherapy: An International Quarterly, 13,* 5–20.

Abramson, L. Y., Metalsky, G. I., & Alloy, L. B. (1989). Hopelessness depression: A theory-based subtype of depression. *Psychological Review, 96,* 358–372.

Akiskal, H. S., Djenderedjian, A. H., Rosenthal, R. H., & Khani, M. K. (1977). Cyclothymic disorder: Validating criteria for inclusion in the bipolar affective group. *American Journal of Psychiatry, 134,* 1227–1233.

Akiskal, H. S., Khani, M. K., & Scott-Strauss, A. (1979). Cyclothymic temperamental disorders. *Psychiatric Clinics of North America, 2,* 527–554.

Alba, J. W., & Hasher, L. (1983). Is memory schematic? *Psychological Bulletin, 93,* 207–231.

Alloy, L. B., & Abramson, L. Y. (2000). Cyclothymic personality. In W. E. Craighead & C. B. Nemeroff (Eds.), *The Corsini encyclopedia of psychology and behavioral science* (3rd ed., vol. 1, pp. 417–418). New York: Wiley.

Alloy, L. B., Abramson, L. Y., Grandin, L., Smith, J., Steinberg, J. A., Whitehouse, W. G., & Hogan, M. E. (2004). *Negative self-referent information processing in bipolar spectrum and normal comparison individuals.* Manuscript in preparation, Temple University.

Alloy, L. B., Abramson, L. Y., Metalsky, G. I., & Hartlage, S. (1988). The hopelessness theory of depression: Attributional aspects. *British Journal of Clinical Psychology, 27,* 5–21.

Alloy, L. B., Abramson, L. Y., Murray, L. A., Whitehouse, W. G., & Hogan, M. E. (1997). Self-referent information processing in individuals at high and low cognitive risk for depression. *Cognition and Emotion, 11,* 539–568.

Alloy, L. B., Abramson, L. Y., Raniere, D., & Dyller, I. M. (1999). Research methods in adult psychopathology. In P. C. Kendall, J. N. Butcher, & G. N. Holmbeck (Eds.), *Handbook of research methods in clinical psychology* (2nd ed., pp. 466–498). New York: Wiley.

Alloy, L. B., Abramson, L. Y., Walshaw, P. D., & Neeren, A. M. (in press). Cognitive vulnerability to unipolar and bipolar mood disorders. *Journal of Social and Clinical Psychology.*

Alloy, L. B., Abramson, L. Y., Walshaw, P. D., Whitehouse, W. G., & Hogan, M. E. (2004, October). *Depressive cognitive styles and bipolar spectrum disorders: A unique Behavioral Approach System (BAS) profile?* Paper presented at the meeting of the Society for Research in Psychopathology, St. Louis, MO.

Alloy, L. B., Abramson, L. Y., Whitehouse, W. G., Hogan, M. E., Tashman, N. A., Steinberg, D. L., Rose, D. T., & Donovan, P. (1999). Depressogenic cognitive styles: Predictive validity, information processing and personality characteristics, and developmental origins. *Behaviour Research and Therapy, 37,* 503–531.

Alloy, L. B., Flannery-Schroeder, E., Safford, S., Floyd, T. D., & Abramson, L. Y. (1999). Lifetime comorbidity in 17–24 year olds with bipolar spectrum disorders. *Bipolar Disorders, 1*(Suppl. 1), 22.

Alloy, L. B., Reilly-Harrington, N., Fresco, D. M., Whitehouse, W. G., & Zechmeister, J. S. (1999). Cognitive styles and life events in subsyndromal unipolar and bipolar mood disorders: Stability and prospective prediction of depressive and hypomanic mood swings. *Journal of Cognitive Psychotherapy: An International Quarterly, 13,* 21–40.

Ambelas, A. (1979). Psychologically stressful events in the precipitation of manic episodes. *British Journal of Psychiatry, 135,* 15–21.

Ambelas, A. (1987). Life events and mania: A special relationship. *British Journal of Psychiatry, 150,* 235–240.

American Psychiatric Association. (1994). *Diagnostic and statistical manual of mental disorders* (4th ed.). Washington, DC: Author.

Aronson, T. A., & Shukla, S. (1987). Life events and relapse in bipolar disorder: The impact of a catastrophic event. *Acta Psychiatrica Scandinavica, 75,* 571–576.

Bebbington, P., Wilkins, S., Jones, P., Foerster, A., Murray, R., Toone, B., & Lewis, S. (1993). Life events and psychosis. Initial results from the Camberwell Collaborative Psychosis Study. *British Journal of Psychiatry, 162,* 72–79.

Beck, A. T. (1967). *Depression: Clinical, experimental, and theoretical aspects.* New York: Harper & Row.

Beck, A. T. (1976). *Cognitive therapy and the emotional disorders.* New York: International Universities Press.

Beck, A. T. (1987). Cognitive models of depression. *Journal of Cognitive Psychotherapy: An International Quarterly, 1,* 5–37.

Bentall, R. P., & Thompson, M. (1990). Emotional Stroop performance and the manic defense. *British Journal of Clinical Psychology, 29,* 235–237.

Bertelsen, A., Harvald, B., & Hauge, M. (1977). A Danish twin study of manic-depressive disorders. *British Journal of Psychiatry, 130,* 330–351.

Bidzinska, E. (1984). Stress factors in affective diseases. *British Journal of Psychiatry, 144,* 161–166.

Blatt, S. J., D'Afflitti, J. P., & Quinlan, D. M. (1976). Experiences of depression in normal young adults. *Journal of Abnormal Psychology, 85,* 383–389.

Brady, K. T., & Lydiard, B. (1992). Bipolar affective disorder and substance abuse. *Journal of Clinical Psychopharmacology, 12,* 17S–22S.

Brown, G. W. (1974). Meaning, measurement, and stress of life events. In B. S. Dohrenwend & B. P. Dohrenwend (Eds.), *Stressful life events: Their nature and effects* (pp. 217–243). New York: Wiley.

Brown, G. W. (1989). Life events and measurement. In G. W. Brown & T. O. Harris (Eds.), *Life events and illness* (pp. 3–48). New York: Guilford.

Brown, G. W., & Harris, T. O. (1978). *Social origins of depression: A study of psychiatric disorder in women.* New York: The Free Press.

Chung, R. K., Langeluddecke, P., & Tennant, C. (1986). Threatening life events in the onset of schizophrenia, schizophreniform psychosis and hypomania. *British Journal of Psychiatry, 148,* 680–686.

Clancy, J., Crowe, R., Winokur, G., & Morrison, J. (1973). The Iowa 500: Precipitating factors in schizophrenia and primary affective disorder. *Comprehensive Psychiatry, 14,* 197–202.

Cochran, S. (1984). Preventing medical noncompliance in the outpatient treatment of bipolar affective disorder. *Journal of Consulting and Clinical Psychology, 52,* 873–878.

Davenport, Y. B., & Adland, M. L. (1982). Postpartum psychoses in female and male bipolar manic-depressive patients. *American Journal of Orthopsychiatry, 52,* 288–297.

Depue, R. A., & Monroe, S. M. (1978). The unipolar–bipolar distinction in the depressive disorders. *Psychological Bulletin, 85,* 1001–1030.

Depue, R. A., Slater, J. F., Wolfstetter-Kausch, H., Klein, D., Goplerud, E., & Farr, D. (1981). A behavioral paradigm for identifying persons at risk for bipolar depressive disorder: A conceptual framework and five validation studies. *Journal of Abnormal Psychology, 90,* 381–438.

Dobson, K. S. (1989). A meta-analysis of the efficacy of cognitive therapy for depression. *Journal of Consulting and Clinical Psychology, 57,* 414–419.

Dunner, D. L., Patrick, V., & Fieve, R. (1979). Life events at the onset of bipolar affective illness. *American Journal of Psychiatry, 136,* 508–515.

Dunner, D. L., Russek, F. D., Russek, B., & Fieve, R. R. (1982). Classification of bipolar affective disorder subtypes. *Comprehensive Psychiatry, 23,* 186–189.

Ehlers, C. L., Frank, E., & Kupfer, D. J. (1988). Social zeitgebers and biological rhythms: A unified approach to understanding the etiology of depression. *Archives of General Psychiatry, 45,* 948–952.

Eich, E., Macaulay, D., & Lam, R. W. (1997). Mania, depression, and mood-dependent memory. *Cognition and Emotion, 11,* 607–618.

Ellicott, A., Hammen, C., Gitlin, M., Brown, G., & Jamison, K. (1990). Life events and the course of bipolar disorder. *American Journal of Psychiatry, 147,* 1194–1198.

Fava, G. A., Savron, G., Grandi, S., & Rafanelli, C. (1997). Cognitive-behavioral treatment of drug resistant major depressive disorder. *Journal of Clinical Psychiatry, 58,* 278–282.

Francis-Raniere, E., Alloy, L. B., & Abramson, L. Y. (2004). *Depressive personality styles and bipolar spectrum disorders: Prospective tests of the event congruency hypothesis.* Manuscript submitted for publication.

Frank, E., Kupfer, D. J., Ehlers, C. L., & Monk, T. H. (1994). Interpersonal and social rhythm therapy for bipolar disorder: Integrating interpersonal and behavioral approaches. *Behavior Therapist, 17,* 143.

Freeman, T. (1971). Observations on mania. *International Journal of Psychology, 52,* 479–486.

French, C. C., Richards, A., & Scholfield, E. J. C. (1996). Hypomania, anxiety and the emotional Stroop. *British Journal of Clinical Psychology, 35,* 617–626.

Geller, B., & DelBello, M. P. (Eds.). (2003). *Bipolar disorder in childhood and early adolescence.* New York: Guilford.

Gitlin, M. J., Cochran, S. D., & Jamison, K. R. (1989). Maintenance lithium treatment: Side effects and compliance. *Journal of Clinical Psychiatry, 50,* 127–131.

Glassner, B., & Haldipur, C. V. (1983). Life events and early and late onset of bipolar disorder. *American Journal of Psychiatry, 140,* 215–217.

Glassner, B., Haldipur, C. V., & Dessauersmith, J. (1979). Role loss and working-class manic depression. *Journal of Nervous and Mental Disease, 167*, 530–541.

Goodwin, F. K., & Jamison, K. R. (1990). *Manic-depressive illness.* New York: Oxford University Press.

Grandin, L. D., Alloy, L. B, & Abramson, L. Y. (2004). *Childhood events and bipolar spectrum disorders.* Manuscript submitted for publication.

Hall, K. S. (1984). *A prospective study of life events and affective episode in a population of manic-depressive patients.* Unpublished doctoral dissertation, Columbia University, New York.

Hall, K. S., Dunner, D. L., Zeller, G., & Fieve, R. R. (1977). Bipolar illness: A prospective study of life events. *Comprehensive Psychiatry, 18*, 497–505.

Hammen, C. (1991). Generation of stress in the course of unipolar depression. *Journal of Abnormal Psychology, 100*, 555–561.

Hammen, C., Ellicott, A., & Gitlin, M. (1992). Stressors and sociotropy/autonomy: A longitudinal study of their relationship to the course of bipolar disorder. *Cognitive Therapy and Research, 16*, 409–418.

Hammen, C., Ellicott, A., Gitlin, M., & Jamison, K. (1989). Sociotropy/autonomy and vulnerability to specific life events in patients with unipolar depression and bipolar disorders. *Journal of Abnormal Psychology, 98*, 154–160.

Hammen, C., & Gitlin, M. (1997). Stress reactivity in bipolar patients and its relation to prior history of disorder. *American Journal of Psychiatry, 154*, 856–857.

Hammen, C., Gitlin, M., & Altshuler, L. (2000). Predictors of work adjustment in bipolar I patients: A naturalistic longitudinal follow-up. *Journal of Consulting and Clinical Psychology, 68*, 220–225.

Harmon-Jones, E., Abramson, L. Y., Sigelman, J., Bohlig, A., Hogan, M. E., & Harmon-Jones, C. (2002). Proneness to hypomania/mania symptoms or depression symptoms and asymmetrical frontal cortical responses to an anger-evoking event. *Journal of Personality and Social Psychology, 82*, 610–618.

Healy, D., & Williams, J. M. G. (1988). Dysrhythmia, dysphoria, and depression: The interaction of learned helplessness and circadian dysrhythmia in the pathogenesis of depression. *Psychological Bulletin, 103*, 163–178.

Hill, C. V., Oei, T. P., & Hill, M. A. (1989). An empirical investigation of the specificity and sensitivity of the Automatic Thoughts Questionnaire and Dysfunctional Attitudes Scale. *Journal of Psychopathology and Behavioral Assessment, 11*, 291–311.

Hirshfeld, D. R., Gould, R. A., Reilly-Harrington, N. A., Morabito, C., Cosgrove, V., Fredman, S., & Sachs, G. S. (1998, November). *Short-term adjunctive cognitive-behavioral group therapy for bipolar disorder: Preliminary results from a controlled trial.* Paper presented at the Association for the Advancement of Behavior Therapy Meeting, Washington, DC.

Hollon, S. D., Kendall, P. C., & Lumry, A. (1986). Specificity of depressogenic cognitions in clinical depression. *Journal of Abnormal Psychology, 95*, 52–59.

Hunt, N., Bruce-Jones, W., & Silverstone, T. (1992). Life events and relapse in bipolar affective disorder. *Journal of Affective Disorders, 25*, 13–20.

Ingram, R. E., Miranda, J., & Segal, Z. V. (1998). *Cognitive vulnerability to depression.* New York: Guilford.

Jamison, K. R., & Akiskal, H. S. (1983). Medication compliance in patients with bipolar disorders. *Psychiatric Clinics of North America, 6*, 175–192.

Johnson, S. L., & Kizer, A. (2002). Bipolar and unipolar depression: A comparison of clinical phenomenology and psychosocial predictors. In I. H. Gotlib & C. L. Hammen (Eds.), *Handbook of depression* (pp. 141–165). New York: Guilford.

Johnson, S. L., & Miller, I. (1997). Negative life events and time to recovery from episodes of bipolar disorder. *Journal of Abnormal Psychology, 106*, 449–457.

Johnson, S. L., & Roberts, J. E. (1995). Life events and bipolar disorder: Implications from biological theories. *Psychological Bulletin, 117*, 434–449.

Joffe, R. T., MacDonald, C. M., & Kutcher, S. P. (1989). Life events and mania: A case-controlled study. *Psychiatry Research, 30*, 213–216.

Just, N., Abramson, L. Y., & Alloy, L. B. (2001). Remitted depression studies as tests of the cognitive vulnerability hypotheses of depression onset: A critique and conceptual analysis. *Clinical Psychology Review, 21*, 63–83.

Keck, P. E., & McElroy, S. L. (1996). Outcome in the pharmacological treatment of bipolar disorder. *Journal of Clinical Pharmacology, 16*(Suppl. 1), 15–23.

Kennedy, S., Thompson, R., Stancer, H., Roy, A., & Persad, E. (1983). Life events precipitating mania. *British Journal of Psychiatry, 142*, 398–403.

Klein, D. N., Depue, R. A., & Slater, J. F. (1985). Cyclothymia in the adolescent offspring of parents with bipolar affective disorder. *Journal of Abnormal Psychology, 94*, 115–127.

Kraepelin, E. (1921). *Manic-depressive insanity and paranoia* (R. M. Barclay, trans.; G. M. Robertson, Ed.). Edinburgh, Scotland: Livingstone.

Leff, J. P., Fischer, M., & Bertelson, A. C. (1976). A cross-national epidemiological study of mania. *British Journal of Psychiatry, 129*, 428–442.

Leonhard, K. (1957). *Aufteilung der endogenen Psychosen* [Differentiation of endogenous psychosis]. Berlin, Germany: Akademieverlag.

Lewinsohn, P. M., Steinmetz, J. L., Larson, D. W., & Franklin, J. (1981). Depression-related cognitions: Antecedent or consequence? *Journal of Abnormal Psychology, 90*, 213–219.

Lyon, H. M., Startup, M., & Bentall, R. P. (1999). Social cognition and the manic defense: Attributions, selective attention, and self-schema in bipolar affective disorder. *Journal of Abnormal Psychology, 108*, 273–282.

Malkoff-Schwartz, S., Frank, E., Anderson, B., Sherrill, J. T., Siegel, L., Patterson, D., & Kupfer, D. J. (1998). Stressful life events and social rhythm disruption in the onset of manic and depressive bipolar episodes. *Archives of General Psychiatry, 55*, 702–707.

McPherson, H., Herbison, P., & Romans, S. (1993). Life events and relapse in established bipolar affective disorder. *British Journal of Psychiatry, 163*, 381–385.

Miklowitz, D. J., & Alloy, L. B. (1999). Psychosocial factors in the course and treatment of bipolar disorder: Introduction to the special section. *Journal of Abnormal Psychology, 108*, 555 557.

Miklowitz, D. J., & Goldstein, M. J. (1997). *Bipolar disorder: A family-focused treatment approach*. New York: Guilford.

Miklowitz, D. J., Goldstein, M. J., & Nuechterlein, K. H. (1995). Verbal interactions in the families of schizophrenic and bipolar affective patients. *Journal of Abnormal Psychology, 104*, 268–276.

Neale, J. M. (1988). Defensive function of manic episodes. In T. F. Oltmanns & B. A. Maher (Eds.), *Delusional beliefs* (pp. 138–156). New York: Wiley.

Newman, C. F., Leahy, R. L., Beck, A. T., Reilly-Harrington, N. A., & Gyulai, L. (2002). *Bipolar disorder: A cognitive therapy approach*. Washington, DC: APA Books.

Nurnberger, J. L., & Gershon, E. S. (1992). Genetics. In E. S. Paykel (Ed.), *Handbook of affective disorders* (2nd. ed., pp. 131–148). New York: Guilford.

O'Connell, R. A. (1986). Psychosocial factors in a model of manic depressive disease. *Integrative Psychiatry, 4*, 150–161.

Otto, M. W., Reilly-Harrington, N. A., Kogan, J. N., Henin, A., & Knauz, R. O. (1999). *Cognitive-behavior therapy for bipolar disorder: Treatment manual*. Unpublished manuscript, Massachusetts General Hospital and Harvard Medical School, Boston, MA.

Pardoen, D., Bauwens, F., Tracy, A., Martin, F., & Mendlewicz, J. (1993). Self-esteem in recovered bipolar and unipolar out-patients. *British Journal of Psychiatry, 163*, 755–762.

Pergui, G., Toni, C., & Akiskal, H. S. (1999). Anxious-bipolar comorbidity: Diagnostic and treatment challenges. *Psychiatric Clinics of North America, 22*, 565–583.

Perris, H. (1984). Life events and depression: Part 2. Results in diagnostic subgroups, and in relation to the recurrence of depression. *Journal of Affective Disorders, 7*, 25–36.

Post, R. (1992). Transduction of psychosocial stress into the neurobiology of recurrent affective disorders. *American Journal of Psychiatry, 149,* 999–1010.

Prien, R. F., & Potter, W. Z. (1990). NIMH workshop report on treatment of bipolar disorder. *Psychopharmacology Bulletin, 26,* 409–427.

Reilly-Harrington, N. A., Alloy, L. B., Fresco, D. M., & Whitehouse, W. G. (1999). Cognitive styles and life events interact to predict bipolar and unipolar symptomatology. *Journal of Abnormal Psychology, 108,* 567–578.

Rosenfarb, I. S., Becker, J., Khan, A., & Mintz, J. (1998). Dependency and self-criticism in bipolar and unipolar depressed women. *British Journal of Clinical Psychology, 37,* 409–414.

Sclare, P., & Creed, F. (1990). Life events and the onset of mania. *British Journal of Psychiatry, 156,* 508–514.

Scott, J., Stanton, B., Garland, A., & Ferrier, I. N. (2000). Cognitive vulnerability in patients with bipolar disorder. *Psychological Medicine, 30,* 467–472.

Smith, A. L., & Weissman, M. M. (1992). Epidemiology. In E. S. Paykel (Ed.), *Handbook of affective disorders* (2nd ed., pp. 111–129). New York: Guilford.

Taylor, S. E., & Crocker, J. (1981). Schematic bases of social information processing. In E. T. Higgins, P. Herman, & M. P. Zanna (Eds.), *The Ontario symposium in personality and social psychology* (Vol. 1, pp. 81–134). Hillsdale, NJ: Lawrence Erlbaum Associates.

Tracy, A., Bauwens, F., Martin, F., Pardoen, D., & Mendlewicz, J. (1992). Attributional style and depression: A controlled comparison of remitted unipolar and bipolar patients. *British Journal of Clinical Psychology, 31,* 83–84.

Weissman, M. M., Bruce, M. L., Leaf, P. J., Florio, L. P., & Holzer, C. E. (1990). Affective disorders. In L. Robins & D. A. Regier (Eds.), *Psychiatric disorders in America* (pp. 53–80). New York: The Free Press.

Weissman, M. M., Leaf, P. J., Tischler, G. L., Blazer, D. G., Karno, M., Bruce, M. L., & Florio, L. P. (1988). Affective disorders in five United States communities. *Psychological Medicine, 18,* 141–153.

Winters, K. C., & Neale, J. M. (1985). Mania and low self-esteem. *Journal of Abnormal Psychology, 94,* 282–290.

Wortman, C. B., & Brehm, J. W. (1975). Response to uncontrollable outcomes: An integration of reactance theory and the learned helplessness model. In L. Berkowitz (Ed.), *Advances in experimental social psychology* (Vol. 8, pp. 277–336). New York: Academic Press.

5

Cognitive Vulnerability to Suicide

Jeremy W. Pettit
University of Houston

Thomas E. Joiner, Jr.
Florida State University

Suicide is a national health epidemic in the United States, responsible for the deaths of approximately 30,000 people annually (Miniño, Arias, Kochanek, Murphy, & Smith, 2002). It is the 11th leading cause of death, surpassing liver disease and hypertension (Miniño et al., 2002). Moreover, suicide is the third leading cause of death among adolescents and young adults (Miniño et al., 2002), the fourth leading cause of death among adults age 25 to 44, and the sixth leading cause of death among children age 5 to 14 (National Center for Health Statistics, 2002). Between 1960 and 1988, the overall national suicide rate increased 17%, and the rate among adolescents increased 200%. Young males in the United States have the highest suicide rate in the world (Blumenthal, 1990). Furthermore, rates among the elderly have sharply increased over the past half-century (Buda & Tsuang, 1990).

There are roughly 30,000 completed suicides each year, but a substantially larger number of individuals attempt, but do not complete, the act. Estimated rates range from 10 (Andreasen & Black, 1995) to as many as 50 attempts (Garland & Zigler, 1993) per completed suicide, including those who eventually complete suicide and those who attempt but never complete suicide. This represents a wide range, but it corresponds to a minimum of 300,000 attempted suicides in the United States alone each year; this number may actually be as high as 1.5 million attempts per year. Recent data estimate that there are 734,000 attempts annually (Miniño et al., 2002), which corresponds to roughly 25 attempts per completion. According to the National Comorbidity Survey, 4.6% of the general population between age 15 and 54 has attempted suicide at least once (Kessler, Borges, & Walters, 1999). Furthermore, 13.5% of the general population reported experiencing suicidal ideation on at least one occasion. Other investigators have reported similar lifetime suicidal ideation rates. For instance, Paykel, Myers, Lindenthal, and Tanner (1974) found a lifetime suicidal ideation rate of 13.3% and a 1-year prevalence rate of 8.9% in the general population. Weissman et al. (1999) found that, across a sample of nine countries, lifetime rates of suicidal ideation ranged from a low of 2.1% (Beirut, Lebanon) to 18.5% (Christchurch, New Zealand). Thus, a substantial percentage of the population experiences suicidal thoughts at one time or another.

These figures indicate that suicidal behavior is an alarmingly common phenomenon, which appears to be increasing each year. So what leads to this ultimate decision—the purposeful resolution to end one's own life? Various causal theories have been espoused, and most mental health professionals adopt a multifactorial approach to understanding the etiology of suicidal behavior. That is, they maintain that suicide may be caused by any of a number of variables, and most likely results from the interaction of multiple causes.

This chapter reviews the evidence for a group of such proposed vulnerabilities to suicide: cognitive vulnerabilities. In psychological terms, cognition has generally referred to mental processes such as thinking, knowing, and remembering (Kassin, 2004). Cognitive vulnerabilities to suicide, therefore, involve patterns of thinking and storing and retrieving information that place an individual at increased risk for suicidal behaviors.

COGNITIVE VULNERABILITIES TO SUICIDALITY

A number of specific cognitive vulnerabilities to suicide have been proposed as parts of larger models of suicidality. In general, these models have included multiple cognitive vulnerabilities. This chapter distinguishes these vulnerabilities into four broad categories: future-oriented cognitions, self-oriented cognitions, interpersonally oriented cognitions, and escape-oriented cognitions. Thus, it does not present theoretical models of cognitive vulnerabilities to suicide separately. Rather, aspects of various models that fall into the four categories are grouped together. Nevertheless, it is important to note that a high degree of overlap exists among these categories, and inclusion in a particular category is not mutually exclusive.

Future-Oriented Cognitions

Future-oriented cognitions refer to thoughts and expectations regarding the occurrence of impending or temporally distant events. According to certain theories of suicidality, individuals' anticipation of future outcomes may place them at an increased risk for suicidal behaviors. The leading models of future-oriented cognitions as vulnerabilities to suicide are reviewed in the following paragraphs.

Theories/Models

Hopelessness. The hopelessness theory of suicidality has concentrated primarily on the role of future-oriented cognitions in placing an individual at risk for suicide. Stemming from the hopelessness theory of depression (Abramson, Metalsky, & Alloy, 1989), the hopelessness theory of suicidality proposes that a variety of suicide-related phenomena (ranging from suicidal ideation to completed suicide) compose a core symptom of hopelessness depression. In short, the hopelessness theory of depression asserts that the vulnerability of a negative cognitive style is a proximal sufficient cause of depression. This vulnerability is comprised of two future-oriented beliefs that serve as the essential components of hopelessness theory: a negative outcome expectancy and a helplessness expectancy. The negative outcome expectancy refers to the expectation that highly desired outcomes will not occur and highly aversive outcomes will occur. The helplessness expectation refers to the belief that the individual can do nothing to change the likelihood of these negative outcomes. Thus, individuals with this particular cognitive vulnerability believe that life events will not occur as they desire, and they are powerless to change the occurrence of such events.

Abramson et al. (1989) posited that attributions made in response to perceived negative life events (or nonoccurrence of positive life events) foster the development of hopelessness and ultimately suicide. In particular, attributions regarding the causes and consequences of negative life events, as well as characteristics about the self, may make individuals more likely to experience hopelessness depression and suicide. Suicide is most likely to occur when an individual holds the perception that negative life events have important consequences, are caused by stable and global factors, and suggest that the individual is somehow flawed or inadequate. These views compose what Abramson et al. labeled a "depressogenic cognitive style." In this model, hopelessness mediates the relation between the depressogenic cognitive style and suicidality.

The hopelessness model of depression and suicide is a diathesis–stress model, with the depressogenic cognitive style serving as the diathesis, and negative life events serving as the stressor. Hence, individuals demonstrating the depressogenic cognitive style should only develop hopelessness depression, and subsequent suicide, in the wake of the triggering effects of negative life events. Furthermore, Abramson et al. noted that specific vulnerabilities exist in the form of cognitive vulnerabilities in a particular content domain. Negative events occurring within the context of one of these content domains place the individual at a specific risk for the development of depression and suicide.

A plethora of empirical research has supported a relation between hopelessness and suicide. Furthermore, a substantial body of work has demonstrated that hopelessness is predictive of suicide (Beck, Brown, Berchick, Stewart, & Steer, 1990; Beck, Kovacs, & Weissman, 1975; Bedrosian & Beck, 1979; Kazdin, French, Unis, Esveldt-Dawson, & Sherick, 1983). For instance, Beck reported relatively high accuracy rates in the prediction of suicide using the Beck Hopelessness Scale (BHS; Beck & Steer, 1993; Beck, Weissman, Lester, & Trexler, 1974) among both psychiatric outpatients (Beck & Steer, 1993) and psychiatric inpatients (Beck, Brown, & Steer, 1989; Beck, Brown, Steer, Dahlsgaard, & Grisham, 1999; Beck, Steer, Epstein, & Brown, 1990; Beck, Steer, Kovacs, & Garrison, 1985). Similarly, Fawcett and colleagues (Fawcett et al., 1987, 1990) reported a moderate degree of success using hopelessness in the prediction of eventual suicide. Additional research suggests that hopelessness is better than depression at distinguishing suicidality (T. E. Ellis & Ratliff, 1986; Minkoff, Bergman, Beck, & Beck, 1973). Given the inherent difficulties in predicting suicide (e.g., low base rate occurrence), Beck and colleagues' findings support the implementation of hopelessness assessment in the prediction of suicide.

Although such findings indicate that hopelessness is indeed predictive of suicide, they do not investigate the pathway introduced by the hopelessness model of suicidality (i.e., individuals with the depressogenic cognitive style will be at increased risk for suicide, and hopelessness mediates this relation). Direct tests of the hopelessness model of suicidality, although sparse, have generally been supportive. The first test of the model by Joiner and Rudd (1995) detected that the presence of a depressogenic cognitive style (i.e., tendency to attribute negative interpersonal events to stable, global causes) predicted stress-related increases in suicidality. Despite confirming the general model of cognitive vulnerability to suicide, the findings did not support the mediational pathway of depressogenic style–hopelessness–suicidality. Hence, Joiner and Rudd found mixed support for the model.

Abramson et al. (1998) provided cogent support for the hopelessness model using a prospective design. As part of their ongoing behavioral high risk two-site prospective design (Cognitive Vulnerability to Depression Project), the authors compared participants designated as high cognitive risk to those designated as low cognitive risk. Over the course of 2½ years, those in the high risk group were more likely to exhibit suicidality than those in the low risk group. Moreover, this was still the case after controlling for other relevant variables such as prior history of suicidality, prior history of major and/or minor depression, borderline and antisocial personality disorders, and parental history of depression. In addition to supporting the general cognitive vulnerability to suicidality model, Abramson et al. specifically delineated and empirically supported the role of hopelessness as a mediator of the relation between depressogenic cognitive style and suicidality.

Abramson and colleagues' (1998) ongoing investigation employs college students making the transition from late adolescence into young adulthood. Consequently, their results may be applicable to both late adolescents and adults. Up to this point, however, the connection between hopelessness and suicidality among children and adolescents has remained unclear (Weishaar, 2000). Researchers have reported positive correlations between suicidal ideation and hopelessness among clinical samples of children and adolescents (e.g., Asarnow & Guthrie, 1982; Carlson & Cantwell, 1982; Esposito, Johnson, Wolfsdorf, & Spirito, 2003; Kazdin et al., 1983; Kazdin, Rogers, & Colbus, 1986; Spirito, Williams, Stark, & Hart, 1988). Nevertheless, Asarnow, Carlson, and Guthrie (1987, as cited in Weishaar, 2000) indicated that when depression is partialed out, the correlation between hopelessness and suicide no longer reaches levels of statistical significance. Other work (e.g., Rich, Kirkpatrick-Smith, Bonner, & Jans, 1992) suggests that hopelessness may be predictive of suicidality among adolescents, consistent with findings among adult samples. Nevertheless, Rudd (1990) found that the relation between depression and suicidal ideation was greater than the relation between hopelessness and suicidal ideation. The findings are conflicted, and so the verdict is still out with reference to the specific role of hopelessness in suicidality among youngsters.

Some have identified potential antecedents to the development of a depressogenic cognitive style. In an investigation of parental characteristics, Alloy et al. (2001) recognized that mothers of individuals with a depressogenic cognitive style were more likely to exhibit negative inferential styles and dysfunctional attitudes. Furthermore, both mothers and fathers of such individuals provided more stable, global attributional feedback for negative events in their child's life, and offered more negative consequence feedback for negative social events in their child's life. Finally, low levels of emotional acceptance and warmth from fathers were more prevalent among individuals displaying a depressogenic cognitive style. Gibb, Alloy, Abramson, Rose, Whitehouse, Donovan, et al. (2001) identified another precursor to a depressogenic cognitive style: childhood emotional maltreatment. Higher levels of self-reported childhood emotional maltreatment were predictive of the later development of a depressogenic cognitive style. In contrast, lower levels of childhood physical maltreatment were associated with a depressogenic cognitive style. Although the mechanism by which developmental emotional maltreatment leads to a depressogenic cognitive style is not known, individuals possessing this style may have internalized their adverse environments and the negative cognitions espoused by their abusers. Of particular relevance to the current discussion, Gibb, Alloy, Abramson, Rose, Whitehouse, and Hogan (2001) also found that childhood emotional maltreatment (but not physical or sexual maltreatment) uniquely predicted suicidal ideation in adulthood, and hopelessness partially mediated this relation.

Thus, a large body of evidence supports the association between hopelessness and suicide, and a smaller amount of empirical data suggests that the hopelessness model is an accurate representation of the development of hopelessness and, in turn, suicidality. As Abramson, Alloy, and colleagues continue to work on the Cognitive Vulnerability to Depression (CVD) Project, the role of hopelessness in suicidality will be further illuminated.

Problem-Solving Skills. Although hopelessness has typically been at the forefront of future-oriented cognitions, another set of cognitions related to future outcomes has also been theoretically linked to suicidality. This kindred cognitive vulnerability involves deficits in problem-solving abilities. Problem-solving abilities, although not consisting entirely of future-focused thoughts, certainly contain a set of cognitions that have a direct bearing on future occurrences. Therefore, we have categorized them as future-oriented cognitions, even though they do not represent "pure" future-oriented cognitions.

A rudimentary paradigm of problem solving emphasizes the importance of three primary steps: representing the problem, generating potential solutions, and evaluating the solutions (A. Ellis & Hunt, 1989; Glass & Holyoak, 1986; see D'Zurilla & Goldfried, 1971, for an alternative model of problem solving). For a number of reasons, suicidal individuals may possess limitations in the application of one or more of these steps. Suicidal individuals have been described as feeling both hopeless and helpless, believing that they are not capable of finding a solution to their predicament, and others will not will not be able to provide respite for them either

(Freeman & Reinecke, 1993). As such, these individuals may be considered "cognitively constricted," or fixated on a given trauma. Due to this state of cognitive constriction, suicidal individuals perceive suicide, a possible solution, as the *only* solution (Leenaars, 1999). These people are unable to generate alternative courses of action or examine the validity of their fixated beliefs (Freeman & Reinecke, 1993). Thus, distressed individuals who display deficiencies in the second step of the problem-solving process (i.e., generating alternative solutions) may be at an increased risk of suicidal behavior.

Despite a limitation in problem-solving skills, some individuals may go through life largely unfettered. Among those who experience significant negative life events, however, meager problem-solving abilities may turn an uncomfortable situation into a potentially deadly situation. The inability to manage elevated levels of stress leaves suicide as the final solution falling within their modest problem-solving repertoire.

In addition to the research on hopelessness, empirical work provides support for the notion that deficits in problem-solving skills may place individuals at increased risk for suicide. These findings apply to children (e.g., Asarnow et al., 1987; Orbach, Rosenheim, & Hary, 1987), adolescents (e.g., Carris, Sheeber, & Howe, 1998; Esposito et al., 2003; King, Segal, Naylor, & Evans, 1993; Rotheram-Borus, Trautman, Dopkins, & Shrout, 1990; Sadowski & Kelley, 1993), and adults (e.g., Pollock & Willams, 1998; Priester & Clum, 1993; Rudd, Rajab, & Dahm, 1994; Schotte & Clum, 1982, 1987), thus supporting the validity of this model across the developmental life span. Moreover, suicidal individuals display deficits in problem-solving abilities in a broad area of life situations, including interpersonal and impersonal tasks (e.g., Asarnow et al., 1987; Levenson, 1974; Mraz & Runco, 1994; Patsiokas, Clum, & Luscomb, 1979), as well as general coping skills (Weishaar, 2000). In particular, evidence suggests that suicidal individuals have difficulty generating solutions to problems (Orbach et al., 1987; Patsiokas et al., 1979; Schotte & Clum, 1987), resist implementing potential solutions (Josepho & Plutchik, 1994; Linehan, Camper, Chiles, Strosahl, & Shearin, 1987; Rotheram-Borus et al., 1990), and resist modifying ineffective solutions (Levenson & Neuringer, 1971). This last point corresponds to the finding that cognitive rigidity serves as a vulnerability to suicidality. Other research corroborates this relation, suggesting that suicidal ideators, attemptors, and completers exhibit elevated levels of cognitive rigidity as compared to nonsuicidal individuals (e.g., Levenson, 1974; Patsiokas et al., 1979). Finally, a small amount of evidence suggests that low social problem-solving skills are more predictive of suicide potential than hopelessness (Chang, 1998). Hence, a relatively large base of empirical work provides evidence that deficient problem-solving abilities in a variety of areas are related to suicide. In contrast, improved problem-solving skills appear to produce the opposite effect (i.e., they lead to lower levels of suicidality; Joiner, Pettit, et al., 2001; Joiner, Voelz, & Rudd, 2001; Rudd et al., 1996).

Given the primarily cross-sectional nature of the data reviewed here, it would be premature to conclude that problem-solving deficits serve as a prospective risk factor for suicidality. Indeed, excluding the treatment studies of Joiner and colleagues (Joiner, Pettit, et al., 2001; Joiner, Voelz, et al., 2001) and Rudd et al. (1996), only two studies cited in the previous paragraph longitudinally assessed the predictive ability of problem-solving deficits (Chang, 1998; Priester & Clum, 1993). Therefore, despite strong evidence for an association between problem-solving deficits and suicidal behavior, the status of problem-solving skills as a vulnerability to suicide remains somewhat unclear at this time.

Looming Vulnerability. A third model of suicidality emphasizing the contribution of future-oriented cognitions focuses on perceived instability and expected rapid change in one's environment. The looming vulnerability model, proposed by Riskind and colleagues (e.g., Riskind, 1997; Riskind, Long, Williams, & White, 2000), posits that the expectation of rapid, aversive change serves as a determinant of anxiety. Riskind et al. (2000) accorded special importance to the perception of change in relation to threatening stimuli or occurrences. In particular, four perceived factors accompanying fluctuation among threats impact the intensity of these threats: *magnitude*, or total amount of change; *velocity*, or speed at which the threat is escalating; *acceleration*, or rate of increase of velocity; and *momentum*, or the combination of velocity and amount of change.

A sense of looming vulnerability involves creating mental representations of intensifying danger. As a result, methods of avoiding or escaping this danger are pursued. According to the theory, escalating and unbearable psychological pain may produce an escape/avoidance response of suicide. Among individuals with a sense of looming vulnerability, the future is perceived as becoming increasingly painful, and the internal pressure to escape escalates. The addition of hopelessness to individuals' sense of looming vulnerability creates the highest levels of desperation, and consequently, the greatest risk for suicide. These individuals view the future as becoming increasingly more painful, and also believe that their situation is unavoidable and unchangeable. In this scenario, looming vulnerability and hopelessness both serve as potential risk factors for suicidality, and the interaction of these two risk factors places individuals at an even increased risk for suicidality.

A large base of empirical evidence supports the looming vulnerability model of anxiety. This is not the focus of this chapter, so that evidence is not reviewed here (see Riskind, 1997, for a review). The model's link to suicide, however, has not yet been directly investigated. Nevertheless, Riskind et al. (2000) offered reason to believe that this model may be applicable to suicide. First, escape from psychological pain, one of the tenets of the looming vulnerability model, appears to be directly related to suicide (e.g., Baumeister, 1990; see later section on escape-oriented cognitions as a vulnerability to suicide). Second, the proposal that the combination of hopelessness and a sense of looming vulnerability elevate suicide risk already has a degree of indirect support, as comorbid anxiety has been found to increase suicidality among depressed and hopeless individuals (Bakish, 1999; Rudd, Dahm, & Rajab, 1993). Finally, a sense of looming vulnerability increases behaviors related to suicidality, such as alcohol and substance abuse.

The looming vulnerability model of suicidality represents a recent and provocative theory in the field of suicidality. Based on theory and solid empirical support in the area of anxiety disorders, this model offers promise as a potential explanation of some suicidal behaviors. Despite its success in predicting anxiety, it has not yet been tested among suicidal individuals. Future research will determine its validity as a cognitive vulnerability to suicide.

Therapeutic and Preventive Implications

Following the logic of the hopelessness model of suicidality, altering the attributional styles of hopeless individuals will lead to a reduction in suicidal behaviors. More specifically, addressing the two future-oriented beliefs of a negative outcome expectancy and a helplessness expectancy may prove beneficial in the treatment of suicidality. Unfortunately, little research has investigated specific treatments targeting such cognitions. Although not posited to be the sole component of treatment, traditional cognitive therapies (e.g., Beck's CT, Ellis' RET) often place an emphasis on altering such maladaptive cognitions. The demonstrated efficacy of such interventions offers a degree of support for the therapeutic application of techniques designed to alter hopeless cognitions. These therapies also address a number of other factors as well, making it difficult to tease out the specific effects of addressing hopelessness.

In contrast to the lack of empirical evidence regarding treatments of hopelessness, those focusing on problem-solving deficits are among the most well-researched suicide interventions. Consistent with the notion that problem-solving deficits place an individual at risk for suicide, treatments targeting problem-solving skill improvements appear to be effective in reducing suicidal symptoms (Rudd et al., 1996; Rudd, 2000; Rudd, Joiner, & Rajab, 2001). Recently, Joiner and colleagues (Joiner et al., 2001a) applied the "broaden and build" model of positive emotions (see

Fredrickson, 1998) to the treatment of suicidality, finding that the acquisition of problem-solving attitudes partly mediated the remission of suicidal symptoms (the presence of positive affect played the other key role in reducing symptoms). Analogously, Joiner, Voelz, et al. (2001) found that suicidal ideation was reduced among individuals who received cognitive behavioral therapy (CBT) with an emphasis on problem solving. Similar results have been obtained by other researchers (Liberman & Eckman, 1981; Salkovskis, Atha, & Storer, 1990), thereby bolstering the efficacy of CBT with a problem-solving component.

In addition to directly reducing suicidal ideation, CBT with a problem-solving focus may indirectly decrease suicidality by reducing related risk factors. For instance, Rudd (2000) reported that such treatment has been found to reduce depression (e.g., Lerner & Clum, 1990; Liberman & Eckman, 1981; Salkovskis et al., 1990), hopelessness (Lerner & Clum, 1990; Patsiokas & Clum, 1985), and loneliness (Lerner & Clum, 1990). Hence, the positive effects of problem-solving treatment may directly impact suicidality, or may be experienced through its influence on related risk factors.

Finally, given the pernicious effects of comorbid anxiety on suicidality among depressed individuals (i.e., increases suicidality over and above hopelessness and depression), methods of reducing anxiety may also be effective in reducing suicidality. Various cognitive techniques for reducing anxiety are available (e.g., Barlow, Pincus, Heinrichs, & Choate, 2003; Barlow, Raffa, & Cohen, 2002; Heimberg, 2002).

Limitations

As has been demonstrated in this brief review, scholarly investigations generally support the validity of two areas of future-related cognitions as vulnerabilities to suicide: hopelessness and problem-solving deficits. A third future-oriented cognition, represented by the looming vulnerability model, has not yet been investigated in the context of suicide. Despite the support for the first two models, however, certain issues limit the extent to which these constructs can be regarded as legitimate vulnerabilities to suicide.

First, in regard to both the hopelessness model and the problem-solving model, a relatively small number of studies has investigated all the theoretical underpinnings of the models. For instance, although many have demonstrated an association between hopelessness and suicide, few have prospectively investigated the developmental sequence of the model (i.e., depressogenic cognitive style interacts with perceived negative life event to produce hopelessness depression, which in turn leads to suicidality). Furthermore, Abramson et al. (1998) and Gibb, Alloy, Abramson, Rose, Whitehouse, and Hogan (2001) provided the only support for the mediational role of hopelessness. Nevertheless, rigorous tests of this model are coming shortly, and should allow for more thorough investigations of the validity of the model.

Second, given the relatively wide focus of therapeutic interventions, determining the amount of improvement brought about specifically by interventions aimed at hopelessness or problem-solving deficits becomes difficult. Unless the theories underlying these two models are applied to treatment in a controlled manner, drawing conclusions about the efficacy of such models is not possible.

Self-Oriented Cognitions

Self-oriented cognitions, broadly speaking, involve individuals' perceptions of themselves as entities. Numerous theories of psychopathology emphasize the role of self-oriented cognitions in the development of psychological disorders. Despite the importance accorded to the "self" in the general field of psychopathology, the specific role of self-oriented cognitions in suicidality remains largely understudied. Rather, the connection between such thought patterns and suicide has typically been indirect, focusing on the relation between self-oriented cognitions and disorders related to suicide (e.g., depression). Consequently, the discussion of self-oriented cognitions as a vulnerability to suicide includes inferences drawn from indirect associations to suicide.

Theories/Models

Catalogical Error. In early work on the etiology of suicide, Shneidman (1957, 1961) posited that erroneous cognitive processes, particularly in reference to the self, may lead an individual to suicidal behavior. Drawing on the rules of logic, Shneidman argued that individuals who decide to kill themselves commit a "catalogical" error in reasoning. Their error is not in the deductive process; rather, it is a semantic error resulting from the ambiguous use of a specific term, usually the self (Lester, 1972). An example of a catalogical error was provided by Shneidman (1957): "If people kill themselves, then they will get attention; I will kill myself: therefore I will get attention" (p. 32). As is evident from this example, such individuals demonstrate a faulty concept of the self. That is, they may view suicide as a means of producing a desired effect on their environment, but they will not be alive to experience the intended benefits of this action. Thus, according to Shneidman, faulty self-oriented cognitions may place an individual at increased risk for carrying out suicidal intentions. Although these dysfunctional cognitions are not viewed as distal vulnerabilities to suicide, they may play a role in leading already distressed individuals to carry out suicidal ideations.

Cognitive Triad. After the seminal work of Shneidman, Beck and colleagues explored the role of self-oriented cognitions in depression, and ultimately suicide, and placed it as one component of the "cognitive triad" (Beck, 1967). The cognitive triad is composed of a negative view of the self as a failure, a negative view of the world as harsh and overwhelming, and a negative view of the future as hopeless (Weishaar, 2000). This section focuses on one element of the triad: the negative view of the self. Beck (1967) proposed that a low self-concept, or viewing oneself as a failure, places an individual at increased risk of depression and suicidality. Unfortunately, relatively little empirical attention has been allocated to this component, and there is as yet no theoretical explanation of why negative self-views promote suicidal behaviors.

Although they have not received the degree of empirical attention ascribed to future-oriented cognitions, self-oriented cognitions still appear to be related to suicide. Beck and colleagues (e.g., Beck, Steer, et al., 1990; Beck & Stewart, 1988) found that negative self-views served as a prospective risk factor for suicidality, even when controlling for depression and hopelessness. Similar work from other researchers has supported this finding (e.g., Wetzel & Reich, 1989). In an investigation on a related negative self-oriented cognition, Brevard, Lester, and Yang (1990) revealed that higher levels of self-blame distinguished suicide completers from nonsuccessful suicide attempts. In addition, high levels of shame, referring to a negative evaluation of the whole self (Lewis, 1971), have been empirically linked to suicide (e.g., Hassan, 1995; Hastings, Northman, & Tangney, 2000; Lester, 1998).

Out of the theoretical proposition that negative self-views predispose an individual to suicidal behaviors, Beck, Steer, et al. (1990) developed a specific measure to identify individuals with low self-concepts: the Beck Self-Concept Test (BST). The BST measures individuals' self-oriented cognitions on a number of personally relevant attributes, including intellectual ability, work efficacy, physical attractiveness, and virtues and vices (Beck, Steer, & Epstein, 1992). It has received moderate support in identifying those at risk for suicide, and is less likely than the Beck Hopelessness Scale to falsely identify individuals who are not at risk. On the other hand, it is also less likely to identify those who are truly at risk for suicide. Given the catastrophic and irreversible nature of suicide, sensitivity is justly accorded more importance than specificity. Thus, the BHS is preferable to the BST alone for the identification of those who may be at risk for suicide. Nonetheless, the work of Beck and others indicates that negative self-oriented cognitions do indeed serve as a vulnerability to suicide.

Self-Discrepancy Theory. A more thoroughly researched model of self-oriented cognitions as a vulnerability to psychopathology is Higgins' (1987) self-discrepancy theory. A self-discrepancy, according to Higgins, is a mismatch between an individual's self-concept and desired self-images. Three self-oriented concepts are important in this model: the "ideal" self; the "ought" self; and the "actual" self, or "self-concept." The ideal self represents what individuals desire to be, the ought self represents what individuals feel they should be, and the actual self/self-concept is the individuals' perception of who they really are. According to the model, perceived incongruities between the three selves lead to symptoms resembling either anxiety or depression. Individuals exhibiting discrepancies between their actual self and ideal self are likely to experience depressivelike symptoms such as sadness and disappointment, whereas those experiencing a mismatch between their actual self and ought self often feel guilty, shameful, fearful, and anxious (Higgins, 1989). The negative consequences of self-discrepancies depend on two factors: the amount of the discrepancy and the accessibility of the discrepancy. In general, the larger the discrepancy, and the more accessible it is, the more likely it will lead to psychopathology.

Self-discrepancy theory, like most etiological models of suicidality, is not specific to suicide. That is, discrepancies in one's "selves" may produce a variety of pathological conditions, some of which are associated with suicide or may even themselves serve as a vulnerability to suicide (e.g., depression). In the latter case, the dysfunctional self-oriented cognitions would not necessarily be a direct vulnerability to suicide, as the mechanism by which suicide occurs involves the development of some other pathological state.

In an investigation of the self-discrepancy theory as applied to suicide, Cornette, Strauman, and Abramson (2004) purported that discrepancies between actual and ideal selves and between actual and ought selves were related to suicidal ideation. Outside of this study, the self-discrepancy theory remains largely uninvestigated in the context of suicidality.

Perfectionism. A final self-oriented cognitive variable that has been theoretically linked to suicide and related disorders is perfectionism. This variable has been construed as the desire to attain idealistic goals without failing (Brouwers & Wiggum, 1993; Slade, Newton, Butler, & Murphy, 1991; Vohs et al., 2001). It therefore involves holding unrealistic standards for oneself and then being highly critical of oneself when these standards are not met. The tendency to maintain perfectionistic self-views has been implicated in suicide, as well as a host of related psychiatric disorders (e.g., depression, Flett, Besser, Davis, & Hewitt, 2003; eating disorders, Vohs et al., 2001; obsessive compulsive disorder, Coles, Frost, Heimberg, & Rheaume, 2003).

Research on perfectionism has not investigated the role of self-orienting cognitions as a vulnerability to suicide per se, but it has demonstrated an association between the two variables. For instance, perfectionistic attitudes regarding oneself have been linked by some studies to suicidal ideation among psychiatric inpatients and alcoholics (Hewitt, Flett, & Weber, 1994; Hewitt, Norton, Flett, Callander, & Cowan, 1998; Ranieri et. al, 1987), but other research failed to replicate this finding (Hewitt, Flett, & Turnbull-Donovan, 1992). Negative self-cognitions, including perfectionism, have also been associated with suicidal ideation among adolescents and children (e.g., Hewitt, Newton, Flett, & Callander, 1997; Kazdin et al., 1983; Overholser, Adams, Lehnert, & Brinkman, 1995). Gould et al. (1998), however, reported that perfectionism did not predict suicide risk among children and adolescents after controlling for psychiatric disorders. These contradictory findings affirm that the role of perfectionism in suicide is not yet clear, and further research will be necessary to delineate if, and under what circumstances, perfectionistic beliefs place an individual at risk for suicide.

Therapeutic and Preventive Implications

In general, maladaptive cognitions regarding the self appear to place an individual at increased risk for suicide. Accordingly, treatments focused on altering the negatively distorted view of the self may reduce the likelihood that a person will exhibit suicidal behaviors. Although empirical work has not explicitly investigated the efficacy of self-perception altering therapies for suicidality, cognitive restructuring of one's self-view is a major ingredient of most forms of cognitive therapy. For instance, as one component of the cognitive triad, negative self-views represent a prime target of cognitive therapy for depression (e.g., Rush & Beck, 1988).

Several techniques have been employed in modifying self-oriented cognitions. One such technique involves hypothesis testing of beliefs held about oneself. In this case, individuals are encouraged to gather evidence to either support or refute various aspects of their negative self-view. This technique is one of the core components of cognitive therapy.

Other techniques may be applied depending on the individual's level of belief certainty. A number of studies have demonstrated that individuals low in belief certainty may alter their belief through the use of a leading questions technique (Dillehay & Jernigan, 1970; Swann, Giuliano, & Wegner, 1982; Swann, Pelham, & Chidester, 1988). This technique draws on rules of communication, and results in answers that confirm the premises of the question (Swann et al., 1988). When applied to the alteration of distorted self-views among suicidal individuals, an example of a leading question might be "Why do others view you as a worthwhile person?" Research in social psychology suggests that people alter their beliefs to conform to their answers to such leading questions (Fazio, Effrein, & Falender, 1981). If this finding applies to suicidal individuals, those low in belief certainty may modify their negative self-views following a leading questions intervention.

For those high in belief certainty, however, the leading questions approach may not be convincing enough to change their firmly entrenched negative self-views (e.g., Swann & Ely, 1984). As Swann et al. (1988) demonstrated, a paradoxical strategy that consists of posing superattitudinal leading questions to such persons may be more effective in altering their beliefs. This strategy places individuals in a paradoxical situation by posing questions that are consistent with, but slightly more extreme, than their negative views. In response, people tend to shift away from their extreme position, even to the point that they are inconsistent with their initial position. For instance, a question such as "Why do you think that you are the most incompetent, worthless person on the planet?" may lead individuals high in belief certainty to respond in a way that highlights the idea that they are not the worst person in the world. It is important to note that these techniques have not been studied in the context of suicide intervention, but general social psychology findings suggest that this approach may be effective.

Limitations

In general, self-oriented cognitions lack empirical support as specific vulnerabilities to suicide. Although some well-controlled studies have demonstrated that negative self-views and self-blame serve as temporal antecedents to suicide (e.g., Beck et al., 1990; Beck & Stewart, 1988), the majority of the research in this area has been correlational. Consequently, we cannot definitively conclude that these cognitions precede suicide, or make an individual more likely to exhibit suicidal behaviors.

Interpersonally Oriented Cognitions

In line with our discussion of self-oriented cognitions, this category could have been labeled "other-oriented" cognitions. Nevertheless, this class of interpersonally oriented cognitions refers to more than simply thoughts or concerns about those in the suicidal individual's environment. Indeed, included in this category are theories focusing on the role of the individual within an interpersonal context. Stated differently, interpersonally oriented cognitions encompass the thoughts, beliefs, and attitudes that suicidal individuals hold regarding significant others in their environment as well as their relationships with these people.

Theories/Models

Altruism and Burdensomeness.   The notion that suicidal behavior may occur in the context of an interpersonal environment was well-developed long before psychology emerged as a scientific discipline. Dating back to ancient times, altruistically motivated suicide involves sacrificing one's own life for the perceived benefit of others, whether it be society as a whole or a selected group of individuals. Such forms of suicide are recalled in ancient (e.g., Sparta's Lycurgus admonished his people to maintain his laws "until his return," then departed to Delphi, where he starved himself to death and thus delayed "his return" infinitely) and modern days (e.g., Japanese "kamikaze" pilots performed suicide missions in World War II for the perceived betterment of their fellow countrymen). In both cases, the suicidal actions may be construed as cognitively focused suicides, in that the behavior was motivated by the individuals' beliefs that the end-result of their deaths would be improved conditions for their kinsmen.

Although the phenomenon of altruistic suicide has existed for millennia, Durkheim's writings (1897) were among the first to promote scientific discourse on the issue. Later, de Cantanzaro (1995) drew on this altruistic view of suicide in the formulation of a sociobiological theory of suicidality. In short, de Cantanzaro argued that a sense of burdensomeness toward kin may erode self-preservational motives, which in turn, fosters suicidality. The logic of this perspective suggests a type of cost–benefit judgment, wherein the cost of one's own suicide is justified by removal of burden from biological kin (Joiner et al., 2002). Thus, this model suggests that perceived liability to one's own gene pool is a precursor of completed suicide.

While investigators of this model have traditionally emphasized the evolutionary-psychological notion of burdensomeness and suicide, this model also fits within the rubric of cognitive vulnerabilities to suicide. More specifically, the cognitive vulnerability involved in this model arises from interpersonal motives. From this perspective, the belief that individuals pose a burden to their loved ones may increase the probability that they will attempt or complete suicide.[1]

Relatively little empirical support exists for the role of interpersonally oriented cognitions as a vulnerability to suicide. This may be due, in part, to recent theories espousing this position (e.g., the burdensomeness model was first presented in by de Catanzaro in 1995). Despite the limited empirical work in this area, the early findings have generally supported the notion that interpersonal variables are linked to suicidality. For instance, de Catanzaro (1995) revealed that a sense of burdensomeness to-

---

[1]We in no way suggest that this belief is rational, or that suicide is a desirable outcome even in the event that an individual does require high levels of attention or care from loved ones.

ward one's family was positively correlated with suicidal symptoms within community and clinical samples. Joiner et al. (2002), in a more stringent test of the model, replicated and extended the findings of de Catanzaro. The authors found that perceived burdensomeness was significantly more predictive of suicide completer status than other relevant variables such as general emotional pain, hopelessness, and the desire to control one's own feelings or to control others. In a second study, a sense of burdensomeness was significantly correlated with lethality of suicide method, whereas the aforementioned other variables were not. Brown, Dahlen, Mills, Rick, and Biblarz (1999) similarly found among a sample of college undergraduates that perceived benefit to kin was negatively predictive of depression and hopelessness. In contrast, Pettit et al. (2002) revealed that burdensomeness was significantly and negatively correlated with lethality of suicide method among Chinese suicide completers. Although this finding contradicts the notion that a perceived sense of burdensomeness serves as a cognitive vulnerability to suicide, the authors argued that the model is theoretically sound when interpreted from a multicultural perspective (i.e., a complete lack of burdensomeness in a collectivistic society such as the People's Republic of China may be indicative of detachment from one's environment, thus increasing the likelihood of suicidality among such individuals). As an aside, this illustrates and emphasizes the importance of developing and interpreting models of behavior from a culturally appropriate perspective.

Overall, a limited amount of empirical data suggests that burdensomeness, and consequently, interpersonally oriented cognitions, may serve as a vulnerability factor for suicide. Nevertheless, future investigations will need to address this area more thoroughly in order to delineate the specific role of these cognitions in suicidality.

Other Interpersonally Oriented Cognitions. In addition to burdensomeness, other interpersonally oriented cognitions have been linked to suicidality. For instance, Beck, Steer, and Brown (1993) proposed that individuals possessing dysfunctional beliefs regarding their relationships with others might be more likely to exhibit suicidal ideation. More specifically, they suggested that sociotropy manifested by acquiescing to the expectations of others, believing that it is important to impress others, and being sensitive to the opinions of others would be characteristics of suicidal individuals. Similarly, other researchers have posited the role of interpersonally focused cognitions in suicidality, including sensitivity to social criticism and socially prescribed perfectionism, defined as the belief that significant others hold unrealistic standards, stringently evaluate, and exert pressure on the individual to be perfect (Hewitt & Flett, 1991; Hewitt et al., 1992; Ranieri et al., 1987).

Beck et al. (1993) found that the interpersonally oriented cognitions regarding interpersonal sensitivity, other's expectations, and impressing others were indeed associated with suicidal ideation. Nevertheless, this association was not predictive once a variety of other relevant variables (e.g., past suicide attempts, hopelessness, and depression) were controlled (as cited in Weishaar, 2000). Thus, interpersonally oriented cognitions appeared to be related to suicide ideation, but their connection with suicidality only existed in the context of other variables.

Hewitt et al. (1992) found that the maladaptive cognitions of socially prescribed perfectionism, referring to others' expectations of the individual, predicted suicidal ideation among psychiatric inpatients. Among hospitalized, adolescent suicide attempters, Boergers, Spirito, and Donaldson (1998) found that socially prescribed perfectionism predicted a desire to die as the primary reason for attempting suicide. Ranieri et al. (1987) also found that suicidal ideators were more likely to exhibit heightened levels of interpersonal sensitivity to criticism, thus providing additional support for the role of interpersonally oriented cognitions in suicidality.

Therapeutic and Preventive Implications

Given the immediate importance of keeping suicidal individuals from prematurely ending their lives, interpersonally oriented cognitions are rarely the primary focus of suicide interventions. Many interventions, nonetheless, address interpersonal cognitions during the course of treatment (e.g., crisis intervention strategies often stress the importance of enhanced social support). Treatments focusing on assisting individuals in reinterpreting interpersonal interactions and overcoming the pressures of socially prescribed perfectionism may lead to a decrease in suicidality. Moreover, challenging beliefs and faulty interpretations regarding burdensomeness may also be an effective way to decrease suicidality. To date, however, this conjecture has not been empirically validated.

Dialectical behavior therapy (DBT; Linehan, 1987), which includes a cognitive component, appears to be effective in improving the interpersonal skills and relationships of individuals with borderline personality disorder, a group at high risk for suicidal behaviors (e.g., Linehan, Tutek, Heard, & Armstrong, 1994). Although the treatment and findings are not specific to interpersonally oriented cognitions, the argument could logically be made that DBT positively impacts such cognitions among suicidal individuals.

The role of perfectionism has been described in both the self-oriented cognitions section as well as the interpersonally oriented cognitions section. In terms of treatment, these two facets of perfectionism may be combined. As mentioned earlier, techniques focusing on cognitive restructuring may be of great benefit to those maintaining maladaptive, perfectionistic beliefs. Unfortunately, this has not yet been tested empirically. Drawing on the findings of the NIMH Treatment of Depression Collaborative Research Program (TDCRP), Blatt (1995) argued that highly perfectionistic individuals may need extensive, long-term treatment. In short, he noted that high levels of perfectionism interfered with therapeutic response to brief treatments of depression, although long-term intensive treatment produced superior responses among individuals holding such views. Consequently, more extensive therapy may be necessary for highly perfectionistic, self-critical patients.

Interpersonal psychotherapy (IPT; Klerman, Weissman, Rounsaville, & Chevron, 1984), focusing on developing appropriate interpersonal skills for dealing with problems such as grief, role issues, and interpersonal deficits, has received support as an efficacious intervention for depression. Through its impact on depression, therefore, it may indirectly reduce suicidality. Once again, however, IPT for suicide has not been subjected to empirical investigation.

Clearly, more research needs to be conducted on treating suicide from an interpersonally oriented standpoint. Basic psychopathology research indicates that these cognitions occur among suicidal individuals, and may exacerbate suicidality. Future work should emphasize the integration of these findings into a testable treatment intervention.

Limitations

In general, the role of interpersonally oriented cognitions as a vulnerability to suicide is still at a theoretical level. Nevertheless, empirical evidence to date does allow us to reasonably conclude that these thought patterns are associated with suicide. Future research is necessary to determine if these cognitions increase the likelihood of suicidality, or they are just concomitants of suicidality.

Similarly, suicide intervention research at present does not permit us to draw firm conclusions regarding treatments centered on interpersonally oriented cognitions. As our understanding of the relation between such cognitions and suicidal behavior continues to develop, treatments will most likely incorporate these findings in a manner that will allow them to be examined in a therapeutic context.

Escape-Oriented Cognitions

The last category of cognitive vulnerabilities to suicide includes cognitions focused on escaping one's current unpleasant state. The notion that suicide involves escape is hardly new, and was included in early theories of suicide (e.g., Menninger, 1938; Freud, as cited by Litman, 1996). More recently, researchers have discussed the presence of escape-oriented cognitions among suicidal individuals, with the most well-developed escape theory of suicide coming from Baumeister (1990).

Theories/Models

Escape Theory of Suicide. Baumeister's provocative escape theory of suicide (Baumeister, 1990; Vohs & Baumeister, 2000) was drawn from his more general escape theory (Baumeister & Sher, 1988). This theory highlights the influence of a number of variables, including cognitive factors, emotional states, and negative life events. In the theory, Baumeister presented a causal chain by which an individual's attempt to escape from aversive self-awareness and negative affect may ultimately lead to self-defeating and even suicidal behaviors.

The first component of the causal chain is the occurrence of a negative life event. The negative life event is simply an experience that falls below the individual's standards or expectations. Thus, it is a discrepancy between a desired outcome and an actual outcome. The individuals' interpretation of the event determines whether they proceed to the second step of the causal chain. This step consists of internal attributions made for the negative life event. That is, rather than attributing the failure to external factors, such individuals attribute the negative occurrence to their own incompetence. This internal attribution of failure leads to an aversive self-awareness, whereby the view of the self as inadequate comes into direct conflict with the drive for self-esteem. Aversive self-awareness, in turn, produces a state of negative affect. The extreme unpleasantness associated with aversive self-awareness and self-directed negative affect motivate the individual to quickly and thoroughly remove the negative state, regardless of the costs and the long-term impact accompanying the removal. This disregard for long-term consequences is termed *cognitive destruction* or *mental narrowing*. Cognitive deconstruction is a state in which the individual is completely focused on the immediate temporal and spatial present. Thus, attention is shifted away from the negative self-blame and is directed toward concrete bodily sensations and physical movements. This deconstructed state also allows the individual to avoid the meaningful thought required to make comparisons between the self and one's standards, thereby minimizing affect. Moreover, it leads to behavioral disinhibition, irrational thought, lack of emotionality, and passivity.

Cognitive deconstruction allows the individual to remain in detached, passive state, unaware of the self in a meaningful manner (Vohs & Baumeister, 2000). This is a transient state, however, giving way to a higher level identity in which the individual once again becomes negatively focused on the self. This pattern of thoughts becomes cyclical, as the individual shifts from cognitive deconstruction to aversive self-awareness. To end this cycle, the individual either accepts the personal failure in a meaningful way, or takes a more lasting action (e.g., suicide) to escape aversive self-awareness.

Little empirical support exists for the role of escape-oriented cognitions in suicidality. Nevertheless, Reich, Newson, and Zautra (1996) found that health declines among the elderly, serving as the proposed negative life occurrence, led to lowered self-esteem and fatalism. These, in turn, resulted in confused thinking and helplessness. Confused thinking, but not helplessness, produced suicidal ideation. This study provides a limited degree of support for the general processes operating in the escape theory. It is important to note, however, that Reich et al. did not test Baumeister's conceptualization of the escape theory per se; rather, they tested a variation of the model that may or may not be representative of the original theory.

Other research, although not investigating models of suicidality, suggests that certain components of the escape model are related to suicide. First, disinhibition, one of the consequences of cognitive deconstruction, has been demonstrated to be present among suicidal individuals (Cantor, 1976; Hendin, 1982, as cited in Vohs & Baumeister, 2000). Comparable findings pertain to passivity, a second consequence of cognitive deconstruction. Research suggests that suicidal individuals engage in passive coping strategies (Linehan et al., 1987) and adopt an external locus of control (Gerber, Nehemkis, Faberow, & Williams, 1981).

Suicide as a Desirable Solution. Several researchers have argued that severely distressed individuals view suicide as a desirable solution to, or escape from, their problems. In general, this trend has been seen among individuals with poor problem-solving skills. Beck, Rush, Shaw, and Emery (1979) noted that when the usual problem-solving approaches are not effective, such individuals resort to suicide as an attractive way to resolve the dilemma.

Although research on the "desirability" of suicide as a solution to one's problems is limited, Orbach et al. (1987) found that suicidal children who were unable to produce solutions for life and death situations were also more likely to display an attraction for death. Linehan and colleagues also pointed out that coping beliefs and the ability to generate solutions to problems are negatively correlated to suicide intent (Linehan et al., 1987; Strosahl, Linehan, & Chiles, 1992).

Therapeutic and Preventive Implications

To our knowledge, no intervention currently addresses escape-oriented cognitions among suicidal individuals. Certain therapies, however, may be amenable to such populations. For instance, treatments assisting individuals in reattributing negative life events may halt progression through the proposed sequence of events leading to suicide. In addition, interventions such as DBT, which assist the distressed individual in managing and dealing with negative affect, may prevent the subsequent state of cognitive destruction.

Among individuals who view suicide as an appealing solution to current dilemmas, treatments addressing limited problem-solving abilities may be effective. That is, by forming alternative solutions, the allure of suicide may diminish, thereby reducing the intent to end one's life. At this point, however, empirical evidence does not provide conclusive support for the possible methods of treatment proposed in this section.

Limitations

Overall, the literature on the role of escape-oriented cognitions in suicide at this point is heavier on theory than empirical data. Some evidence suggests that escape-focused cognitions may predispose an individual to suicidality, but more evidence and more rigorous investigations will be needed before concluding that escape-oriented cognitions serve as a vulnerability for suicide. Analogously, no investigations have explored potential treatments based on the notion of escape-oriented cognitions. As findings come from future investigations of the escape theory, treatment interventions may incorporate the relevant information in a manner that will allow empirical scrutiny.

This chapter has presented four broad areas of cognitive vulnerabilities to suicide: future-oriented cognitions, self-oriented cognitions, interpersonally oriented cognitions, and escape-oriented cognitions. Within these categories, the theories, evidence, therapeutic implications, and limitations have been reviewed regarding a number of specific vulnerabilities. Within the future-oriented category, hopelessness and problem-solving deficits appear to be the most well-studied and validated vulnerabilities to suicide. Among self-oriented cognitions, the negative self-view component of Beck's cognitive triad, self-discrepancies, perfectionism, and the catalogical error represent potential vulnerabilities to suicide, although some areas have not yet received adequate research attention to be designated as vulnerabilities. Interpersonally oriented cognitions, also due to a scarcity of research, lack empirical validation as vulnerabilities to suicide. However, burdensomeness, generally maladjusted views of one's social relation to others, and socially prescribed perfectionism hold promise as possible vulnerabilities. Finally, components of Baumeister's escape theory of suicide and the perception of suicide as a desirable solution may serve as escape-oriented cognitions predisposing an individual to suicide.

In general, these proposed cognitive factors require further validation before they can conclusively be designated as vulnerabilities to suicide, as opposed to correlates. A vulnerability factor, or risk factor, must meet the criteria of both covariance and temporal precedence (Kazdin, 1999). Currently, hopelessness and problem-solving deficits meet these criteria. Other variables such as negative self-views and perfectionism have a moderate amount of support as vulnerabilities to suicide. Further research is required to conclusively designate the remainder of these variables.

A major limitation exists in the knowledge of how to effectively prevent or treat suicidality. A recent chapter on science and the practice of clinical suicidology reported that only 23 randomized or controlled studies targeting suicidality existed at the time of the writing (Rudd, 2000). This number included both intervention and treatment studies. Only 8 of these 23 studies emphasized the importance of cognitions in the treatment of suicidality. Each of these employed a variant of cognitive behavioral therapy, with a primary focus on problem solving. Although the results of these studies are promising in their support of CBT (6 of 8 found support for the use of CBT with a problem-solving component), a void clearly exists in the outcome research on suicidality treatments in general, and in research on cognitively focused techniques in particular.

As stated earlier, the material presented suggests that a number of cognitive factors play a role in suicidality. With the exception of problem-solving skills, however, it appears as though many of these factors have not been integrated into a formulizable, testable treatment of suicidality. Outcome research addressing this issue will be key to developing and validating more effective methods of treatment.

Despite the lack of research on the treatment of suicide, a promising finding is that cognitive therapy generally reduces suicidality. In contrast to the benefits of therapy, premature termination of cognitive therapy and inadequate response to treatment have been identified as indicators of increased risk for suicide (Dahlsgaard, Beck, & Brown, 1998). This finding is not specific to interventions focused on a given cognitive domain (e.g., self-oriented, future-oriented, etc.); rather, it suggests that, to a certain extent, generalized forms of cognitive therapy are effective in the treatment of suicidality. Nevertheless, matching an individual's particular cognitive "weakness area" to a specific treatment may be an area of promising investigation in the future. Before that happens, however, a few criteria must be met: The specific role of cognitive vulnerabilities must be more clearly understood, methods of identifying areas of cognitive maladjustment must be developed and validated, and the efficacy of treatments for these cognitive deficits must be clearly demonstrated. Obviously, much work remains before these criteria are sufficiently met. Through rigorous empirical investigation, and continued theoretical modification, we feel that this represents an achievable, and certainly worthwhile, goal.

REFERENCES

Abramson, L. Y., Alloy, L. B., Hogan, M. H., Whitehouse, W. G., Akhavan, S., & Chiara, A. (1998). Suicidality and cognitive vulnerability to depression among college students: A prospective study. *Journal of Adolescence, 21*, 1–13.

Abramson, L. Y., Alloy, L. B., Hogan, M. H., Whitehouse, W. G., Gibb, B. E., Hankin, B. L., & Cornette, M. M. (2000). The hopelessness theory of suicidality. In T. E. Joiner & M. D. Rudd (Eds.), *Suicide science: Expanding the boundaries* (pp. 17–32). New York: Kluwer Academic.

Abramson, L. Y., Metalsky, G. I., & Alloy, L. B. (1989). Hopelessness depression: A theory-based subtype of depression. *Psychological Review, 96*, 358–372.

Alloy, L. B., Abramson, L. Y., Hogan, M. W., Whitehouse, W. G., Rose, D. T., Robinson, M. S., Kim, R. S., & Lapkin, J. B. (2000). The Temple–Wisconsin Cognitive Vulnerability to Depression (CVD) Project: Axis I and II psychopathology in the parents of individuals at high and low cognitive risk for depression. *Journal of Abnormal Psychology, 109*(3), 403–418.

Alloy, L. B., Abramson, L. Y., Tashman, N. A., Berrebbi, D. S., Hogan, M. E., Whitehouse, W. G., Crossfield, A. G., & Morocco, A. (2001). Developmental origins of cognitive vulnerability to depression: Parenting, cognitive, and inferential feedback styles of the parents of individuals at high and low cognitive risk for depression. *Cognitive Therapy and Research, 25*(4), 397–423.

Andreasen, N. C., & Black, D. W. (1995). *Introductory textbook of psychiatry*. Washington, DC: American Psychiatric Press.

Asarnow, J. R., Carlson, G. A., & Guthrie, D. (1987). Coping strategies, self-perceptions, hopelessness, and perceived family environments in depressed and suicidal children. *Journal of Consulting and Clinical Psychology, 55*, 361–366.

Asarnow, J. R., & Guthrie, D. (1989). Suicidal behavior, depression, and hopelessness in child psychiatric inpatients. *Journal of Clinical Child Psychology, 18*, 129–136.

Bakish, D. (1999). The patient with comorbid anxiety and depression: The unmet need. *Journal of Clinical Psychiatry, 60*(2), 20–24.

Barlow, D. H., Pincus, D. B., Heinrichs, N., & Choate, M. L. (2003). Anxiety disorders. In G. Stricker & T. A. Widiger (Eds.), *Handbook of psychology: Clinical psychology* (pp. 119–147). New York: Wiley.

Barlow, D. H., Raffa, S. D., & Cohen, E. M. (2002). Psychosocial treatments for panic disorders, phobias, and generalized anxiety disorder. In P. E. Nathan & J. M. Gorman (Eds.), *A guide to treatments that work* (pp. 301–335). London: Oxford University Press.

Baumeister, R. F. (1990). Suicide as escape from self. *Psychological Review, 97*(1), 90–113.

Baumeister, R. F., & Sher, S. J. (1988). Self-defeating behavior patterns among normal individuals: Review and analysis of common self-destructive tendencies. *Psychological Bulletin, 104*(1), 3–22.

Beck, A. T. (1967). *Depression: Clinical, experimental, and theoretical aspects*. New York: Harper & Row.

Beck, A. T., Brown, G. K., Berchick, R. J., Stewart, B. L., & Steer, R. A. (1990). Relationship between hopelessness and ultimate suicide: A replication with psychiatric outpatients. *American Journal of Psychiatry, 147*, 190–195.

Beck, A. T., Brown, G. K., & Steer, R. A. (1989). Prediction of eventual suicide in psychiatric inpatients by clinical ratings of hopelessness. *Journal of Consulting and Clinical Psychology, 57*(2), 309–310.

Beck, A. T., Brown, G. K., Steer, R. A., Dahlsgaard, K. K., & Grisham, J. R. (1999). Suicide ideation at its worst point: A predictor of eventual suicide in psychiatric outpatients. *Suicide and Life-Threatening Behavior, 29*(1), 1–9.

Beck, A. T., Kovacs, M., & Weissman, A. (1975). Hopelessness and suicidal behavior: An overview. *Journal of the American Medical Association, 234*, 1146–1149.

Beck, A. T., Rush, A. J., Shaw, B. F., & Emery, G. (1979). *Cognitive therapy of depression.* New York: Guilford.

Beck, A. T., & Steer, R. A. (1993). *Manual for the Beck Hopelessness Scale.* New York: Psychological Corporation.

Beck, A. T., Steer, R. A., & Brown, G. (1993). Dysfunctional attitudes and suicidal ideation in psychiatric outpatients. *Suicide and Life-Threatening Behavior, 23*(1), 11–20.

Beck, A. T., Steer, R. A., & Epstein, N. (1992). Self-concept dimensions of clinically depressed and anxious outpatients. *Journal of Clinical Psychology, 48*(4), 423–432.

Beck, A. T., Steer, R. A., Epstein, N., & Brown, G. (1990). The Beck Self-Concept Test. *Psychological Assessment: A Journal of Consulting and Clinical Psychology, 2*(2), 191–197.

Beck, A. T., Steer, R. A., Kovacs, M., & Garrison, B. (1985). Hopelessness and eventual suicide: A 10-year prospective study of patients hospitalized with suicide ideation. *American Journal of Psychiatry, 142*, 559–563.

Beck, A. T., & Stewart, B. (1988). *The self-concept as a risk factor in patients who kill themselves.* Unpublished manuscript, Center for Cognitive Therapy, Philadelphia.

Beck, A. T., Weissman, A., Lester, D., & Trexler, L. (1974). The measurement of pessimism: The Hopelessness Scale. *Journal of Consulting and Clinical Psychology, 42*, 861–865.

Bedrosian, R. C., & Beck, A. T. (1979). Cognitive aspects of suicidal behavior. *Suicide and Life-Threatening Behavior, 9*(2), 87–96.

Blatt, S. J. (1995). The destructiveness of perfectionism: Implications for the treatment of depression. *American Psychologist, 50*(12), 1003–1020.

Blumenthal, S. J. (1990). An overview and synopsis of risk factors, assessment, and treatment of suicidal patients over the life cycle. In S. J. Blumenthal & D. J. Kupfer (Eds.), *Suicide over the life cycle: Risk factors, assessment and treatment of suicidal patients* (pp. 685–733). Washington, DC: American Psychiatric Press.

Boergers, J., Spirito, A., & Donaldson, D. (1998). Reasons for adolescent suicide attempts: Associations with psychological functioning. *Journal of the American Academy of Child & Adolescent Psychiatry, (12)*, 1287–1293.

Brevard, A., Lester, D., & Yang, B. (1990). A comparison of suicide notes written by suicide completers and suicide attempters. *Crisis, 11*, 7–11.

Brouwers, M., & Wiggum, C. D. (1993). Bulimia and perfectionism: Developing the courage to be imperfect. *Journal of Mental Health Counseling, 15*, 141–149.

Brown, R. M., Dahlen, E., Mills, C., Rick, J., & Biblarz, A. (1999). Evaluation of an evolutionary model of self-preservation and self-destruction. *Suicide and Life-Threatening Behavior, 29*(1), 58–71.

Buda, M., & Tsuang, M. T. (1990). The epidemiology of suicide: Implications for clinical practice. In S. J. Blumenthal & D. J. Kupfer (Eds.), *Suicide over the life cycle: Risk factors, assessment and treatment of suicidal patients* (pp. 17–37). Washington, DC: American Psychiatric Press.

Cantor, P. C. (1976). Personality characteristics found among youthful female suicide attempters. *Journal of Abnormal Psychology, 85*, 324–329.

Carlson, G. A., & Cantwell, D. P. (1982). Suicidal behavior and depression in children and adolescents. *Journal of the American Academy of Child Psychiatry, 21*, 361–368.

Carris, M. J., Sheeber, L., & Howe, S. (1998). Family rigidity, adolescent problem-solving deficits, and suicidal ideation: A mediational model. *Journal of Adolescence, 21,* 459–472.

Chang, E. C. (1998). Cultural differences, perfectionism, and suicidal risk in a college population: Does social problem solving still matter? *Cognitive Therapy and Research, 22*(3), 237–254.

Coles, M. E., Frost, R. O., Heimberg, R. G., & Rheaume, J. (2003). "Not just right experiences": Perfectionism, obsessive-compulsive features and general psychopathology. *Behaviour Research and Therapy, 41*(6), 681–700.

Cornette, M. M., Strauman, T. J., & Abramson, L. Y. (2004). *Self-discrepancy theory and suicidal ideation: Ideal, ought, and future self-belief patterns in vulnerability to suicidal thought.* Manuscript in preparation.

Dahlsgaard, K. K., Beck, A., T., & Brown, G. K. (1998). Inadequate response to therapy as a predictor of suicide. *Suicide and Life-Threatening Behavior, 28*(2), 197–204.

de Catanzaro, D. (1995). Reproductive status, family interactions, and suicidal ideation: Surveys of the general public and high-risk groups. *Ethology & Sociobiology, 16,* 385–394.

Dillehay, R. C., & Jernigan, L. R. (1970). The biased questionnaire as an instrument of opinion change. *Journal of Personality and Social Psychology, 15,* 144–150.

Durkheim, E. (1897). *Le suicide: Etude de socologie* [Suicide: A study in sociology]. Paris: F. Alcan.

D'Zurilla, T. J., & Goldfried, M. R. (1971). Problem-solving and behavior modification. *Journal of Abnormal Psychology, 78,* 107–126.

Ellis, A., & Hunt, R. R. (1989). *Fundamentals of human memory and cognition* (4th ed.). Dubuque, IA: W. C. Brown.

Ellis, T. E., & Ratliff, K. G. (1986). Cognitive characteristics of suicidal and nonsuicidal psychiatric inpatients. *Cognitive Therapy and Research, 10*(6), 625–634.

Esposito, C., Johnson, B., Wolfsdorf, B. A., & Spirito, A. (2003). Cognitive factors: Hopelessness, coping, and problem solving. In A. Spirito & J. C. Overholser (Eds.), *Evaluating and treating adolescent suicide attempters: From research to practice* (pp. 89–112). San Diego: Academic Press.

Fawcett, J., Scheftner, W., Clark, D. C., Hedeker, D., Gibbons, R., & Coryell, W. (1987). Clinical predictors of suicide in patients with major affective disorders: A controlled prospective study. *American Journal of Psychiatry, 144,* 35–40.

Fawcett, J., Scheftner, W., Fogg, L., Clark, D. C., Young, M. A., Hedeker, D., & Gibbons, R. (1990). Time-related predictors of suicide in major affective disorder. *American Journal of Psychiatry, 147,* 1189–1194.

Fazio, R. H., Effrein, E. A., & Falender, V. J. (1981). Self-perceptions following social interaction. *Journal of Personality and Social Psychology, 41,* 232–242.

Flett, G. L., Besser, A., Davis, R. A., & Hewitt, P. L. (2003). Dimensions of perfectionism, unconditional self-acceptance, and depression. *Journal of Rational-Emotive and Cognitive Behavior Therapy, 21*(2), 119–138.

Fredrickson, B. L. (1998). What good are positive emotions? *Review of General Psychology, 2,* 300–319.

Freeman, A., & Reinecke, M. A. (1993). *Cognitive therapy of suicidal behavior.* New York: Springer.

Garland, A. F., & Zigler, E. (1993). Adolescent suicide prevention: Current research and social policy implications. *American Psychologist, 48*(2), 169–182.

Gerber, K. E., Nehemkis, A. M., Faberow, N. L., & Williams, J. (1981). Indirect self-destructive behavior in chronic hemodialysis patients. *Suicide and Life-Threatening Behavior, 11,* 31–42.

Gibb, B. E., Alloy, L. B., Abramson, L. Y., Rose, D. T., Whitehouse, W. G., Donovan, P., Hogan, M. E., Cronholm, J., & Tierney, S. (2001). History of childhood maltreatment, negative cognitive styles, and episodes of depression in adulthood. *Cognitive Therapy and Research, 25*(4), 425–446.

Gibb, B. E., Alloy, L. B., Abramson, L. Y., Rose, D. T., Whitehouse, W. G., & Hogan, M. E. (2001). Childhood maltreatment and college students' current suicidal ideation: A test of the hopelessness theory. *Suicide and Life-Threatening Behavior, 31*(4), 405–415.

Glass, A. L., & Holyoak, K. J. (1986). *Cognition* (2nd ed.). New York: Random House.

Gould, M. S., King, R., Greenwald, S., Fisher, P., Schwab-Stone, M., Kramer, R., Flisher, A. J., Goodman, S., Canino, G., & Shaffer, D. (1998). Psychopathology associated with suicidal ideation and attempts among children and adolescents. *Journal of the American Academy of Child and Adolescent Psychiatry, 37*(9), 915–923.

Hassan, R. (1995). *Suicide explained*. Victoria, Australia: Melbourne University Press.

Hastings, M. E., Northman, L. M., & Tangney, J. P. (2000). Shame, guilt, and suicide. In T. E. Joiner & M. D. Rudd (Eds.), *Suicide science: Expanding the boundaries* (pp. 67–79). New York: Kluwer Academic.

Heimberg, R. G. (2002). Cognitive-behavioral therapy for social anxiety disorder: Current status and future directions. *Biological Psychiatry, 51*(1), 101–108.

Hendin, H. (1982). *Suicide in America*. New York: Norton.

Hewitt, P. L., Flett, G. L., & Turnbull-Donovan, W. (1992). Perfectionism and suicide potential. *British Journal of Clinical Psychology, 31,* 181–190.

Hewitt, P. L., Flett, G. L., & Weber, C. (1994). Dimensions of perfectionism and suicide ideation. *Cognitive Therapy and Research, 18*(5), 439–460.

Hewitt, P. L., & Flett, G. L. (1991). Perfectionism in the self and social contexts: Conceptualization, assessment, and association with psychopathology. *Journal of Personality and Social Psychology, 60*(3), 456–470.

Hewitt, P. L., Newton, J., Flett, G. L., & Callander, L. (1997). Perfectionism and suicide ideation in adolescent psychiatric patients. *Journal of Abnormal Child Psychology, 25*(2), 95–101.

Hewitt, P. L., Norton, R., Flett, G. L., Callander, L., & Cowan, T. (1998). Dimensions of perfectionism, hopelessness, and attempted suicide in a sample of alcoholics. *Suicide and Life-Threatening Behavior, 28*(4), 395–406.

Higgins, E. T. (1987). Self-discrepancy: A theory relating self and affect. *Psychological Review, 94,* 319–340.

Higgins, E. T. (1989). Self-discrepancy theory: What patterns of self-beliefs cause people to suffer? In L. Berkowitz (Ed.), *Advances in experimental social psychology* (Vol. 22, pp. 93–136). New York: Academic Press.

Joiner, T. E., Jr., & Rudd, M. D. (1995). Negative attributional style for interpersonal events and the occurrence of severe interpersonal disruptions as predictors of self-reported suicidal ideation. *Suicide and Life-Threatening Behavior, 25,* 297–304.

Joiner, T. E., Jr., Pettit, J. W., Perez, M., Burns, A. B., Gencoz, T., Gencoz, F., & Rudd, M. D. (2001). Can positive emotion influence problem-solving attitudes among suicidal adults? *Professional Psychology: Research and Practice, 32,* 507–512.

Joiner, T. E., Jr., Voelz, Z. R., & Rudd, M. D. (2001). For suicidal young adults with comorbid depressive and anxiety disorders, problem-solving treatment may be better than treatment as usual. *Professional Psychology: Research and Practice, 32*(3), 278–282.

Joiner, T., Pettit, J. W., Walker, R. L., Voelz, Z. R., Cruz, J., Rudd, M. D., & Lester, D. (2002). Perceived burdensomeness and suicidality: Two studies on the suicide notes of those attempting and those completing suicide. *Journal of Social and Clinical Psychology, 21,* 531–545.

Josepho, S. A., & Plutchik, R. (1994). Stress, coping, and suicide risk in psychiatric inpatients. *Suicide and Life-Threatening Behavior, 24*(1), 48–57.

Kassin, S. (2004). *Psychology*. Essex, England: Pearson Education Limited.

Kazdin, A. E. (1999). Current (lack of) status of theory in child and adolescent psychotherapy research. *Journal of Clinical Child Psychopathology, 28*(4), 533–543.

Kazdin, A. E., French, N. H., Unis, A. S., Esveldt-Dawson, K., & Sherick, R. B. (1983). Hopelessness, depression, and suicidal intent among psychiatrically disturbed inpatient children. *Journal of Consulting and Clinical Psychology, 51,* 504–510.

Kazdin, A. E., Rogers, A., & Colbus, D. (1986). The Hopelessness Scale for Children: Psychometric characteristics and concurrent validity. *Journal of Consulting and Clinical Psychology, 54,* 241–245.

Kessler, R. C., Borges, G., & Walters, E. E. (1999). Prevalence of and risk factors for lifetime suicide attempts in the National Comorbidity Survey. *Archives of General Psychiatry, 56,* 617–626.

King, C. A., Segal, H. G., Naylor, M., & Evans, T. (1993). Family functioning and suicidal behavior in adolescent inpatients with mood disorders. *Journal of the American Academy of Child and Adolescent Psychiatry, 32,* 1198–1206.

Klerman, G. L., Weissman, M. M., Rounsaville, B. J., & Chevron, E. S. (1984). *Interpersonal psychotherapy of depression.* New York: Basic Books.

Leenaars, A. A. (1999). Rational suicide: A psychological perspective. In J. L. Werth (Ed.), *Contemporary perspectives on rational suicide* (pp. 135–141). Philadelphia: Brunner/Mazel.

Lerner, M., & Clum, G. (1990). Treatment of suicide ideators: A problem-solving approach. *Behavior Therapy, 21,* 403–411.

Lester, D. (1972). *Why people kill themselves.* Springfield, IL: Thomas.

Lester, D. (1998). The association of shame and guilt with suicidality. *Journal of Social Psychology, 138,* 535–536.

Levenson, M. (1974). Cognitive characteristics of suicide risk. In C. Neuringer (Ed.), *Psychological assessment of suicide risk* (pp. 150–163). Springfield, IL: Thomas.

Levenson, M., & Neuringer, C. (1971). Problem-solving behavior in suicidal adolescents. *Journal of Consulting and Clinical Psychology, 37,* 433–436.

Lewis, H. B. (1971). *Shame and guilt in neurosis.* New York: International Universities Press.

Liberman, R., & Eckman, T. (1981). Behavior therapy vs. insight-oriented therapy for repeated suicide attempters. *Archives of General Psychiatry, 38,* 1126–1130.

Linehan, M. M. (1987). Dialectical behavior therapy for borderline personality disorder: Theory and method. *Bulletin of the Menninger Clinic, 51*(3), 261–276.

Linehan, M. M., Camper, P., Chiles, J., Strosahl, K., & Shearin, E. (1987). Interpersonal problem-solving and parasuicide. *Cognitive Therapy and Research, 11,* 1–12.

Linehan, M. M., Tutek, D. L., Heard, H. L., & Armstrong, H. E. (1994). Interpersonal outcome of cognitive behavioral treatment for chronically suicidal borderline patients. *American Journal of Psychiatry, 151*(12), 1771–1776.

Litman, R. E. (1996). Sigmund Freud on suicide. In J. T. Maltsberger & M. J. Goldblatt (Eds.), *Essential papers on suicide. Essential papers in psychoanalysis* (pp. 200–220). New York: New York University Press.

Menninger, K. A. (1938). *Man against himself.* Oxford, England: Harcourt Brace.

Minkoff, K., Bergman, E., Beck, A., & Beck, R. (1973). Hopelessness, depression, and attempted suicide. *American Journal of Psychiatry, 130,* 455–459.

Miniño, A. M., Arias, E., Kochanek, K. D., Murphy, S. L., & Smith, B. L. (2002). Deaths: Final data for 2000. *National Vital Statistics reports, 50*(15). Hyattsville, MD: National Center for Health Statistics.

Mraz, W., & Runco, M. A. (1994). Suicide ideation and creative problem-solving. *Suicide and Life-Threatening Behavior, 24*(1), 38–47.

National Center for Health Statistics. (2002). *Monthly Vital Statistics Report, 47*(19). Retrieved February 18, 2005, from http://www.cdc.gov/nchs/fastats/suicide.htm

Orbach, I., Rosenheim, E., & Hary, E. (1987). Some aspects of cognitive functioning in suicidal children. *Journal of the American Academy of Child and Adolescent Psychiatry, 25*(2), 181–185.

Overholser, J., Adams, D., Lehnert, K., & Brinkman, D. (1995). Self-esteem deficits and suicidal tendencies among adolescents. *Journal of the American Academy of Child and Adolescent Psychiatry, 34,* 919–928.

Patsiokas, A. T., & Clum, G. A. (1985). Effects of psychotherapeutic strategies in the treatment of suicide attempters. *Psychotherapy, 22,* 281–290.

Patsiokas, A. T., Clum, G. A., & Luscomb, R. L. (1979). Cognitive characteristics of suicide attemptors. *Journal of Consulting and Clinical Psychology, 47,* 478–484.

Paykel, E. S., Myers, J. K., Lindenthal, J. J., & Tanner, J. (1974). Suicidal feelings in the general population: A prevalence study. *British Journal of Psychiatry, 124,* 460–469.

Pettit, J. W., Lam, A. G., Voelz, Z. R., Walker, R. L., Joiner, T. E., Jr., Lester, D., & He, Z. X. (2002). Perceived burdensomeness and lethality of suicide method among suicide completers in the People's Republic of China. *Omega: Journal of Death and Dying, 45*(1), 57–67.

Pollock, L. R., & Williams, J. M. G. (1998). Problem solving and suicidal behavior. *Suicide and Life-Threatening Behavior, 28*(4), 375–387.

Priester, M. J., & Clum, G. A. (1993). The problem-solving diathesis in depression, hopelessness, and suicide ideation: A longitudinal analysis. *Journal of Psychopathology and Behavioral Assessment, 15,* 239–254.

Ranieri, W. F., Steer, R. A., Lavrence, T. I., Rissmiller, D. J., Piper, G. E., & Beck, A. T. (1987). Relationship of depression, hopelessness, and dysfunctional attitudes to suicide ideation in psychiatric inpatients. *Psychological Reports, 61,* 967–975.

Reich, J., Newson, J. T., & Zautra, A. J. (1996). Health downturns and predictors of suicidal ideation: An application of the Baumeister model. *Suicide and Life-Threatening Behavior, 26*(3), 282–291.

Rich, A. R., Kirkpatrick-Smith, J., Bonner, R. I., & Jans, F. (1992). Gender differences in psychosocial correlates of suicidal ideation among adolescents. *Suicide and Life-Threatening Behavior, 22,* 364–373.

Riskind, J. H. (1997). Looming vulnerability to threat: A paradigm for anxiety. *Behavior Research and Therapy, 35*(8), 685–702.

Riskind, J. H., Long, D. G., Williams, N. L., & White, J. C. (2000). Desperate acts for desperate times: Looming vulnerability and suicide. In Joiner & Rudd (Eds.), *Suicide science: Expanding the boundaries* (pp. 105–115). New York: Kluwer Academic.

Rotheram-Borus, M. J., Trautman, P. D., Dopkins, S. C., & Shrout, P. E. (1990). Cognitive style and pleasant activities among female adolescent suicide attempters. *Journal of Consulting and Clinical Psychology, 58,* 554–561.

Rudd, M. D. (1990). An integrative model of suicidal ideation. *Suicide and Life-Threatening Behavior, 20*(1), 16–30.

Rudd, M. D. (2000). Integrating science into the practice of clinical suicidology: A review of the psychotherapy literature and a research agenda for the future. In R. W. Maris, S. S. Canetto, J. L. McIntosh, & M. M. Silverman (Eds.), *Review of suicidology 2000* (pp. 47–83). New York: Guilford.

Rudd, M. D., Dahm, P. F., & Rajab, M. H. (1993). Diagnostic comorbidity in persons with suicidal ideation and behavior. *American Journal of Psychiatry, 150*(6), 928–834.

Rudd, M. D., Joiner, T. E., Jr., & Rajab, M. H. (2001). *Treating suicidal behavior: An effective, time-limited approach.* New York: Guilford.

Rudd, M. D., Rajab, M. H., & Dahm, P. F. (1994). Problem-solving appraisal in suicide ideators and attempters. *American Journal of Orthopsychiatry, 64,* 136–149.

Rudd, M. D., Rajab, M. H., Orman, D. T., Stulman, D. A., Joiner, Jr., T. E., & Dixon, W. (1996). Effectiveness of an outpatient problem-solving intervention targeting suicidal young adults: Preliminary results. *Journal of Consulting and Clinical Psychology, 64,* 179–190.

Rush, A. J., & Beck, A. T. (1988). Cognitive therapy of depression and suicide. In S. Lesse (Ed.), *What we know about suicidal behavior and how to treat it* (pp. 283–306). Northvale, NJ: Aronson.

Sadowski, C., & Kelley, M. L. (1993). Social problem solving in suicidal adolescents. *Journal of Consulting and Clinical Psychology, 61*, 121–127.

Salkovskis, P., Atha, C., & Storer, D. (1990). Cognitive-behavioral problem solving in the treatment of patients who repeatedly attempt suicide: A controlled trial. *British Journal of Psychiatry, 157*, 871–876.

Schotte, D. E., & Clum, G. A. (1982). Suicide ideation in a college population: A test of a model. *Journal of Consulting and Clinical Psychology, 46*, 690–696.

Schotte, D. E., & Clum, G. A. (1987). Problem solving skills in suicidal psychiatric patients. *Journal of Consulting and Clinical Psychology, 55*, 49–54.

Shneidman, E. S. (1957). The logic of suicide. In E. S. Shneidman & N. L. Faberow (Eds.), *Clues to suicide* (pp. 31–40). New York: McGraw-Hill.

Shneidman, E. S. (1961). Statistical comparisons between attempted and committed suicides. In N. L. Faberow & E. S. Shneidman (Eds.), *The cry for help* (pp. 19–47). New York: McGraw-Hill.

Slade, P. D., Newton, T., Butler, N. M., & Murphy, P. (1991). An experimental analysis of perfectionism and dissatisfaction. *British Journal of Clinical Psychology, 30*, 169–176.

Spirito, A. Williams, C., Stark, L. J., & Hart, K. (1988). The Hopelessness Scale for Children: Psychometric properties and clinical utility with normal and emotionally disturbed adolescents. *Journal of Abnormal Child Psychology, 16*, 445–458.

Strosahl, K. D., Chiles, J. A., & Linehan, M. M. (1992). Prediction of suicide intent in hospitalized parasuicides: Reasons for living, hopelessness, and depression. *Comprehensive Psychiatry, 33*(6), 366–373.

Swann, W. B., Jr., & Ely, R. J. (1984). A battle of wills: Self-verification versus behavioral confirmation. *Journal of Personality and Social Psychology, 46*, 1287–1302.

Swann, W. B., Jr., Giuliano, T., & Wegner, D. M. (1982). Where leading questions can lead: The power of conjecture in social interaction. *Journal of Personality and Social Psychology, 42*, 1025–1035.

Swann, W. B., Jr., Pelham, B. W., & Chidester, T. R. (1988). Change through paradox: Using self-verification to alter beliefs. *Journal of Personality and Social Psychology, 54*(2), 268–273.

Vohs, K. D., & Baumeister, R. F. (2000). Escaping the self consumes self-regulatory resources: A self-regulatory model of suicide. In T. E. Joiner & M. D. Rudd (Eds.), *Suicide science: Expanding the boundaries* (pp. 33–41). New York: Kluwer Academic.

Vohs, K. D., Voelz, Z. R., Pettit, J. W., Bardone, A. M., Katz, J., Abramson, L. Y., Heatherton, T. F., & Joiner, T. E., Jr. (2001). Perfectionism, body dissatisfaction, and self-esteem: An interactive model of bulimic symptom development. *Journal of Social and Clinical Psychology, 20*(4), 476–497.

Weishaar, M. E. (2000). Cognitive risk factors in suicide. In R. W. Maris, S. S. Canetto, J. L. McIntosh, & M. M. Silverman (Eds.), *Review of suicidology 2000* (pp. 112–139). New York: Guilford.

Weissman, M. M., Bland, R. C., Canino, G. J., Greenwald, S., Hwu, H. G., Joyce, P. R., Karam, E. G., Lee, C. K., Lellouch, J., Lepine, J. P., Newman, S. C., Rubio-Stipec, M., Wells, J. E., Wickramaratne, P. J., Wittchen, H. U., & Yeh, E. K. (1999). Prevalence of suicide ideation and suicide attempts in nine countries. *Psychological Medicine, 29*(1), 9–17.

Wetzel, R. D., & Reich, T. (1989). The cognitive triad and suicide intent in depressed inpatients. *Psychological Reports, 65*, 1027–1032.

6

Cognitive Vulnerability to Mood Disorders: An Integration

Saskia K. Traill
Ian H. Gotlib
Stanford University

Cognitive models of mood disorders (Abramson, Seligman, & Teasdale, 1978; Beck, 1963, 1964, 1967; Beck & Young, 1985; Bower, 1981; Teasdale & Dent, 1987) have provided the impetus for a large body of empirical research aimed at identifying and evaluating cognitive vulnerabilities to these disorders. In early work in this area, investigators relied on self-report methodologies to assess cognitive functioning in depressed individuals. More recently, researchers increasingly have utilized information-processing tasks to conduct more sophisticated assessments. The four preceding chapters in this book are timely reviews of contemporary methodologies and studies examining cognitive vulnerability to mood disorders. Considered collectively, they suggest several future directions for research in this area.

Each chapter describes cognitive vulnerability to a form of psychopathology by focusing on diathesis–stress formulations. Reference to diathesis–stress models was first made more than 40 years ago in formulations of schizophrenia (e.g., Bleuler, 1963; Rosenthal, 1963), in which the diathesis, or vulnerability to developing the disorder, was genetic. More recently, such models have been applied to understanding the development of depressive disorders from a cognitive perspective (Abramson, Metalsky, & Alloy, 1989; Beck, 1987; Monroe & Simons, 1991). In these formulations, the diathesis is not genetic, but rather is some form of cognitive dysfunction. In the preceding chapters, cognitive diathesis–stress formulations are posited to lead to depressive episodes in unipolar depression (chaps. 2 and 3, this vol.), bipolar depression (chap. 4, this vol.), and possibly to suicide (chap. 5, this vol.).

The importance of investigating cognitive vulnerabilities stems from a theme that runs consistently through a number of cognitive theories of mood disorders: At some point, usually early in individuals' lives, events occur that leave them vulnerable to developing a mood disorder in the face of specific types of emotional adversity or life stressors. In particular, two of the diathesis–stress models discussed in the preceding chapters are the primary cognitive models used today to understand mood disorders: hopelessness theory and Beck's schema theory. Given the emphasis of these diathesis–stress formulations on cognitive vulnerability and life stress, the appropriate and accurate assessment of these two constructs is clearly of critical importance to the validity and the utility of the models.

This chapter raises and examines a number of questions concerning exactly what is being measured in studies of cognitive vulnerability. It contends that, within the framework of diathesis–stress formulations, it is unclear from the findings of these studies whether or not investigators are actually attaining their goal of measuring pure diatheses or pure stressors; rather, it is likely that researchers are inadvertently assessing the interaction of diatheses and stressors. This issue is discussed in terms of the assessment of cognitive vulnerability to depressive episodes in unipolar depression and bipolar disorder. In many cases, investigators are probably not assessing diatheses independent of stress. Furthermore, if they are to do so, researchers may need to include appropriate mood induction procedures in their studies that serve to activate, or prime, cognitive vulnerabilities. A more explicit consideration of the empirical separation of diatheses and stressors will strengthen the conclusions that can be drawn from studies examining the role of cognition in depression.

ASSESSING VULNERABILITY

Researchers have spent decades attempting to measure vulnerability to mood disorders, particularly to episodes of depression. In empirically assessing diathesis–stress models, it is critical that the measurement of vulnerabilities, or diatheses, be distinguished from the assessment both of stress and of the interaction between diatheses and stress. The preceding four chapters described a number of different assessment procedures in the context of various diathesis–stress models. In particular, they focused on the diathesis–stress formulations of two major theories: hopelessness theory and Beck's schema theory. We turn now to a consideration of these theories, of the diatheses each theory would expect to be able to measure, and of the methodologies used to measure those diatheses.

Hopelessness Theory

Alloy et al. (chap. 2, this vol.), Ingram et al. (chap. 3, this vol.), and Pettit and Joiner (chap. 5, this vol.) all describe the concept of hopelessness depression. Based in part on Abramson, Seligman, and Teasdale's (1978) helplessness theory, which itself is based on Seligman's (1975) original learned helplessness theory, Abramson, Metalsky, and Alloy (1989) formulated a hopelessness theory of depression. According to this theory, depressed individuals are characterized by a set of expectations about the world that are maladaptive or depressotypic. Specifically, hopelessness theory posits that depressed people have a negative view of the future based on attributes they assigned events of the past. In the original learned helplessness theory, the experience of uncontrollable negative events was posited to lead to the expectation that future negative events are also uncontrollable, therefore reducing the likelihood that one will act on these events. In hopelessness theory, the same expectations hold, but in addition, the individual also develops negative cognitions about the event. Negative events are seen as stable, which means they will not change; as internal, which means they are due to one's own misdoings; and as global, which means they permeate the individual's environment. Similarly, the individual is posited to make the opposite attributions about positive events: They are seen as unstable, external, and specific. Beliefs about the extent of the consequences of negative events are also posited to be a part of negative cognitive style, as are beliefs about the implications of negative events on the self-concept. Together, this pattern of attributions is hypothesized to lead to a sense of hopelessness, which creates a vulnerability to depression.

It is clear from the helplessness/hopelessness perspective that measuring cognitive style is critical in assessing vulnerability to depression. Indeed, from this perspective cognitive style is the diathesis for depression. To the extent that these negative styles are accessible to the individual's conscious processes, to the individual's awareness, researchers should be able to assess vulnerability to hopelessness using self-report methodologies. The Cognitive Vulnerability to Depression (CVD) Project does just that, using the Dysfunctional Attitudes Scale (Weissman & Beck, 1978) and a modification of the Attribution Style Questionnaire called the Cognitive Styles Questionnaire (Alloy et al., 2000). In the CVD project, individuals who obtain a high composite score on these two measures are categorized as being at high cognitive risk for depression.

Alloy and her colleagues characterize vulnerability as "particular negative cognitive styles [that] increase an individual's likelihood of developing episodes of depression after experiencing a negative life event" (chap. 2, this vol.). In fact, this is proposed to explain both hopelessness depression and Beck's schema theory. As Alloy et al. note, the most important evidence for demonstrating that cognitive style is a vulnerability factor is showing that it predicts future episodes of depression. Importantly, the CVD assessment of risk does predict future onset of depression, both first and recurrent episodes, even after initial level of depressive symptomatology is controlled. Alloy et al. argue that the predictive value of negative cognitive style supports the conceptualization of this construct as a vulnerability factor for depression.

Ingram et al. (chap. 4, this vol.) elucidate the contention of the major cognitive theories of depression that cognitive vulnerabilities are "latent" until they are activated by a stressful event. Specific vulnerabilities may differ from one another in this regard. For example, whereas schemas and dysfunctional attitudes or beliefs must generally be activated before they can be measured, it is less clear that cognitive style also requires activation before it can be assessed. Because students in the CVD project were categorized as high risk in part on the basis of an assessment of their level of dysfunctional attitudes, it is important to consider the possibility that at the initial assessment these high risk students were already experiencing the effects of a life stressor. In this project, participants were assigned to high or low cognitive risk groups independent of their mood at the time that they completed the cognitive questionnaires (Alloy & Abramson, 1999). Following Ingram et al.'s reasoning, the fact that the participants who scored high on the self-report cognitive vulnerability measures were sufficiently aware of their maladaptive cognitive functioning to explicitly endorse dysfunctional cognitions raises the possibility that they had already experienced a negative event that activated these negative cognitions and permitted their reporting. In other words, the conscious self-reporting of the processes that comprise a negative cognitive style in these participants may reflect a diathesis–stress interaction, in which low severity stressors are already beginning to create cognitive dysfunctions through their interaction with the vulnerability, rather than the cognitive vulnerability itself. Conceptualized in this way, the cognitive style measured in the CVD project may not be the intended pure diathesis, but rather the interaction of the diathesis with stress that has already occurred.

Another possible interaction between diathesis and stress involves the actual process of completing the questionnaires. Requiring a participant to think about hypothetical negative events, such as not getting into any colleges, or not having a date for a school dance, may itself function as a mildly activating stressor. If this is the case, then completing the questionnaires may serve as a prime for the cognitive diatheses they are trying to assess. To test this possibility, researchers might measure changes in automatic processing as a function of completing these questionnaires, or the psychophysiological effects on the participants of completing these questionnaires. Without this type of research, it is difficult to know if there may be possible reactive effects on cognitive functioning as a result of completing questionnaires assessing dysfunctional cognitions.

If high scores on the cognitive styles questionnaire are indeed due, at least in part, to the interaction between diathesis and stress, then one way to examine this confound is to carefully assess current life stress for each participant and to control statistically for concurrent stressors when assessing diatheses. Although this would clearly be a conservative test of cognitive vulnerability hypotheses, the findings would be more conclusive in their support of cognitive theories of depression. In fact, in the CVD project, Alloy, Abramson, and their colleagues assessed life stress every 6 weeks for the first 2½ years of follow-up, using two different measures of life stress. We very much look forward to their reports of the predictive value of self-reported cognitive vulnerability controlling for life stress.

One important issue, therefore, concerns the interpretation of high scores on self-report measures of cognitive diatheses in the absence of an explicit manipulation designed to make the diathesis accessible to measurement. A related issue concerns the interpretation of low scores on these measures. It is possible that there are two distinct groups of individuals who obtain low scores on self-report measures of cognitive diatheses. If diatheses must be activated before they can be assessed, then there will be individuals who possess cognitive vulnerabilities but who, because they have not experienced a significant life stressor to activate these vulnerabilities, will report low levels of maladaptive cognitions and, consequently, be categorized as being at low cognitive risk for depression. In addition, individuals who are not at high cognitive risk for depression will also obtain low scores on the measures of cognitive diatheses. One way to assess this possibility and differentiate these two groups of low scoring individuals would be to develop and administer to them analog stressors in the laboratory, and then use an idiographic approach to select as high cognitive risk for depression those individuals whose cognitive status changed as a function of exposure to the stressor.

Again, this issue may be less central to the hopelessness theory than to Beck's schema theory (described later) because it may not be necessary to posit that the diathesis in the hopelessness theory must be activated by some event before it is accessible to self report. Nevertheless, being clear that the assessment is for purely diatheses, as opposed to an interaction of diathesis and stressor, is crucial to increasing understanding of how to identify high risk individuals for further study and, eventually, for appropriate prevention programs. Alloy and colleagues' demonstration that cognitive style predicts future onset of depression even after controlling for initial depressive symptomatology is compelling, and suggests that cognitive styles are important in understanding the development of episodes of mood disorder. As Pettit and Joiner (chap. 5, this vol.) indicate, self-reported levels of hopelessness are associated with risk for suicide, although this has not yet been demonstrated with negative cognitive style. Future studies investigating the relations among cognitive style, suicidality, and suicide may similarly benefit by considering whether self-reported negative cognitive styles indicate a pure diathesis or an interaction between diatheses and negative life stressors that have already occurred. These different conceptions may suggest different prevention strategies for individuals who appear to be at risk for suicidality, and may also help to elucidate the nature of the associations among depressive symptomatology, hopelessness, and suicidality discussed by Pettit and Joiner (chap. 5, this vol.).

Beck's Schema Theory

Alloy et al. (chap. 4, this vol.), Ingram et al. (chap. 3, this vol.), and Pettit and Joiner (chap. 5, this vol.) discuss Beck's (1963, 1967) cognitive theory of depression. Essentially, Beck posited that experiences in early childhood lead to stable depressive schemas, which subsequently become activated in the face of negative life events. Once the schemas are activated, dysfunctional cognitive content and processes continue to interact with adverse environmental experience, leading to a downward spiral into a clinically significant depressive episode. Schemas may be characterized by maladaptive cognitions, such as dysfunctional attitudes or beliefs; by a negative cognitive style, as described in hopelessness theory; or by maladaptive cognitive processes, such as selective attention and memory for negative stimuli. Moreover, schemas include not only complex structures, or filters, for classifying external stimuli, but also "structuralized logical elements," such as assumptions, syllogisms, and premises that lead individuals to draw specific types of conclusions about external events (Beck, 1964, p. 563). Beck suggested that the negative affect that derives from these erroneous conclusions about the self, the world, and the future can lead to further cognitive distortions, and the ongoing interactions between negative affect and dysfunctional cognitive processes, style, and content contribute to the development and exacerbation of depressive episodes.

As noted earlier, researchers began to assess schemas in depressed persons using self-report questionnaires or interviews. Certainly, these instruments can measure cognitions that are accessible to the individual's awareness, dysfunctional attitudes and beliefs, or cognitive styles of which the individual is aware. Importantly, however, with the notable exception of the CVD project, investigations using these instruments have not been particularly successful in predicting future episodes of depression based on self-reports of dysfunctional cognitions (see Abramson et al., 2002; Barnett & Gotlib, 1988; and Ingram, Miranda, & Segal, 1998, for reviews of this literature). In some respects, this is not surprising. Questionnaires and interviews are reasonable measures to use to assess "controlled," or "effortful," cognitive processing (Hartlage, Alloy, Vazquez, & Dykman, 1993). Beck's theory, however, conceptualizes schemas as involving "automatic" processing. Because this type of functioning occurs at a level outside people's awareness, individuals do not have easy access to the content of their schemas and, therefore, are unable to give valid self-reports of their schematic functioning. Consequently, important aspects of the individual's cognitive functioning that are theorized to represent risk factors for depression will not be measured by the administration of questionnaires and interviews. Moreover, if people's responses to questionnaires assessing the nature of their schemas are not necessarily accurate, the association between these responses and subsequent functioning is unlikely to be systematic.

Given these limitations of self-report and interview methodologies, other forms of schema assessment have been developed. As Ingram et al. (chap. 3, this vol.) note, schemas influence the way in which people process information in their environment. Schemas direct attention to certain classes of stimuli and facilitate memory for specific kinds of information. This focus on the importance of information processing in assessing schemas has led to the development and adaptation of methodologies utilized in experimental cognitive psychology to measure attention and memory functioning. More specifically, investigators interested in the relation between information processing and depression have examined biases of depressed individuals in attention to, and memory for, depressotypic emotional stimuli (e.g., Gotlib, Krasnoperova, Neubauer, & Joormann, 2004; Gotlib, Kasch, et al., 2004). Interestingly, Alloy and her colleagues (chap. 2, this vol.) report that high cognitive risk, as assessed by two self-report questionnaires, interacted with high negative self-referent information processing to predict depression. This finding suggests that it may be the interaction of self-reported cognitive style and schematic functioning, assessed through information-processing procedures, that predicts change in depressive symptoms. If this finding is replicated in future research, then it highlights the importance of considering both controlled and automatic cognitive functioning in understanding depression.

In the same way that cognitive style may not be accessible to measurement unless the beliefs or attitudes are activated by exposure to a stressor, it is possible that biases in information processing are activated in the presence of negative mood (see Gotlib & Krasnoperova, 1998). As Ingram et al. (chap. 3, this vol.) indicate, in diathesis–stress models cognitive risk factors "are largely inactive until the individual encounters adversity." To model this adversity in the laboratory, investigators have developed and conducted what have become known as "priming studies," in which these putative cognitive diatheses are activated by inducing a transient negative mood in the participants. Because these diatheses are hypothesized to remain latent until they are activated by negative emotions, they are not expected to be easily accessible to measurement in the absence of this activation. Moreover, because only people at risk for depression are hypothesized to have these diatheses, inducing a transient negative mood in individuals without the cognitive diathesis for depression is not expected to lead them to exhibit biases in their processing of negative information.

Ingram et al. (chap. 3, this vol.) describe a number of studies in which investigators attempted to activate cognitive vulnerabilities in at-risk individuals by inducing negative mood in the laboratory and found differences in information processing between those individuals who are susceptible to depression and those who are not (see Gotlib et al., 2005). As was the case with self-report measures of cognitive dysfunction, one implication of the results of these studies is that nondepressed individuals who exhibit biases in attention and/or memory in the absence of any explicit mood or stress manipulation may have already experienced stressors or elevations in negative mood of sufficient intensity permit the assessment of these cognitive processes.

An important question raised by the four preceding chapters concerns the extent to which diathesis–stress formulations that are used to explain the onset of unipolar depression are generalizable to explain episodes of depression in mood disorders other than Major Depressive Disorder. Of particular interest is whether or not cognitive models for depression can be extended to explain the development of depressive episodes in bipolar disorder. Alloy et al. (chap. 4, this vol.) assert that bipolar depressive episodes are similar to unipolar depressive episodes. From this perspective, one would predict that individuals at risk for developing bipolar disorder, or for experiencing a depressive episode in their bipolar disorder, would exhibit negative cognitions similar to those that have been found in self-report and information-processing assessments of individuals at risk for unipolar depression. Interestingly, as Alloy et al. point out, bipolar depressed individuals do appear to show biases on information-processing tasks similar to those exhibited by unipolar depressed individuals, but are characterized by a different pattern of responses on self-report and interview measures.

A related question that arises from the research in bipolar disorders concerns the kinds of diatheses that would be expected in individuals at risk for developing manic episodes. If both depressive and manic episodes in individuals who are diagnosed with bipolar disorder are tied in some way to the experience of stressful events, then it is possible that there is a negative cognitive vulnerability that underlies manic episodes in a manner similar to that hypothesized for depressive episodes. In this context, it is noteworthy that Alloy, Reilly-Harrington, Fresco, Whitehouse, and Zechmeister (1999) found that hypomanic individuals who had never experienced an episode of depression reported different negative self-perceptions, dysfunctional attitudes, and negative attribution styles than did bipolar individuals who had experienced previous episodes of depression. Given this pattern, it is not clear whether hypomanic individuals are characterized by information-processing vulnerabilities; further research in this area is warranted. In this context, Johnson and her colleagues examined differences in cognitive factors that are involved in the onset of depressive episodes versus manic episodes in individuals with bipolar disorder (see Johnson & Fingerhut, 2004; Johnson & Kizer, 2002).

Thus, the use of mood-priming paradigms with individuals who are statistically at risk for developing mood disorders may help to distinguish between symptoms and vulnerabilities for depressive episodes in both unipolar depression and bipolar disorder. Studies examining these constructs in children of bipolar parents, in individuals who have remitted from depressive episodes, and in individuals at risk for experiencing hypomanic episodes will be helpful in delineating how diathesis–stress models for depression may be extended beyond Major Depressive Disorder (see Gotlib et al., 2005). It may also be the case that the methodologies used to examine the comprehensiveness of diathesis–stress models will help to refine cognitive theories of psychopathology, and contribute to the development of other theories of mood disorders.

ASSESSING STRESS

A parallel to the measurement of vulnerability in diathesis–stress models of mood disorders, and of depressive episodes in particular, is the assessment of stress in individuals who are susceptible to developing depression. Many investigators use self-report questionnaires in attempting to measure levels of stress. A number of researchers have found that individuals with unipolar depression or bipolar disorder report experiencing a stressful life event prior to the onset of a depressive episode (e.g., Johnson & Kizer, 2002; Monroe & Hadjiyannakis, 2002). Consistent with a diathesis–stress model of depression, these findings have been interpreted as demonstrating that negative life events can interact with preexisting vulnerabilities to cause a depressive episode. It is important to recognize, however, that diatheses can affect both the generation and the measurement of life stress (Hammen, 1991; Monroe & Simons, 1991). Consideration of the possible interactions between the two aspects of the diathesis–stress model may help to clarify and refine current theories about mechanisms of developing depression, particularly from a developmental perspective, and may suggest directions for future research.

In diathesis–stress models, cognitive vulnerabilities are hypothesized to interact with environmental stressors to affect the way individuals think about, feel about, and interpret the world. Therefore, in the presence of even a relatively minor life stressor or a transient negative mood, individuals at high cognitive risk for depression would be expected to react differently and more negatively than would low cognitive risk individuals. This negative reaction could exacerbate the impact of stressors, cause benign situations to become negative, or actually contribute to the generation of negative events. Considered from this perspective, finding higher levels of life stress among vulnerable or depressed individuals may reflect the inadvertent assessment of a diathesis rather than the measurement of independent external stressors. Consistent with this possibility, Hammen (1991) observed that women who had experienced an episode of depression (either as part of bipolar disorder or as unipolar depression) reported the same number of independent life events as healthy, normal controls, but reported significantly more dependent life events (i.e., those in which the individual played some role).

Thus, self-report assessments of major life events that are not independent of the individual may actually be measuring a combination of diathesis and stress. Alloy et al. (chap. 4, this vol.) note that both retrospective and prospective reports of bipolar individuals suggest that episodes are often preceded by negative life events. They point out that these studies are characterized by methodological limitations: Participants may use life events to explain the cause of their disorders; memory for life events may diminish over time; episode onset dates may be imprecise; some studies lack appropriate comparison groups; and, finally, many studies do not differentiate between dependent and independent life events. In addition, cognitive vulnerabilities may affect not only the reporting, but the very experience of these events, making otherwise benign experiences feel more negative and more stressful. In addition, Ingram et al. (chap. 3, this vol.) review findings showing how an association between personality characteristics and specific kinds of life stress may reflect the effects of personality characteristics on life stress, or the effect of cognitive diatheses causing life stress in areas of an individual's life that are particularly salient or important.

We look forward to reports of the CVD prospective assessment of life stress. As noted earlier, project life stress was assessed every 6 weeks for the first 2½ years of follow-up. Stress was assessed using both the Life Events Questionnaire (LEQ; Alloy & Clements, 1992; Needles & Abramson, 1990) and a stress interview. These convergent assessment procedures were implemented to prevent confounds of symptoms and events in depressed individuals; this design may also limit confounds of vulnerabilities and events in nondepressed individuals, and is therefore particularly important. Nevertheless, there is always the possibility that the findings of this assessment may not reflect the measurement of pure stress, but rather the interaction of a diathesis and life stress.

This formulation of the interaction of diatheses with stress to produce more stress is also important in the context of the developmental conclusions drawn by Alloy et al. (chap. 2, this vol.). Alloy et al. indicate that the mothers of high risk individuals reported more negative consequence feedback than did mothers of low risk individuals, and they suggest on the basis of this finding that children may develop negative cognitive styles through receiving negative feedback from their parents. Alloy et al. also reveal that "participants' cognitive risk status fully mediated the relation between reported levels of childhood emotional maltreatment and the occurrence of [depression] during the first 2.5 years of follow-up." Although Alloy et al.'s conclusions concerning the role of cognitive risk status as mediating the association between childhood maltreatment and subsequent depression, and the development of negative cognitive styles through receiving negative feedback from parents, are intriguing, it is important that future research examine the role played by already existing cognitive vulnerabilities in contributing to the early stressful environment.

Moreover, even when stressors are independent of a cognitive diathesis, the presence of a diathesis may affect self-reports of life stress. For example, individuals whose diathesis leads them to interpret events as negative may experience a mild earthquake as a life-threatening situation, whereas a neighbor may not even encode the earthquake as a life event of any consequence. Even before individuals become depressed, the same "tyrannical self" that contributes to the maintenance of depressive episodes (Ingram et al., chap. 3, this vol.) may influence their reporting on a life stress questionnaire or interview; they may remember negative events better than do nonvulnerable people; they may remember the events as more negative and experience current life stressors as more negative than they might if they were less vulnerable. Self-report methodologies, such as the Life Experiences Questionnaire, cannot calibrate scale anchors for everyone who responds to these instruments. Combining these questionnaires with follow-up interviews to review stated answers, as Abramson, Alloy, and their colleagues are doing in the CVD project, will help to reduce the possibility of participants' overreporting of severity. "Over-*perception*" of severity, that is, the experience of an event as more severe than it was, may be harder to tease apart, and may be a function not of the stressor per se, but of the diathesis to experience stress as severe. Brown and Harris' (1978) Life Events and Difficulties Schedule (LEDS), and more recent modifications of the LEDS (Monroe & Roberts, 1990), including the stress interview used in the CVD project, contain more contextual analyses of the events that can be coded by a team of investigators to reduce confounds of differential perceptions of life stress.

Explicit comparisons of self-report measures of stress with the contextualized, interview-based assessments of stress may help to disentangle the nature of the relation between life stress and cognitive vulnerability. Because in the CVD project stress was measured in the 6-month follow-up assessment using both self-report and interview procedures, it is possible in that project to examine discrepancies between self-reports of stressful events and events that are identified and rated as stressful through an interview. In fact, unpublished analyses of those data suggest that individuals who are labeled as high risk both experienced more stressful events and reported them accurately on the self-report questionnaire. Furthermore, those individuals were no more likely than their low risk counterparts to report experiencing life events on the questionnaire that were not coded as such by the interview (Safford, Crossfield, Alloy, & Abramson, 2004). These analyses represent an important step in validating different methods used to collect information about life stress, and also reveal intriguing areas for future exploration of the association between life stress and psychopathology.

In discussing the assessment of stress, we have focused on the prototypical situation in which an individual who is vulnerable to depression experiences an acute, severe, life stressor and subsequently develops a depressive episode. This does not mean that stressors must be acute or severe discrete events in order to affect the likelihood that an individual will develop an episode of depression. In fact, there is evidence to suggest that low grade but chronic stressors are more prevalent than are major, severe, life events, and they also explain more of the demographic and clinical characteristics of mood disorders (e.g., Pearlin & Lieberman, 1979; Turner, Wheaton, & Lloyd, 1995). Certainly, it can be more difficult to separate the independence of chronic stressors from vulnerability factors than is the case for severe life events. For example, socioeconomic status has been found to be associated with the prevalence of depression (Kessler et al., 1994), but it is difficult to establish a clear model to explain the relation between vulnerability to depression and financial difficulties. Nevertheless, lifetime chronic stress clearly plays an important role in the development and course of mood disorders, and the role of these stressors must be considered in continuing to develop theories of diathesis–stress models for mood disorders.

ASSESSING THE DIATHESIS–STRESS INTERACTION

The previous sections discussed the difficulties inherent in empirically separating cognitive diatheses and stress. As difficult as it may be to distinguish vulnerability from stress in empirical tests of diathesis–stress models of mood disorders, it is critical that we persist in this endeavor and attempt to gain a more comprehensive understanding of the nature of the relation between these two constructs. In particular, studies that examine the effects of experimentally manipulated stressors in individuals who vary in their level of vulnerability to mood disorder may provide important information about the interaction of diatheses and stressors.

Investigators have attempted to address the issue of separating diathesis from stress in a number of different ways. One strategy, for example, is to covary mood scores when assessing diatheses in an attempt to reduce the impact of mood symptoms, which presumably are the result of interactions of diatheses and stress. For example, in the CVD project, Abramson and Alloy and their colleagues covaried initial scores on the Beck Depression Inventory so that the depressive symptoms and diagnoses assessed at Time 2 would be more likely to be due to vulnerabilities assessed at Time 1 than to Time 1 depressive symptoms. Although this strategy may indeed reduce extra-experimental interactions between vulnerabilities and stressors, it is not clear precisely what it is that is being covaried. The Beck Depression Inventory assesses sad mood, eating, sleep disturbance, disappointment, guilt, and so on, so it is certainly not only mood that is being covaried. And the fact that there may not be concordance between Time 1 and Time 2 symptoms further blurs exactly what is being covaried. It is important for future research to assess more precisely what should be controlled for when using this methodology.

Another procedure used by investigators to separate vulnerability from stress involves presenting participants with a stressor experimentally in the laboratory. Analog stressors have the advantage of being more controlled than those in the environment, and more temporally restricted, in that experimenters can assess the individual immediately following the stressor and during the recovery. Ingram et al. (chap. 3, this vol.) describe the methodologies and results of priming studies, which introduce mild, transient stressors (in this case, mood inductions) in order to measure diatheses in participants. The underlying formulation is that diatheses can only be assessed accurately after they have been activated by a stressor. This procedure may be less important for studies of currently or remitted depressed individuals, who may come into an experiment already experiencing some level of diathesis activation (Judd et al., 2000). For never-disordered individuals who are known to be at higher risk, however (e.g., the children of disordered parents), diatheses may not be measurable until they are activated by some form of stress. For these samples, the development of paradigms that may identify those at particular risk without having to wait for negative life events to occur outside of the laboratory may facilitate the implementation of prevention programs and increase their effectiveness (cf. Gotlib et al., 2005).

In assessing diatheses in bipolar disorder, the need for appropriate analog stressors becomes more complex. As Alloy et al. (chap. 4, this vol.) point out, assessing the vulnerability to manic episodes may rely on inducing a transient negative or euphoric mood, or even an irritable mood in children. Studies designed to identify which of these mood stressors most consistently activates diatheses may provide important information about bipolar disorder in general, about different subtypes of bipolar disorder, and about the similarity of depressive episodes in bipolar disorder and unipolar depression (see Johnson & Fingerhut, 2004; Johnson & Kizer, 2002).

Finally, in the context of Alloy at al.'s (chap. 2, this vol.) discussion of recent research examining personality characteristics, such as autonomy and sociotropy, as diatheses for mood disorders, there is a strong need for careful consideration of precisely how to induce a stressor appropriately in the laboratory. More concretely, it might be expected that the diatheses of sociotropic individuals would be activated only in the presence of sociotropic stressors, and the diatheses of autonomous individuals to be activated only in response to threats to their autonomy. In the former case, social rejection might activate diatheses, whereas in the latter case, failure to complete a task or negative feedback about academic performance would be expected to activate diatheses. The potential importance of considering whether specific analog stressors are appropriate for assessing different subtypes of depression clearly highlights the complexities involved in adequately investigating diathesis–stress models of depression.

The likely confounding of cognitive diatheses and life stress in studies of the development of depressive disorders may make it seem overwhelming for researchers to attempt to distinguish between these two constructs. Indeed, they are intertwined even at a theoretical level. For example, Beck suggested that cognitive diatheses or schemas are formed early in life by the experience of adverse events. But it is not clear precisely how schemas are formed. That is, would everyone who experiences those adverse events develop diatheses, or would only those individuals who are susceptible to developing the diathesis form the relevant schemas. Is there, in effect, a diathesis for developing a diathesis? Although it will undoubtedly be difficult, the importance of separating diathesis from stress is a critical task for researchers interested in understanding this debilitating group of disorders. It is our hope that investigators will continue to consider the ways in which stress and diatheses may interact, both in the laboratory using various experimental assessments and in the naturalistic environment. With a clearer understanding of these processes, it will be easier to intervene with individuals who are at elevated risk for these disorders.

ACKNOWLEDGMENTS

Preparation of this chapter was facilitated by National Institute of Mental Health grant MH59259 awarded to Ian H. Gotlib.

REFERENCES

Abramson, L. Y., Alloy, L. B., Hankin, B. L., Haeffel, G. J., MacCoon, D. G., & Gibb, B. E. (2002). The cognitive vulnerability–stress models of depression in a self-regulatory and psychobiological context. In I. H. Gotlib & C. L. Hammen (Eds.), *Handbook of depression* (3rd ed., pp. 268–294). New York: Guilford.

Abramson, L. Y., Metalsky, G. I., & Alloy, L. B. (1989). Hopelessness depression: A theory-based subtype of depression. *Psychological Review, 96*, 358–372.

Abramson, L. Y., Seligman, M. E., & Teasdale, J. D. (1978). Learned helplessness in humans: Critique and reformulation. *Journal of Abnormal Psychology, 87*(1), 49–74.

Alloy, L. B., & Abramson, L. Y. (1999). The Temple–Wisconsin Cognitive Vulnerability to Depression Project: Conceptual background, design, and methods. *Journal of Cognitive Psychotherapy, 13*(3), 227–262.

Alloy, L. B., Abramson, L. Y., Hogan, M. E., Whitehouse, W. G., Rose, D. T., Robinson, M. S., Kim, R. S., & Lapkin, J. B. (2000). The Temple–Wisconsin Cognitive Vulnerability to Depression Project: Lifetime history of Axis I psychopathology in individuals at high and low cognitive risk for depression. *Journal of Abnormal Psychology, 109*, 403–418.

Alloy, L. B., & Clements, C. M. (1992). Illusion of control: Invulnerability to negative affect and depressive symptoms after laboratory and natural stressors. *Journal of Abnormal Psychology, 101*(2), 234–245.

Alloy, L. B., Reilly-Harrington, N. A., Fresco, D. M., Whitehouse, W. G., & Zechmeister, J. S. (1999). Cognitive styles and life events in subsyndromal unipolar and bipolar mood disorders: Stability and prospective prediction of depressive and hypomanic mood swings. *Journal of Cognitive Psychotherapy: An International Quarterly, 13*, 21–40.

Barnett, P. A., & Gotlib, I. H. (1988). Psychosocial functioning and depression: Distinguishing among antecedents, concomitants, and consequences. *Psychological Bulletin, 104*(1), 97–126.

Beck, A. T. (1963). Thinking and depression: I. Idiosyncratic content and cognitive distortions. *Archives of General Psychiatry, 9*(4), 324–333.

Beck, A. T. (1964). Thinking and depression: II. Theory and therapy. *Archives of General Psychiatry, 10*(6), 561–571.

Beck, A. T. (1967). *Depression: Clinical, experimental, and theoretical aspects.* Philadelphia: University of Pennsylvania Press.

Beck, A. T. (1987). Cognitive models of depression. *The Journal of Cognitive Psychotherapy: An International Quarterly, 1*, 5–37.

Beck, A. T., Rush, A. J., Shaw, B. F., & Emery, G. (1979). *Cognitive therapy of depression.* New York: Guilford.

Beck, A. T., & Young, J. E. (1985). Depression. In D. Barlow (Ed.), *Clinical handbook of psychological disorders: A step-by-step treatment manual* (pp. 206–244). New York: Guilford.

Bleuler, M. (1963). Conception of schizophrenia within the last fifty years and today. *Proceedings of the Royal Society of Medicine, 56,* 945–952.

Bower, G. H. (1981). Mood and memory. *American Psychologist, 36*(2), 129–148.

Brown, G. W., & Harris, T. O. (1978). *Social origins of depression: A study of psychiatric disorder in women.* New York: The Free Press.

Gotlib, I. H., Kasch, K. L., Traill, S., Joormann, J., Arnow, B., & Johnson, S. L. (2004). Coherence and specificity of information-processing biases in depression and social phobia. *Journal of Abnormal Psychology, 113,* 386–398.

Gotlib, I. H., & Krasnoperova, E. (1998). Biased information processing as a vulnerability factor for depression. *Behavior Therapy, 29*(4), 603–617.

Gotlib, I. H., Krasnoperova, E., Neubauer, D. L., & Joormann, J. (2004). Attentional biases for negative interpersonal stimuli in clinical depression. *Journal of Abnormal Psychology, 113,* 127–135.

Gotlib, I. H., Traill, S. K., Montoya, R. L., Joormann, J., & Chang, K. (2005). Attention and memory biases in the offspring of parents with Bipolar Disorder: Indications from a pilot study. *Journal of Child Psychology and Psychiatry, 46,* 84–93.

Hammen, C. (1991). Generation of stress in the course of unipolar depression. *Journal of Abnormal Psychology, 100*(4), 555–561.

Hartlage, S., Alloy, L. B., Vazquez, C., & Dykman, B. (1993). Automatic and effortful processing in depression. *Psychological Bulletin, 113,* 247–278.

Ingram, R. E., Miranda, J., & Segal, Z. V. (1998). *Cognitive vulnerability to depression.* New York: Guilford.

Johnson, S. L., & Fingerhut, R. (2004). Negative cognitive styles predict the course of bipolar depression, not mania. *Journal of Cognitive Psychotherapy, 18,* 149–162.

Johnson, S. L., & Kizer, A. (2002). Psychosocial factors in the course of unipolar and bipolar depression. In I. Gotlib & C. Hammen (Eds.), *Handbook of depression* (3rd ed., pp. 141–165). New York: Guilford.

Judd, L. J., Hagop, S. A., Zeller, P. J., Paulus, M., Leon, A. C., Maser, J. D., Endicott, J., Coryell, W., Kunovac, J. L., Mueller, T. I., Rice, J. P., & Keller, M. B. (2000). Psychosocial disability during the long-term course of unipolar major depressive disorder. *Archives of General Psychiatry, 57,* 375–380.

Kessler, R. C., McGonagle, K. A., Zhao, S., Nelson, C. B., Hughes, M., Eshleman, S., Wittchen, H.-U., & Kendler, K. S. (1994). Lifetime and 12-month prevalence of *DSM–III–R* psychiatric disorders in the United States: Results from the National Comorbidity Survey. *Archives of General Psychiatry, 51,* 8–19.

Monroe, S. M., & Hadjiyannakis, K. (2002). The social environment and depression: Focusing on severe life stress. In I. Gotlib & C. Hammen (Eds.), *Handbook of depression* (3rd ed., pp. 314–340). New York: Guilford.

Monroe, S. M., & Roberts, J. E. (1990). Special issue: IIV. Advances in measuring life stress. *Stress Medicine, 6*(3), 209–216.

Monroe, S. M., & Simons, A. D. (1991). Diathesis–stress theories in the context of life stress research: Implications for the depressive disorders. *Psychological Bulletin, 110*(3), 406–425.

Needles, D. J., & Abramson, L. Y. (1990). Positive life events, attributional style, and hopefulness: Testing a model of recovery from depression. *Journal of Abnormal Psychology, 99*(2), 156–165.

Pearlin, L. I., & Lieberman, M. A. (1979). Social sources of emotional distress. In R. Simmons (Ed.), *Research in community and mental health* (pp. 17–48). Greenwich, CT: JAI Press.

Rosenthal, D. (1963). A suggested conceptual framework. In D. Rosenthal (Ed.), *The Genain quadruplets* (pp. 505–516). New York: Basic Books.

Safford, S. M., Crossfield, A. G., Alloy, L. B., & Abramson, L. Y. (2004). *Negative cognitive style, depression, and the reporting of negative life events: Harsh environment, stress generation, or reporting bias?* Manuscript under editorial review.

Seligman, M. E. P. (1975). *Helplessness: On depression, development and death.* San Francisco: Freeman.

Teasdale, J. D., & Dent, J. (1987). Cognitive vulnerability to depression: An investigation of two hypotheses. *British Journal of Clinical Psychology, 26*(2), 113–126.

Turner, R. J., Wheaton, B., & Lloyd, D. A. (1995). The epidemiology of social stress. *American Sociological Review, 60*(1), 104–125.

Weissman, A. N., & Beck, A. T. (1978). *Development and validation of the Dysfunctional Attitude Scale.* Toronto, Canada: American Educational Research Association Annual Convention.

Wittchen, H.-U., & Kendler, K. S. (1994). Lifetime and 12-month prevalence of *DSM–III–R* psychiatric disorders in the United States: Results from the National Comorbidity Study. *Archives of General Psychiatry, 51*(1), 8–19.

II

ANXIETY DISORDERS

A Unique Vulnerability Common to All Anxiety Disorders: The Looming Maladaptive Style

John H. Riskind
George Mason University

Nathan L. Williams
University of Arkansas

Despite a surge of interest, cognitive vulnerability research on anxiety disorders has lagged behind both advances in the depression literature and work on proximal factors in anxiety (e.g., attention and memory bias). Of the work that has been done on distal vulnerabilities, much focuses on nonspecific and general factors (e.g., perceptions of uncontrollability) that cut across many disorders. As a case in point, perceptions of uncontrollability are associated with depression or even schizophrenia. Accordingly, such research reveals little about any cognitive vulnerabilities common to anxiety disorders but not to depression or other disorders. Other work focuses on very narrow cognitive vulnerabilities that distinguish particular anxiety disorders from each other (e.g., anxiety sensitivity in panic). There has been relatively little research, however, on *general* vulnerability factors that increase risk *across* anxiety disorders, but not depression and other disorders.

This chapter summarizes the most recent advances of our ongoing Cognitive Vulnerability to Anxiety Project (CVA project). The CVA project is designed to complement research on cognitive mechanisms in specific anxiety disorders in that we have focused on a *superordinate cognitive vulnerability* that is postulated to be common to anxiety disorders but not depression. This common vulnerability applies to many particular aspects (e.g., information processing, appraisal, learning history) and types of anxiety disorders (e.g., social phobia, SP; generalized anxiety disorder, GAD; obsessive-compulsive disorder, OCD; and posttraumatic stress disorder, PTSD). Further, this cognitive vulnerability is expected, in conjunction with lower level "disorder-specific" cognitive mechanisms, to confer higher risk for the occurrence of specific anxiety disorders (e.g., responsibility in OCD, catastrophic misinterpretations in panic, worry in GAD).

COMMON AND UNIQUE COGNITIVE VULNERABILITIES TO ANXIETY

Cognitive vulnerabilities to anxiety disorders warrant high research priority because of the prevalence and economic cost of the anxiety disorders. Data from the National Comorbidity Study (NCS) indicate a lifetime prevalence rate of 24.9% and an annual prevalence rate of 17.2% for one of the anxiety disorders, and this total does not include data for PTSD or OCD (Kessler et al., 1994). Further, anxiety disorders were more common than any other class of disorders in the NCS. The anxiety disorders are the single largest and most financially costly class of mental health problems in the United States. For example, anxiety disorders cost an estimated $46.6 billion in 1990 alone in direct and indirect costs (Dupont et al., 1996). Moreover, anxiety disorders are associated with heightened co-occurrence of other Axis I disorders (e.g., Brown, Campbell, Lehman, Grisham, & Mancill, 2001), myriad "unexplained" physical symptoms and chronic health conditions (e.g., Roy-Byrne & Katon, 2000), and a poorer quality of life than nonanxiety disordered patients (Leon, Portera, & Weissman, 1995). An even larger percentage of the population suffers from subclinical anxiety, which may contribute to a range of social, occupational, and health difficulties, including high blood pressure and heart disease, ulcers, lost productivity, impaired sleep, and interpersonal discomfort.

Recent research in the anxiety literature on cognitive vulnerabilities has begun to examine the mechanisms that produce liability for specific types of anxiety disorders (e.g., anxiety sensitivity in panic, or inflated responsibility in OCD). Although knowledge of such disorder-specific mechanisms is important to achieve a full understanding of the cognitive etiology of anxiety disorders, it is equally important to identify common cognitive vulnerability factors. Such common factors are implicit in both cognitive models of anxiety (e.g., Beck & Emery, 1985) and current diagnostic classification of anxiety disorders. For example, the *DSM–IV* reflects the assumption that anxiety disorders have shared, as well as unique, symptoms. It is evident that variables such as trait anxiety and neuroticism are elevated in nearly all anxiety disorders (e.g., Rachman, 1998; Zuckerman, 1999), but represent *nonspecific* vulnerability factors (e.g., Bieling, Antony, & Swinson, 1998).

As depicted in Fig. 7.1, the "general liability" that individuals might have to developing a specific anxiety disorder should be increased by the

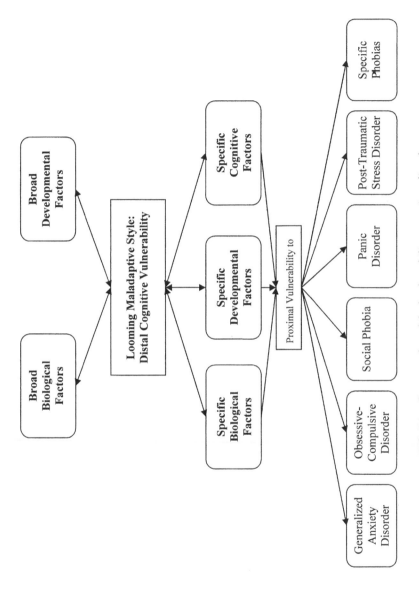

FIG. 7.1.   Conceptual model of vulnerability to anxiety disorders.

177

presence of a superordinate cognitive vulnerability to anxiety disorders, such as the *looming maladaptive style* (Riskind & Williams, 1999a, 1999b; Riskind, Williams, Gessner, Chrosniak, & Cortina, 2000; Williams, Shahar, Riskind, & Joiner, 2004). In conjunction with this broad cognitive vulnerability, additional hyperspecific etiological factors, including those that are cognitive, developmental, or biological, are believed to interact to determine the resultant anxiety disorder(s). These can include lower level disorder-specific cognitive mechanisms that are specific to each anxiety disorder (e.g., inflated beliefs about responsibility in OCD), as well as those that are nonspecific (e.g., beliefs about the uncontrollability of threat). The model conceptualizes this common cognitive vulnerability as a distal, superordinate characteristic style of threat/harm appraisal and elaboration that interacts with the disorder-specific cognitive mechanisms that are central to each anxiety disorder (e.g., predicting social rejection in SP, overestimating responsibility and negative significance in OCD, worry and catastrophizing in GAD, etc.). Ultimately, an adequate cognitive model of anxiety must account for both the common cognitive vulnerability factors and the disorder-specific cognitive mechanisms in each disorder, as well as the interactions between such factors.

THE COGNITIVE VULNERABILITY TO ANXIETY PROJECT

The CVA project was designed to systematically examine a common cognitive vulnerability that is postulated to increase liability to anxiety and anxiety disorders but not depression. This research centers around the cognitive model of anxiety called the *model of looming vulnerability* (Riskind, 1997; Riskind & Williams, 1999a, 1999b; Williams, Shahar, et al., 2004). Like other cognitive models of anxiety (e.g., Beck & Emery, 1985), this model assumes that exaggerated appraisals of threat contribute to the onset, exacerbation, and maintenance of anxiety and its disorders (Riskind, 1997). However, this model of anxiety differs in important ways from other cognitive models in its conceptualization of threat. The next sections elaborate on the model of cognitive vulnerability proposed in the looming vulnerability model (LVM) and summarize the main research findings pertinent to the model.

THE LOOMING VULNERABILITY MODEL OF ANXIETY

According to the looming vulnerability model, the quintessential instance of danger in the phenomenology of anxiety is characterized in terms of mental representations of dynamically intensifying danger and rapidly rising risk. In this way, the LVM differs from the standard cognitive model of anxiety (e.g., Beck & Emery, 1985), in that the model focuses on *dynamic danger content* (e.g., qualities such as the velocity and gathering momentum of threat), rather than on static predictions of threat. The static estimates featured in most cognitive theories of anxiety (e.g., "single-point" estimates of the likelihood or severity of harm; Beck & Emery, 1985) provide a bare picture of the anxious individual's perceptions of threat, constituting a dim reflection and lifeless extract of the anxious individual's phenomenological experience. Thus, the LVM assumes that the phenomenology of danger is dynamic, like a motion picture, rather than static like a photograph. Mental scenarios depict dangers as unfolding and increasing and not static. This is an important conceptual modification of the standard cognitive formulation of anxiety that affords important points of refinement, expansion, and modification for theory, assessment, and treatment. For example, our conceptual modification provides a more fine-grained analysis of the underlying cognitive mechanisms that explicate the attentional bias associated with anxiety, as well as anxious individuals' lack of habituation to fear-relevant stimuli (Riskind, 1997; Riskind, Williams, et al., 2000; Williams, Riskind, Olatunji, & Elwood, 2004).

In the LVM, the universal threat-related cognitive content of anxiety is captured by the core theme of rapidly intensifying danger or rising risk as one projects the self into an anticipated future. This core threat-related content shares an evolutionary continuity with fear responses observed in other species (e.g., fish, fowl, crabs, and primates) in response to rapidly intensifying or approaching "looming" threats (see Riskind, 1997, for a review of ethological and developmental studies). As pointed out later, once this innate threat/harm appraisal mechanism is elaborated into a durable cognitive style, it interacts with environmental events, stressors, and lower order cognitive mechanisms to determine what type of anxiety will likely result.

According to the LVM, anxiety occurs when individuals experience an acute subjective state of looming vulnerability in which danger seems to be increasing and unfolding from instant to instant toward some catastrophic end, creating a sense of rapidly rising risk. At times, such state elicitations of looming vulnerability accurately reflect reality (e.g., when facing an oncoming freight train), at other times they have a moderate but still vague reality basis (e.g., there are intensifying problems in a relationship); and, at still other times, these state elicitations reflect internally generated scenarios that have little basis in reality (e.g., based only on partial or ambiguous environmental information). Thus, looming vulnerability can occur either as a result of an objective stimulus configuration or as the result of an acquired cognitive bias, or it can occur out of an interaction of both. Once activated, the sense of looming vulnerability is a critical phenomenological component of threat that sensitizes anxious individuals to threat movement and signs of intensifying danger in their environments, biases their cognitive processing, and renders their anxiety to be more persistent and less likely to habituate (Riskind, 1997; Riskind, Williams, et al., 2000; Williams, Riskind, Olatunji, & Tolin, 2004).

THE LOOMING MALADAPTIVE STYLE

Although the sense of looming vulnerability can be experienced simply as a state elicitation, it can also develop into a more durable cognitive pattern as a result of exposure to certain antecedent conditions (e.g., developmental or attachment patterns, negative life events). From their learning histories, some individuals develop a characteristic style of threat/harm appraisal, anticipation, and elaboration such that they construct mental scenarios of potential threats as rapidly unfolding, approaching, or increasing in harm or danger. This *looming maladaptive style* (LMS; referred to also as the "looming cognitive style") is assumed to function as a danger schema and to produce the typical dynamic cognitive phenomenology of intensifying danger and rapidly rising risk seen in pathological anxiety. At the same time, the LMS is presumed to remain relatively latent until activated by requisite environmental stimuli (i.e., potential threat stimuli). Consequently, the LMS is assumed to produce a schematic processing bias for threat information in cognitively vulnerable individuals, even when such individuals are not currently anxious.

Given that several recent studies have emphasized the relation between catastrophizing and anxiety (e.g., Davey & Levy, 1998; Vasey & Borkovec, 1992), two important demarcations appear necessary. First, it seems important to distinguish between the LMS and catastrophizing about threat or danger. In our conceptual framework, the LMS acts as an overarching danger schema that is the underlying or distal mechanism that leads to proximal and lower order ideational activity, such as catastrophizing, for specific threat situations. Further, the LMS differs from catastrophizing in that it emphasizes the perceived velocity and rate of change involved in catastrophic cognitions, rather than simply the imagined outcomes of catastrophic cognitions. Concordant with this view, recent research provides evidence that the LMS predicts residualized gains in the extent to which individuals engage in catastrophizing over time (Riskind & Williams, 1999b). The reverse was not true, however, in that catastrophizing does not predict changes in the LMS over time. These findings suggest that the LMS is a stable individual difference that acts to increase vulnerability to later catastrophizing and anxiety while remaining conceptually and psychometrically distinct.

Second, given that recent research highlights the potent role of catastrophic cognitions in the genesis of panic attacks (e.g., Clark, 1988), one may wonder why the LMS does not unequivocally lead to panic reactions. Research suggests that the LMS only serves as a catalyst for panic reactions when the individual experiences stimulus-specific forms of looming vulnerability to bodily sensations, or to the sequel of somatic sensations (e.g., Riskind & Chambliss, 1999). In other types of anxiety, the fear component does not produce a full-blown panic attack because the focus of the looming danger is external to the individual (e.g., a spider), unrelated to somatic sensations (e.g., social rejection), vague or diffuse (e.g., abstract worry about financial concerns), or because self-protective responses are utilized to neutralize or cope with the perceived threat.

ELABORATED SCHEME OF THE PSYCHOLOGICAL REPERCUSSIONS OF THE LMS

The painful repercussions of the LMS are postulated to reverberate throughout the whole of the individuals cognitive, affective, physiological, and behavioral systems through a series of etiological chains that are related to anxiety. As presented in Fig. 7.2, these etiological chains begin with the LMS (the distal vulnerability) and proceed through intermediate and proximal cognitions and information processing to self-protective responses.

Initial Processing

Once the hypothesized LMS is developmentally established, the cognitively vulnerable individual's information processing is filtered through and systematically biased by this putative style of threat/harm appraisal and elaboration. The LMS is assumed to function as a danger schema that pervasively biases the processing of threat-related information (e.g., selective attention, encoding, retrieval, interpretation; Riskind, Williams, et al., 2000; Williams, Riskind, Olatunji, & Tolin, 2004). In addition, the cognitive repercussions of the LMS on information processing are assumed to "trickle down" and affect the whole scope of the individuals' ideational material related to threat elaboration, including their associations, expectations, predictions, fantasies, and dreams.

The person's schema-driven mental representations of rapidly intensifying danger are also likely to lead to an increase in hypervigilance and an attentional bias for threat (e.g., Williams, Riskind, Olatunji, & Tolin, 2004).

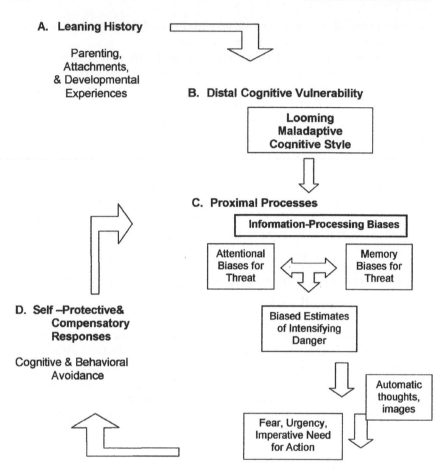

FIG. 7.2.   Etiological model of the looming maladaptive style as a cognitive
vulnerability to anxiety.

For example, the inflated sense that potential dangers are advancing, escalating in risk, unforeseeable, and everpresent should naturally lead the
person to scour the surrounding environment for any potential indicators
of danger. As suggested by the literature on perceptual processes, individuals allocate attention to perceived changes in stimuli that are more
salient or novel (i.e., that are perceived as looming), than to stimuli themselves (Gibson, 1979). Thus, cognitively vulnerable individuals, who experience a chronic state of looming vulnerability, are likely to develop an
attentional bias for threat and to exhibit heightened states of vigilance,
even in the absence of objectively threatening information. Quite the opposite would occur if sources of risk were expected to be stable factors that
have permanence and continuity. If risk was not rising or intensifying,

then the incentive for individuals to have an attentional bias or hypervigilance for threat would be significantly reduced.

Sense of Urgent Threat and Imperative Need for Action

The mental representations of intensifying danger generated by the LMS routinely induce a more intense feeling of fear and personal vulnerability and lead to an increased sense of time urgency and *imperative need for action*. As the anticipated prospect of headlong or rapid destruction seemingly builds within the cognitively vulnerable individuals' mental representations of threat, their level of anxiety and urgency to neutralize or cope with the perceived threat inimically escalates. This point is illustrated with the analogy of individuals who were to misperceive a car that is objectively traveling at 10 miles an hour toward them as traveling at 70 miles an hour. They would have a disturbing sense that they had no time to waste, and indeed, have insufficient time to prepare for, or prevent, the possibility of harm. Such feelings of rapidly escalating threat could catalyze intense feelings of fear and a perceived need to seek desperate, often extreme and rigid, measures to avoid the threat.

In this way, the mental representations of dynamically intensifying or approaching threat generated by the LMS may quickly lead from the initial appraisal of potential threat (e.g., an ambiguous cue), to biased elaborations of the temporal and spatial progression and ultimate consequences of such threat, to an imperative sense of urgency to utilize self-protective or compensatory response. For example, cognitively vulnerable persons might notice a rather mundane "absent" look in a lover, or behavior of other people in a social performance situation, and envision a rapidly rising risk of being rejected; or they might hear an engine noise while driving their cars and mentally simulate a state of rapidly intensifying peril. Whether or not the mental representations of rapidly intensifying danger are accurate, the danger is perceived as more time urgent, more imperative, and consequently more fear inducing.

Self-Protective Behaviors

The sense of rapidly rising risk is likely to naturally evoke greater distress and lead cognitively vulnerable individuals to engage in various *self-protective behaviors*. When direct action is possible, cognitively vulnerable individuals may engage in behavioral avoidance. When direct action is not possible or when there are no instrumental responses immediately available or a lack of sufficient time to prepare for the possibility of countering the prospect of harm, the person may engage in cognitive avoidance behaviors.

Feeling chronically pressed by time and threatened by an imperative need for action on so many fronts, cognitively vulnerable individuals are likely to select "default" coping strategies that have the benefit of being fast acting, but the liabilities of being extreme and often unnecessary (Williams, 2002; Williams & Riskind, 2004b). Typically, this results in "coping rigidity" (i.e., a narrow tendency to use highly restricted avoidance coping strategies across situations, which includes both behavioral and cognitive avoidance; Williams, 2002; Williams & Riskind, 2004b). Research from several recent studies reveals a strong association between the LMS and an avoidant coping style, even when the individual's level of anxiety is statistically controlled. Moreover, this research consistently reveals a strong association between the LMS and decreased coping flexibility (e.g., Williams, 2002; Williams & Riskind, 2004b).

Building on recent research on the role of worry in pathological anxiety, it is assumed that worry can be characterized as another self-protective process (e.g., Borkovec, 1994) such that fear-related imagery is translated into less distressing verbal or linguistic form (Borkovec & Inz, 1990). To this end, results of a recent mentation sampling study provide evidence that higher levels of the LMS are associated with a predominance of imagery-based mental activity during anticipation of an upcoming stressor, whereas worry is associated with a predominance of lexical activity (Williams, McDonald, & Riskind, 2004). Additionally, worry, as well as more abstract metacognitive activities such as metaworry (i.e., worry about the degree to which one is worrying; Wells, 1995) can absorb so much of the vulnerable person's mental capacity that these activities may reduce the amount of attention that the person can allocate to managing frightening mental representations. In some cases, events can be moving so quickly that worry and metaworry cannot provide adaptive, short-term coping options that serve to lessen, or transform, mental representations of rapidly intensifying danger. Once this threshold is reached, the individual is likely to engage in wishful thinking or thought suppression as the primary avoidance strategy. Evidence for these links has been found in several studies (e.g., Riskind & Williams, 2005; Williams, Riskind, Olatunji, & Tolin, 2004).

Cognitively vulnerable persons are being challenged on so many fronts by prospects of intensifying dangers such that they can become taxed and depleted in cognitive and emotional resources (Baumeister, Dale, & Sommer, 1998) and suffer a state of "cognitive *overload*" (Wegner, 1994). As a consequence of feeling wearied by an incessant need for vigilance, caution, and self-protective action, cognitively vulnerable individuals are liable to have fewer mental resources with which to engage in successful mood regulation or to successfully cope with potential threats. These general impairments in the capacity for mental and emotional control, coupled with their schematic processing bias to mentally represent threats as rapidly intensifying, may increase cognitively vulnerable individuals' liability to all forms of anxiety disorder. Evidence has been obtained for this impairment of mental control in a series of recent studies (e.g., Williams, Riskind, Olatunji, & Elwood, 2004).

Bidirectional Feedback Loops

Finally, the etiological chains related to anxiety often involve bidirectional reciprocal feedback loops in which individuals' maladaptive avoidance or neutralizing behavior helps to maintain their distorted mental representations of intensifying danger and their beliefs that they are indeed limited in coping options. Further, the LMS coupled with the inflexible use of cognitive avoidance strategies (e.g., worry) may lead to mental representations of increasingly abstract and diffuse threats that are difficult to challenge or counter. As a consequence, a "confirmation-bias" may be created such that the individuals' faulty primary and secondary appraisals are not only maintained, but also strengthened (e.g., by self-produced "evidence," or "illusory correlations"), thereby catalyzing a slip into a vicious dysfunctional spiral toward pathological anxiety.

SUICIDE AS EXTREME AVOIDANCE COPING

As described elsewhere, suicidality can represent an extreme instance of "self-protective" defensive reactions to rapidly intensifying danger (Riskind, Long, Williams, & White, 2000). Whereas depression, or more exactly, hopelessness, seems to represent the main psychological factor in suicide (e.g., Abramson et al., 1998), recent work suggests that *comorbid anxiety* (and states of looming vulnerability) can further exacerbate suicide risk (for a review see Riskind, Long, et al., 2000). Consistent with escape theories of suicide (Baumeister, 1990; Shneidman, 1989), the LVM of anxiety conceptualizes suicide as being motivated by the desire to avoid rapidly rising and intolerable psychological pain in living. Particularly at risk for suicide are individuals who perceive their life circumstances as progressively worsening and/or intensifying in risk and psychological pain, and who may perceive their situations as hopeless. For example, consider the haunting image of the suicidal stock traders who hurled themselves from high buildings because of the crash of 1929. Such individuals not only saw their current situations as irrevocable, they saw their futures as rapidly becoming more painful, creating a sense of urgency and desperation to escape. Their behavior was motivated by a need to avoid the rapidly rising and inexorable risk of pain. Thus, a *fusion* of hopelessness and looming vulnerability is likely to provide an impelling state that is responsible for producing the most intense desperation and suicidality.

COGNITIVE VULNERABILITY TO ANXIETY:
ITS DEVELOPMENTAL ORIGINS

The model characterizes early experience and development as critical to the formation of the LMS and a common cognitive liability to future anxiety disorders. For example, the LMS may have its roots in faulty modeling and parenting, unresolved childhood fears, or insecure attachment experiences. Some individuals are brought up, from their earliest remembrance, being exposed to events and experiences that promote the development of the cognitive vulnerability. Moreover, some of their most "self-defining" or "life-defining" memories may be laden with such representations of intensifying danger. For example, it is not unusual for anxious clinical patients to recall alarming childhood memories of scenarios that involve "looming entrapment," such as emotional memories of listening to an abusive or drunken parent taking step by step up of a set of stairs to verbally harass or physically injure them (Riskind & Williams, 1999a).

Several lines of relevant empirical research suggest a role for the developmental learning history in creating a cognitive liability to later anxiety. The first line of relevant research indicates that parental anxiety contributes to a vulnerability to anxiety, over and beyond the effects of genetic factors (e.g., Judd, 1965). It is likely that faulty parental modeling or parenting behaviors that involve excessive control or promote avoidance of anxiety-eliciting situations may lead to the development of the LMS. A second line of relevant research suggests that behavioral inhibition and negative emotional reactivity may contribute to the development of the LMS and later vulnerability to anxiety (e.g., Kagan, Reznick, & Snidman, 1987). In this developmental trajectory, behaviorally inhibited and emotionally reactive children may limit their exposure to anxiety-eliciting or novel situations, and consequently retain exaggerated beliefs about the magnitude and severity of environmental threat and underestimations of their own ability to cope with threat.

A third line of research indicates that negative life events of childhood, including parental maltreatment, abuse (physical, sexual, or emotional), neglect, and poor grades could be tied to the development of cognitive vulnerability to anxiety and later risk of anxiety (e.g., Berstein, Garfinkel, & Hoberman, 1989; Tweed, Schoenbach, & George, 1989). It has been suggested that it is not just the incidence of negative life events, but also the controllability with which such events were appraised that contribute to cognitive risk for anxiety (e.g., Chorpita & Barlow, 1998; Rapee, 1991). Given the fact that uncontrollability is a nonspecific factor, linked to both anxiety and depression, consider that anxiety is particularly related to perceived uncontrollability over rapidly intensifying future danger, whereas depression is related to perceived uncontrollability that is tinged with the hopeless permanence of past losses.

A fourth line of relevant research suggests that faulty attachment relationships are likely to contribute to the development of a cognitive vulnerability to anxiety. According to Ainsworth, Blehar, Waters, and Wall's (1978) model of childhood attachment, an anxious/ambivalent attachment reflects the infants' perceptions of the caregiver as inconsistent in responding to their needs, particularly during times of distress. Several recent studies in the CVA project provide evidence that insecure attachment styles (Williams & Riskind, 2004a), impaired parental bonding (Riskind et al., 2004), and retrospective reports of maternal attachment insecurity (Riskind et al., 2004) may represent developmental antecedents of the LMS.

The occurrence of negative events or situations (e.g., faulty modeling, abuse, maltreatment, attachment disruptions) can have a profound effect on the child's developing cognitive-affective schemas and can profoundly influence the information processing. Although any significant negative events or disruptions during childhood have the potential to produce vulnerability to later pathology, it is possible that the quality of the child's subjective interpretation of these disruptions will determine the specific type of vulnerability that is created (e.g., anxiety vs. depression). The extent and quality of these disruptions varies across individuals such that some may experience the loss of a key attachment figure (i.e., an avoidant attachment style resulting from a host of factors ranging from neglect to death), whereas others may experience a sense of ambivalence toward the permanence of the attachment figure (i.e., an anxious-ambivalent attachment style resulting from inconsistent care). Consistent with these predictions, cognitive vulnerability to anxiety has been associated with an anxiety dimension of adult romantic attachment, whereas cognitive vulnerability to depression has been associated with an avoidant dimension of adult romantic attachment (Williams & Riskind, 2004a). Moreover, because much of the integration of childhood experience occurs with the development of formal operational thought in early adolescence, intervening experience between the time of the event and the time at which the event is interpreted and integrated within the self-concept may play a role in determining the resultant vulnerability.

THE GENERALITY AND SPECIFICITY OF THE LMS TO ANXIETY DISORDERS

In the model, the universal aspects of anxiety and its cognitive phenomenology are captured by the theme of looming vulnerability or rapidly intensifying or approaching anticipated future threat. To this end, the sense of looming vulnerability to a potentially uncontrollable threat is viewed both as a *necessary cause* of the experience of anxiety (i.e., it must be above a minimal threshold for any anxiety to occur), and a *sufficient cause* for the experience of anxiety (i.e., its occurrence guarantees the anxiety → self-protective response sequence).

The LMS, as a schema-driven, evolutionarily based process of threat/harm appraisal, elaboration, and anticipation, is likely to increase the probability and frequency of such states of looming vulnerability, and thus confer heightened risk for developing an anxiety disorder. The actual form of the disorder(s) that emerges depends on the interaction of the overarching LMS with situational factors (e.g., specific traumas or learning histories) that create "lower order" and more proximal disorder-specific cognitive mechanisms (e.g., inflated responsibility for the suppression of threatening intrusive thoughts in OCD). In some cases, individuals may have a "stimulus-specific" form of looming vulnerability without developing the LMS. For example, some persons with specific phobias may have a restricted, stimulus-specific looming style (e.g., for representing spiders or social rejections as rapidly approaching or rising in risk). But, in the majority of cases, we postulate that the general LMS cross-situationally biases the ways in which individuals mentally represent the temporal and spatial progression of a range of possible dangers (e.g., spreading contamination, or impending social rejections; e.g., Riskind, Williams, et al., 2000; Williams, Shahar, et al., 2004).

PANIC DISORDER

In current cognitive models, panic is viewed as an acute "alarm reaction" in response to catastrophic cognitions about bodily sensations or about the threat of having future panic attacks (Antony & Barlow, 1996; Clark, 1988). The proximal cognitions that are believed to induce panic typically involve catastrophic misinterpretations of bodily sensations (e.g., faintness, heart palpitations) or anxiety reactions as much more threatening than they really are (e.g., as having a heart attack; Clark, 1988). The trait of anxiety sensitivity appears to be central to panic disorder, such that individuals evidence fears of anxiety symptoms that are based on beliefs that these symptoms have harmful or catastrophic consequences.

The model includes several processes by which the LMS is likely to confer vulnerability to the development of panic disorder. First, cognitively vulnerable individuals, because of the impaired mental and emotional control that they are likely to suffer, may find it more difficult to cope effectively with catastrophic cognitions (e.g., "rationally respond" to them) and thereby engage in faulty compensatory strategies (e.g., Riskind & Williams, 1999a). Second, individuals with the LMS are more likely to mentally play out scenarios in which relatively mundane physical sensations may lead to looming catastrophes, such as hospitalization or death. In many cases, the individual's learning history contains experience with self or significant others who have befallen illness or injury, which becomes a focal point of their LMS. Third, individuals with the LMS are likely to evidence heightened sensitivity and/or hypervigilance for signs of potential threats. These consequences of the LMS can be transmitted, through stimulus-specific forms of looming vulnerability, to fear of the threat of rapidly intensifying bodily sensations (e.g., Riskind & Chambless, 1999). Finally, results of a recent study suggest that both the LMS and anxiety sensitivity contribute uniquely to the prediction of general anxiety symptoms and anxiety-related constructs such as worry (Williams & Reardon, 2004).

GENERALIZED ANXIETY DISORDER

Cognitive perspectives on generalized anxiety disorder (GAD) have suggested that the hyperactivation of danger schemata produces negative automatic thoughts that involve overestimates of danger and elicit somatic distress (e.g., Beck & Clark, 1997). Recent models have extended these perspectives by including additional cognitive processes that are initiated by threatening automatic thoughts and images (Borkovec, 1994; Wells, 1995). Following the proximal automatic thoughts/images, individuals are postulated to engage in compensatory neutralization responses such as maladaptive worry. These models have suggested that worry represents either a type of cognitive avoidance that reduces the emotional and somatic distress evoked by danger-related imagery (e.g., Borkovec & Inz, 1990), or a process that absorbs cognitive capacity and results in less available resources for lower level processing of fear (Wells, 1995). Worry has also been related to catastrophizing and an "automatic questioning style" (e.g., a "what if x happens" style of thinking) that leads to further distortion of threat-related appraisals (e.g., Borkovec & Inz, 1990; Riskind, 1997b).

The LMS is likely to confer vulnerability to GAD by impairing mental control mechanisms required to deal with upsetting thoughts, increasing hypervigilance for threat-related information, and leading individuals to engage in faulty, catastrophic, looming mental simulations of even relatively mundane events or stimuli (Riskind & Williams, 2005). Further, the schematic processing bias produced by the LMS would likely increase recall and cognitive accessibility for threatening material, as well as distort the individual's initial appraisals of threat. To this end, results of a recent mentation sampling study (similar to the Borkovec & Inz, 1990, study) provide evidence that the LMS is associated with a predominance of imagery-based mental experience (Williams, McDonald, & Riskind, 2004).

Thus, cognitively vulnerable individuals are likely to experience more fear-related dynamic imagery that leads to the overutilization of worry as a self-protective process.

SOCIAL PHOBIA

In cognitive models of social phobia, maladaptive proximal cognitions and cognitive processes related to the threat of potential public embarrassment, criticism, or scrutiny is seen as central to the production of acute fear responses (Roth, Fresco, & Heimberg, chap. 10, this vol.). According to the LVM, the LMS is likely to confer vulnerability to social phobia by mechanisms similar to those already described, which when coupled with early formative experiences involving acceptance or worthiness based on perfection lead the individual to envision rapidly intensifying danger of humiliating social rejection or catastrophe in social and performance situations (e.g., Riskind & Mizrahi, 2000; Williams, Shahar, et al., 2004). Again, the individual suffers from impaired mental control mechanisms that make it difficult to dismiss thoughts or images about failure in such situations and that consequently may increase both worry and metaworry about performance in these situations.

OBSESSIVE-COMPULSIVE DISORDER

Cognitive models of obsessive-compulsive disorder (OCD) have included that exaggerated appraisals about the overimportance of intrusive thoughts and inflated personal responsibility to prevent such thoughts or their consequences as central to both the experience of distress and the urge to engage in activities such as compulsive behavior, neutralizing, thought suppression, reassurance seeking, and avoidance (Rachman et al., chap. 9, this vol.; Rachman, 1997; Salkovskis, Shafran, Rachman, & Free-ston, 1999). Research has amply indicated that individuals with OCD commonly attach exaggerated negative significance to their intrusive thoughts and regard them as horrific, repugnant, threatening, and/or dangerous. Moreover, such individuals typically demonstrate paradoxical increases in intrusive thoughts associated with their efforts at cognitive avoidance (e.g., Salkovskis et al., 1999).

As with the other anxiety disorders, the LMS is likely to confer vulnerability to obsessive-compulsive disorder by producing a cognitive load that impairs the person's mental control resources. Cognitively vulnerable individuals who more generally overestimate the magnitude and severity of threat in the environment and experience higher levels of anxiety and distress should have more difficulty suppressing thoughts (e.g., Williams, Riskind, Olatunji, & Elwood, 2004). This tendency would likely manifest in ascribing higher levels of negative significance to intrusive thoughts and images, increased difficulty with thought suppression and neutralization, and greater risk for the development of obsessional thinking. Appraisals of rapidly rising risk are an important antecedent condition that is likely to increase the negative significance that individuals attach to their intrusive thoughts, as well as the responsibility for suppressing the thoughts or their consequences (Riskind, Abreu, Strauss, & Holt, 1997; Williams, Riskind, Olatunji, & Elwood, 2004). Thus, individuals who experience intrusive thoughts that involve content depicting rapidly unfolding action or outcomes may be more likely to experience increased responsibility and perfectionistic concerns, and ascribe greater import to intrusive thoughts, the controllability of such thoughts, and the threat that such thoughts represent (see Riskind, Williams, & Kyrios, 2002, for a review).

POSTTRAUMATIC STRESS DISORDER

Cognitive models of posttraumatic stress disorder (PTSD) have generally emphasized the individuals' failures to incorporate or process traumatic experiences into their conceptual systems or the meaning that individuals make out of traumatic experience (see Feeny & Foa, chap. 11, this vol.). In an attempt to separate the self from the catalyzing traumatic experience, or to prevent their assumptive systems from being shattered, these individuals engage in self-protective processes, such as cognitive avoidance, which have the benefit of maintaining the desired separation of self from experience, but the liability of requiring enormous cognitive resources and taxing the individual's cognitive system. The LMS is likely to confer vulnerability to the development of PTSD after exposure to traumatic events in several ways. First, this style is likely to place an additional cognitive load on the individual and make efforts at effective coping and emotion regulation more difficult (Riskind et al., 2000). Second, the LMS is likely to provide a mental filter that schematically biases and molds the individual's fearful predictions about the rapidly rising risk that similar frightful events will reoccur. Such fearful predictions include both the rapidly intensifying danger of "re-victimization" (e.g., by events such as being raped or physically assaulted anew), and of "re-traumatization" (e.g., by subjective responses such as being engulfed anew by the same frightful body sensations). In the latter instance, the LMS may amplify the detrimental effects of lower level mechanisms such as anxiety sensitivity and metaworry that lead persons to fear their bodily sensations and anxiety reactions. Evidence of a link of the LMS to PTSD is provided by a recent study with college students (Williams, Shahar, et al., 2004) and a study of young adult female survivors of sexual assault, in which females high in the LMS reported significantly higher levels of general anxious symptoms and PTSD-specific symptoms (Williams & Elwood, 2004).

RESEARCH FINDINGS OF THE CVA PROJECT

This section summarizes the main findings of the CVA project that provide evidence for the predictions generated by the LVM. Over the past decade, numerous studies conducted as part of our project have examined the validity of the LMS and, more generally, the LVM of anxiety (e.g., Riskind, 1997; Riskind, Williams, et al., 2000; Riskind & Maddux, 1993; Riskind, Moore, & Bowley, 1995; Riskind & Wahl, 1992, Riskind & Williams, 1999a, 1999b; Riskind & Williams, 2005; Williams, 2002; Williams, Shahar, et al., 2004; Williams et al., 2004a, 2004b). These studies have employed a variety of methodologies to investigate the validity of the LVM, including self-report assessments, computer-simulated movement of objects (e.g., moving spiders vs. moving rabbits), the presentation of videotaped scenarios (e.g., a campus mugging, possible contamination scenarios, etc.), and the presentation of moving and static visual images. Further, these studies have investigated a range of cognitive-clinical processes (e.g., anxiety, thought suppression, coping styles, uncontrollability, catastrophizing, worry, attachment styles, memory bias, etc.) across a wide range of stimuli (e.g., individuals with mental illness, individuals with HIV, contamination, spiders, weight gain, social and romantic rejection, performance mistakes, etc.) and a diversity of populations (e.g., individuals with subclinical obsessive-compulsive disorder, social phobia, generalized anxiety disorder, posttraumatic stress disorder, panic disorder, depression, specific phobias, and subclinical eating disorders).

These studies have provided uniformly consistent evidence for the looming vulnerability formulation (Riskind, 1997; Riskind, Williams, et al., 2000). Several studies, using videotaped or computer-generated stimuli or scenarios, have found evidence that phobic individuals exaggerate the extent to which their feared stimuli (spiders or germs) are changing, advancing, or moving rapidly forward toward them (e.g., Riskind, Kelly, Moore, Harmon, & Gaines, 1992; Riskind & Maddux, 1993; Riskind et al., 1995; Williams, Riskind, Olatunji, & Tolin, 2004). Moreover, these studies indicate that perceptions of looming danger predict stimulus-specific levels of anxiety, even when controlling for stimulus-specific fear. The reverse was not true, however. For example, spider phobics exhibit a bias to imagine spiders as rapidly approaching or likely to approach them (Riskind et al., 1992; Riskind et al., 1995), even when controlling for their level of spider-phobia. Individuals with subclinical obsessive-compulsive disorder exhibit a specific sense of rapidly intensifying danger to contamination (i.e., representing germs as rapidly approaching or spreading; Riskind et al., 1997). Comparable associations exist between a sense of looming vulnerability and fears of Auto-Immune Deficiency Syndrome (Riskind & Maddux, 1994), fears of the public for psychiatric patients (Riskind & Wahl, 1992), and fears of performance mistakes by socially anxious professional musicians (Riskind & Mizrahi, 2000).

Evidence also supports the assumption that a sense of looming vulnerability acts to instigate or exacerbate anxiety, and it is not just a correlate of anxiety. For example, several studies have *experimentally manipulated* looming movement. Riskind and colleagues (1992) examined the effects of such a manipulation by presenting research participants with videotaped scenarios in which tarantulas and rabbits either moved toward the camera, moved away, or were still. The importance of looming vulnerability was evidenced by the fact that the looming movement of tarantulas enhanced fear and threat-related cognitions and did this far more than it did for neutral stimuli like rabbits. The importance of looming vulnerability for fear was shown by the fact that these effects were far stronger for the high-fear-of-spider participants than for the low-fear participants.

Based on these, and similar studies using experimental methods, Riskind and colleagues devised a self-report questionnaire, the Looming Maladaptive Style Questionnaire (LMSQ), to assess the extent to which individuals appraise threat as rapidly rising in risk, progressively worsening, or actively accelerating and speeding up (i.e., exhibit the LMS; Riskind et al., 1992; Riskind, Williams, et al., 2000). Participants are presented with six brief vignettes describing different types of stressful situations, and asked to complete a three-item list of questions for each vignette. The stressful situations include threat of illness, risk of physical injury, romantic rejection, public speaking, and social humiliation.

Numerous studies in our CVA project provide support for the convergent validity of the LMS, indicating that higher scores on the LMSQ are related to higher levels of anxiety as measured on the Beck Anxiety Inventory and the Spielberger trait and state anxiety scales ($r = .39-.49$), and have found usually consistent evidence that the LMS is significantly associated with several correlates of anxiety, including worry, thought suppression, and behavioral avoidance (e.g., Riskind, Williams, et al., 2000; Williams, Shahar, et al., 2004). However, it is important to point out that the LMS is not simply another measure or proxy for trait anxiety. For example, Riskind, Williams, and colleagues (2000) demonstrated with structural equation modeling that whereas the LMS and anxiety are correlated, their measurement properties clearly distinguish between them. Likewise, studies have shown that the LMS, although correlated with measures of anxiety sensitivity, neuroticism, negative affect, or negative life events, can clearly be distinguished from these variables, and the LMS predicts distinct variance in anxiety over and above that predicted by these measures (Riskind, Williams, et al., 2000; Williams & Reardon, 2004; Williams, Shahar, et al., 2004). These findings are critical because they provide evidence that the LMS assesses a cognitive construct that has incremental value in predicting distinct and significant variance in anxiety, even when other variables such as neuroticism or negative affectivity are controlled.

Remarkably consistent evidence has also been found for the discriminant validity of the LMS, suggesting that scores on the LMSQ can differentiate between anxiety and depression (despite the high correlation between these). That is, the significant correlation between the LMS and anxiety remains highly significant when the variance due to depression is statistically controlled, whereas the correlation between LMS and depression is reduced to nonsignificance when the variance due to anxiety is controlled (Williams, Shahar, et al., 2004). These findings on discriminant validity are unique because past investigators have found it difficult to find self-report measures of presumed cognitive characteristics of anxiety that are not also strongly correlated with depression, and this is especially the case in nonclinical populations (Riskind, 1997; Riskind et al., 1992). Equally important are results indicating that the proposed cognitive vulnerability predicts significant unique variance in anxiety, even when relevant cognitive variables are controlled. That is, the claim that the cognitive vulnerability has incremental value is upheld by the fact that it predicts significant variance in anxiety measures beyond the effects accounted for by static predictions of unpredictability, uncontrollability, likelihood, or imminence of threat (e.g., Riskind et al., 2000).

A cluster of studies has also supported the temporal stability of the LMS and its predictive validity as a cognitive vulnerability measure. In one recent longitudinal study, results suggested a high degree of temporal stability for the LMS ($r = .82$), as measured by the LMSQ, over an 8-week time period (e.g., Williams, 2002). Further, in several other longitudinal studies (with follow-ups ranging from 1 week to 4 months in duration), the cognitive vulnerability significantly predicted residualized gains in anxiety and anxiety-relevant constructs when controlling for baseline levels of anxiety (e.g., Riskind & Williams, 1999b; Riskind, Williams, et al., 2000; Williams, 2002; Williams & Riskind, 2004).

A group of short-term prospective studies also supports the postulated effects of the cognitive vulnerability on self-protective responses. These studies have shown that the LMS seems to stimulate worry over time intervals ranging from 1 week (Riskind, Williams, et al., 2000) to 6 weeks (Riskind, in press), after controlling for initial levels on standard measures of pathological worry. Similarly, several studies have confirmed predictions that the LMS predicts residualized gains in thought suppression of threatening material over time. These results converge with a recent study using experimental methods (Williams, Riskind, Olatunji, & Elwood, 2004) in which cognitively vulnerable individuals reported significantly more intrusive thoughts on an instructed thought suppression task. Indeed, the LMS was the single strongest predictor of thought intrusions and distress. Finally, a recent field study with college athletes found that the cognitive vulnerability predicted residualized gains in wishful thinking in the week immediately before, and just after, competition with other college teams (Murphy, Riskind, & Williams, 2000). Thus, several studies have uncovered strong evidence that the cognitive vulnerability is related to self-protective strategies.

COGNITIVE VULNERABILITY TO ANXIETY DISORDERS

An additional cluster of studies supports the relevance of the LMS to a variety of different anxiety disorders. For example, Riskind and Williams (2005) showed that scores for the LMS were significantly more elevated in a community sample of patients with GAD, than in a sample of patients with depressive disorders or normal controls. Riskind, Gessner, and Wolzon (1999) found in a study of inpatients in a detoxification unit for alcohol and substance abuse that those who were diagnosed with GAD had significantly higher scores on the LMS than similar patients who did not have GAD. Williams, Shahar, and colleagues (2004) reported similar results in a sample of college students screened with a measure of GAD, as well as significant associations between the LMS and measures used for screening OCD, social phobia, simple phobias, and PTSD. Riskind and Mizrahi (2000) offered evidence that professional musicians who had higher performance anxiety tended to envision public performances in terms of a rapidly intensifying danger of making humiliating mistakes. Similarly, Riskind and Chambless (1999) indicated that the sense of looming vulnerability to the rapid intensification of somatic symptoms predicted significant variance in panic symptoms and agoraphobic cognitions, beyond the effects of other relevant variables.

LMS AND SCHEMATIC PROCESSING BIAS

The extent to which the LMS produces a schematic processing bias has been examined in several studies investigating its effects on memory. These studies examined memory for lexical and visual threat-related stimuli on both explicit memory tasks (which make direct reference to studied materials) and implicit memory tasks (which make no direct reference to such materials). First, results of a study using a homophone task suggested that the LMS is significantly and uniquely related to the tendency to process and interpret ambiguous verbal information (e.g., "dye" vs. "die") in a threatening manner (e.g., Riskind, Williams, et al., 2000).

As demonstrated by the results of structural equation modeling depicted in Fig. 7.3, the standardized coefficient representing the path between the LMS and the homophone measure was significant, whereas the coefficient representing the path between anxiety and the homophone measure was not. Moreover, elimination of the path between the LMS and the homophone measure resulted in a significant decrement in model fit, whereas elimination of the path from anxiety to the homophone variable did not. A second set of analyses conducted to distinguish the effects of the LMS from likelihood estimates and the latent anxiety variable on the prediction of homophone spelling revealed a similar outcome: Only the path between the LMS and the homophone measure was significant and it was only the elimination of this path that produced a significant decrement in model fit.

These results indicate that the LMS produces a schematic bias for ambiguous information that cannot be accounted for by static expectations of threatening situations (e.g., likelihood estimates). Further, they imply that anxiety may primarily exert an effect on schematic processing via the LMS. Finally, these results were all replicated in even a low anxiety sample, based on a median split of the participants performed on the latent anxiety variable. Thus, these results suggest that the LMS produces a schematic bias in implicit memory, even for individuals who are demonstrably not currently anxious. These results are particularly exciting because they support the postulated role of the LMS as a cognitive vulnerability that can affect information processing, much like what has been found for the depressive explanatory style.

Riskind, Williams, and colleagues (2000) investigated the effects of the LMS on memory for visual threat-related stimuli using a laboratory task in which a series of visual images were presented. Participants were presented with 45 neutral (e.g., fish), positive (e.g., flowers), or threatening visual images (e.g., a house fire or auto crash) and asked to rate the extent to which each image was threatening to ensure attention to the stimuli. We included two measures of explicit memory (a free recall task, a frequency estimation task), and a measure of implicit memory (a word stem completion task). Structural equation modeling replicated the pattern of the preceding study. Again, the standardized coefficient representing the path between the LMS and the dependent variables was significant, whereas the coefficient representing the path between latent anxiety and these de-

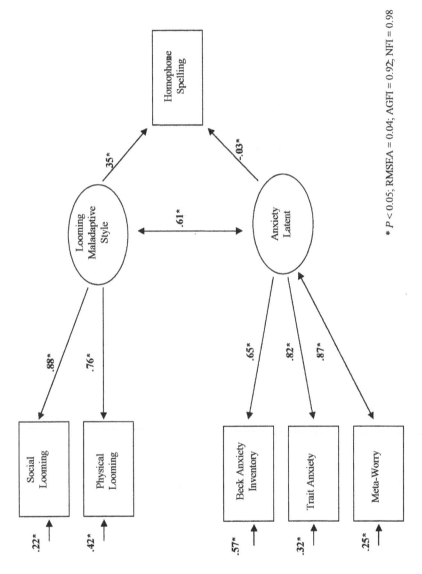

FIG. 7.3. Structural Model of homophone prediction for the LMS and latent anxiety.

*P < 0.05; RMSEA = 0.04; AGFI = 0.92; NFI = 0.98

197

pendent variables was not. Further, omission of the path from the LMS to each of these dependent variables resulted in a significant decrease in model fit, whereas elimination of the path between anxiety and the dependent variables did not. The findings of this study, which have been replicated, indicate that cognitively vulnerable individuals do not suppress anxiety-provoking stimuli shortly after being oriented toward them, but rather are absorbed by them.

Williams, Riskind, Olatunji, and Elwood (2004) investigated the schematic processing effects of the cognitive vulnerability for visual stimuli that differed in both their valence (threatening, neutral, positive) and their level of movement (moving vs. static). A series of visual images were presented on computer, some moving and some static (e.g., a video clip of an accident occurring vs. a picture of a wrecked car). Participants rated each image for level of threat on computer and their reaction times were recorded in milliseconds, and then they completed the series of memory tasks used in the previous study. The more cognitively vulnerable subjects evidenced faster reaction times when presented with moving stimuli (regardless of valence) and faster reaction times for threatening stimuli (regardless of movement). Moreover, high LMS subjects recalled more moving than static images and recalled more threatening than neutral or positive images.

Taken together, these converging sets of findings provide strong evidence that cognitively vulnerable individuals exhibit a pervasive bias for threat-related information in schematic information processing, and this occurs across several different types of laboratory tasks. The results suggest that the LMS is associated with heightened vigilance for threat-related information and for movement, heightened accessibility of cognitive danger schemas, and a systematic bias that is manifested in both implicit and explicit memory.

Furthermore, these results have underscored the important differences between the LVM and the standard cognitive model of anxiety. In general, the standard cognitive model conceptualizes the mental representation of threat in terms of probability estimates about aversive outcomes and their consequences, whereas our model focuses on dynamic mental representations of the rapidity with which danger is intensifying. Like the LVM, Gray's (cf. 1987) theory of anxiety would view the dynamic nature of a threat stimulus as important for maintaining activation of the Behavioral Inhibition System that generates anxiety. Indeed, Gray listed novel stimuli as inputs that activate the Behavioral Inhibition System because they are perceived as unfamiliar or unpredictable. The person does not easily habituate to novel stimuli because this system is activated by "mismatches" or violations of expectations. To the extent that a threat is perceived as changing, the expectations that the person has formed about the environment are less applicable and generate anxiety.

IMPLICATIONS OF THE LOOMING VULNERABILITY MODEL: DIFFERENTIATION OF ANXIETY AND DEPRESSION

Recent investigators have suggested that anxiety and depression represent the same disorder, emphasizing findings that highlight overlap in affective, cognitive, and biological features. However, we hesitate to accept such a conclusion and staunchly disagree with its logical basis. In much the same way that the 97% overlap in DNA sequences does not demonstrate that chimps and human beings are indistinguishable, the overlap between anxiety and depression does not unequivocally demonstrate that anxiety and depression are synonymous. Moreover, there seem to be significant differences between both sets of comparisons (chimps vs. humans & anxiety vs. depression) when they are examined with more refined levels of discrimination. Our CVA project, together with similar research on depression (see Alloy et al., chap. 2, this vol.), provides strong empirical evidence for distinguishing between anxiety and depression via a focus on cognitive content and cognitive processes.

DIFFERENCES BETWEEN THE LOOMING VULNERABILITY AND STANDARD COGNITIVE MODELS OF ANXIETY

The conceptual modification in our model, highlighting the role of rapidly intensifying danger in anxiety, represents a significant advance over the standard cognitive model. These findings are unique in showing that the LMS is strongly, but rather precisely, correlated with anxiety but not depression in both clinical and nonclinical samples. Such evidence of discriminant validity stands in contrast to past results that have indicated that anxiety-related cognitions (i.e., threat cognitions) are often as highly correlated with depression as with anxiety symptoms. The LVM also has implications for assessment and treatment, and could facilitate improved treatment outcome and efficacy. For example, cognitive behavioral therapy has demonstrated efficacy in treating anxiety disorders, but its success with some disorders, such as GAD (Riskind, 1997; Riskind & Williams, 1999a) and OCD (Rachman et al., chap. 9, this vol.), has been moderate and many patients do not respond to current cognitive protocols. Further, even the most efficacious cognitive treatments may benefit from consideration of looming vulnerability and the LMS, particularly when working with resistant clients or clients for whom standard cognitive treatment is not producing the expected gains (Riskind & Williams, 1999a).

CLINICAL IMPLICATIONS

The set of etiological chains that we propose for anxiety in the LVM provide multiple points for therapeutic or preventative intervention. The framework implies that immediate, temporary relief may be provided by cognitive interventions that target the proximal aspects of dysfunctional thinking about intensifying danger, whereas more durable improvement may be provided by changing underlying cognitive vulnerabilities, such as the LMS. As depicted in Fig. 7.4, the typical utterances of anxious patients reflect this sense of looming vulnerability to threat in their dysfunctional automatic thoughts. As is evident from this clinical material, automatic thinking in anxious patients is characterized not only by overestimations of danger, but also by a sense of rapidly rising risk and intensifying danger as one projects the self into some anticipated future. Moreover, the LMS seems to predispose individuals to interpret mundane and ambiguous situations in threatening ways and leads to hypervigilance for threat-related information.

The term *looming management* refers to the various therapeutic clinical uses of the LVM (Riskind & Williams, 1999a). As described in Riskind and Williams, clinicians can address the content and quality of dynamic representations of intensifying danger, particularly imagery-based components, rather than only address the individual's biased way of looking at static predictions or outcomes of potential threats, as implied by the standard cognitive-clinical model. For example, in a sample of subclinical obsessive compulsives, Riskind and colleagues (1997) provided evidence that teaching such individuals to freeze or arrest their mental representations of "looming" contaminants can reduce their level of anxiety.

As Riskind and Williams (1999a) proposed, the clinician could modify the variable of *distance* (either physical or temporal), stretching out or lengthening patients' perceptions of distance from danger in their dynamic mental representation. A second variable the therapist can try to

"My position in my firm is not very secure.
My bosses are looking at me, saying 'Is he crazy?' "
"The clock is ticking away. Any day now my client could sue me."
"You can lose everything at any moment."
"The rug can be yanked from beneath you at any time."
"Change is always dangerous. There are higher expectations with changes.
There is insurmountable work to be done."
"My fears of death, danger, etc., are essentially a fear of change."
Example from Beck's Cognition Checklist
"I am going to have an accident."

FIG. 7.4.   Utterances of patients with generalized anxiety disorder.

modify is *motion*. For example, by using imagery-based techniques and other cognitive-behavioral interventions, the clinician could attempt to interrupt or arrest the forward movement of seemingly intensifying danger. A third variable a therapist could modify is *speed*, or the velocity with which anxious patients perceive potential threat to be intensifying, moving, or changing for the worst. The variable of speed can often be modified using behavioral experiments, hypothesis testing, imagery, or other methods, the end goal of which are to reduce the patient's perceptions of the rapid rise or approach of potential threat. For instance, a patient with social phobia can be instructed to "test" the objective escalation of risk in social situations. Finally, the therapist can modify the patients' perspectives on the role of the self as *target of threat*—rather than observer. This technique can reduce the self-focused nature of perceiving threat and increase their objectivity.

In addition to focusing on the variables involved in anxious patients' mental representations of dynamically intensifying danger, the therapist could attempt to reduce coping rigidity in several ways (e.g., Williams, 2002; Williams & Riskind, 2004b). For example, if anxious patients understand that generating dynamic representations in which potential threats are rapidly intensifying leads to a sense of inflated urgency and a constriction in their possible avenues of coping, then they may be more likely to be able to effectively use the aforementioned strategies. Second, the therapist can help anxious patients to generate proactive coping strategies to neutralize potentially intensifying threats, and to use rehearsal exercises to modify their coping flexibility (their ability to reevaluate and apply multiple coping strategies in response to changes in the veridical conditions of threat; Williams, 2002). Hence, the LVM of anxiety, and the LMS more specifically, are likely to have implications for developing more refined case conceptualizations and increasingly effective treatment strategies for the range of anxiety disorders.

This research conducted in our CVA project makes several unique contributions to our understanding of dysfunctional cognitive processes in anxiety. First, the empirical data so far indicate that the LMS may constitute a distinctive cognitive vulnerability for anxiety and it fills the same distinctive niche for anxiety as the depressive explanatory style does for depression. Second, evidence has supported the key proposition that the LMS is an overarching cognitive vulnerability that is common to many particular aspects of anxiety and anxiety disorders (e.g., PD, SP, OCD, GAD, and PTSD; Williams, Shahar, et al., 2004). Moreover, considerable research indicates that the LMS is linked to many of the specific cognitive mechanisms involved in different anxiety disorders (e.g., exaggerated responsibility, anxiety sensitivity, etc.). Third, and related to the previous points, the LMS produces a strong schematic processing bias for threat-related information, even when people are demonstrably not currently anxious.

Although the CVA project has entered an exciting new phase in research on cognitive vulnerability to anxiety, there are several future challenges. Although there is strong evidence to support the role of the LMS in many particular forms of anxiety disorder, much additional work on clinical populations is necessary. Second, whereas work has begun to examine the interactions between the LMS and specific mechanisms implicated in the pathogenesis of particular disorders (e.g., links from LMS to responsibility in OCD), more steps in this direction are needed. Third, it is essential to have studies that use behavioral high risk designs (similar to those used by the Temple–Wisconsin Cognitive Vulnerability to Depression Project; see Alloy et al., chap. 2, this vol.) to examine the prospective development of anxiety disorders in cognitively vulnerable individuals who have the LMS. Fourth, future research may benefit from the inclusion of additional information-processing tasks (e.g., tasks of preattentive bias, signal detection, or priming) that can provide added ways to test predictions of the LVM. In addition, little is known about whether or not there is a synergistic interaction between objectively assessed stressful events and the cognitive vulnerability (which the model implicitly predicts). We are also pursuing several suggestive findings that indicate the existence of a possible subtype of anxiety symptoms related to the LMS (i.e., "looming vulnerability anxiety"), analogous to "hopelessness depression" as a subtype of depression.

Much remains to be learned about the developmental antecedents (e.g., attachment styles, parenting styles, self-defining and emotional memories) and personality correlates (e.g., harm avoidance, as in Gray, 1987) of the LMS, as well as the possible role it plays in enhancing fear conditioning. For example, the LVM suggests that individuals with the cognitive vulnerability are likely to be more "psychologically prepared" for rapid and persisting fear conditioning (Riskind, 1997)—particularly when the fear-relevant stimuli involved are presented in dynamic states of intensification and/or motion (i.e., such individuals are already prone to appraise fear-relevant stimuli as rapidly intensifying in danger). Additionally, research is required to examine the physiological mechanisms that accompany the LMS and the experience of looming vulnerability. Finally, it may be important to examine the possible moderating effects that different self-protective responses (e.g., worry or other cognitive avoidance strategies) have on the impact of the cognitive vulnerability on information-processing and fear reactions. For example, several studies in the CVA project provide intriguing evidence that worry or metaworry can attenuate or even eliminate the typical effects of the LMS on future anxiety and fear-related schematic processing biases. That is, individuals who "pay a price" by engaging in pathological worry may avoid the fear-related symptoms associated with this cognitive vulnerability. Alternatively, a coping repertoire characterized by coping flexibility may operate as an adaptive protective factor against anxiety and worry.

REFERENCES

Abramson, L. Y., Alloy, L. B., Hogan, M. E., Whitehouse, W. G., Cornette, M., Akharan, S., & Chiara, A. (1998). Suicidality and cognitive vulnerability to depression among college students: A prospective study. *Journal of Adolescence, 21*, 473–487.

Ainsworth, M. S., Blehar, M. C., Waters, E., & Wall, S. (1978). *Patterns of attachment: A psychological study of the Strange Situation*. Hillsdale, NJ: Lawrence Erlbaum Associates.

Antony, M. M., & Barlow, D. M. (1990). Emotion theory as a framework for explaining panic attacks and panic disorder. In R. M. Rapee (Ed.), *Current controversies in the anxiety disorders* (pp. 55–76). New York: Guilford.

Baumeister, R. F. (1990). Suicide as escape from self. *Psychological Review, 97*, 90–113.

Baumeister, R. F., Dale, K., & Sommer, K. L. (1998). Freudian defense mechanisms and empirical findings in modern social psychology: Reaction formation, projection, displacement, undoing, isolation, sublimation, and denial. *Journal of Personality, 66*, 1081–1124.

Beck, A. T., & Clark, D. A. (1997). An information processing model of anxiety: Automatic and strategic processes. *Behaviour Research and Therapy, 35*, 49–58.

Beck, A. T., & Emery, G. (1985). *Anxiety disorders and phobias: A cognitive perspective*. New York: Basic Books.

Berstein, G. A., Garfinkel, B. D., & Hoberman, H. M. (1989). Self-reported anxiety in adolescents. *American Journal of Psychiatry, 146*, 384–386.

Bieling, P. J., Antony, M. M., & Swinson, R. P. (1998). The Stait-Trait Anxiety Inventory, Trait version: Structure and content re-examined. *Behaviour Research and Therapy, 36*, 777–778.

Borkovec, T. D. (1994). The nature, functions, and origins of worry. In G. C. L. Davey & F. Tallis (Eds.), *Worrying: Perspectives on theory assessment, and treatment* (pp. 5–34). New York: Wiley.

Borkovec, T. D., & Inz, J. (1990). The nature of worry in generalized anxiety disorder: A predominance of thought activity. *Behaviour Research and Therapy, 28*, 153–158.

Brown, T. A., Campbell, L. A., Lehman, C. L., Grisham, J. R., & Mancill, R. B. (2001). Current and lifetime comorbidity of the *DSM–IV* anxiety and mood disorders in a large clinical sample. *Journal of Abnormal Psychology, 110*, 585–599.

Chorpita, B. F., & Barlow, D. H. (1998). The development of anxiety: The role of control in the early environment. *Psychological Bulletin, 124*, 3–21.

Clark, D. M. (1988). A cognitive model of panic attacks. In S. Rachman & J. Maser (Eds.), *Panic: Psychological perspectives* (pp. 71–89). Hillsdale, NJ: Lawrence Erlbaum Associates.

Davey, G. C., & Levy, S. (1998). Catastrophic worrying: Personal inadequacy and a perseverative iterative style as features of the catastrophizing process. *Journal of Abnormal Psychology, 107*, 576–586.

Dupont, R. L., Rice, D. P., Miller, L. S., Shiraki, S. S., Rowland, C. R., & Harwood, H. J. (1996). Economic costs of anxiety disorders. *Anxiety, 2*, 167–172.

Gibson, J. J. (1979). *The ecological approach to visual perception*. Boston: Houghton-Mifflin.

Gray, J. A. (1987). *Psychology of fear and stress* (2nd ed.). Cambridge, England: Cambridge University Press.

Judd, L. L. (1965). Obsessive-compulsive neurosis in children. *Archives of General Psychiatry, 12*, 136–143.

Kagan, J., Reznick, S., & Snidman, N. (1987). The physiology and psychology of behavior inhibition in children. *Development Psychology, 58*, 1459–1473.

Kessler, R. C., McGonagle, K. A., Zhao, S., Nelson, C. B., Hughes, M., Eshleman, S., Wittchen, H., & Kendler, K. S. (1994). Lifetime and 12-month prevalence of *DSM–III–R* psychiatric disorders in the United States: Results from the National Comorbidity Survey. *Archives of General Psychiatry, 51*, 8–19.

Leon, A. C., Portera, L., & Weissman, M. M. (1995). The social costs of anxiety disorders. *British Journal of Psychiatry, 166*, 19–22.

Murphy, B., Riskind, J. H., & Williams, N. L. (2000). *Cognitive vulnerability and avoidance in college athletes.* Unpublished manuscript.

Rachman, S. (1998). *Anxiety.* East Sussex, England: Psychology Press.

Rachman, S. (1997). A cognitive theory of obsessions. *Behavioral Research and Therapy, 35*, 793–802.

Rapee, R. M. (1991). Psychological factors involved in generalized anxiety. In R. M. Rapee & D. H. Barlow (Eds.), *Chronic anxiety, generalized anxiety disorder, and mixed anxiety-depression* (pp. 76–94). New York: Guilford.

Riskind, J. H. (1997). Looming vulnerability to threat: A cognitive paradigm for anxiety. *Behaviour Research and Therapy, 35*(5), 386–404.

Riskind, J. H. (in press). *Looming and loss: Cognitive factors in emotional dysfunction.* New York: Plenum.

Riskind, J. H., Abreu, K., Strauss, M., & Holt, R. (1997). Looming vulnerability to spreading contamination in subclinical OCD. *Behaviour Research and Therapy, 35*(5), 405–414.

Riskind, J. H., & Chambless, D. L. (1999). *Exploring cognitive antecedents of panic: Effects of looming vulnerability, perceived control, and causal attributions.* Unpublished manuscript.

Riskind, J. H., Gessner, T. D., & Wolzon, R. (1999). *Cognitive vulnerability to alcohol dependence in an inpatient sample: Implications of the looming maladaptive style.* Unpublished manuscript.

Riskind, J. H., Kelly, K. Moore, R., Harman, W., & Gaines, H. (1992). The looming of danger: Does it discriminate focal phobia and general anxiety from depression? *Cognitive Therapy and Research, 16*, 1–20.

Riskind, J. H., Long, D. G., Williams, N. L., & White, J. C. (2000). Desperate acts for desperate times: Looming vulnerability and suicide. In T. Joiner & D. M. Rudd (Eds.), *Suicide science: Expanding the boundaries* (pp. 105–115). New York: Plenum.

Riskind, J. H., & Maddux, J. E. (1994). The loomingness of danger and the fear of AIDS: Perceptions of motion and menace. *Journal of Applied Social Psychology, 24*(5), 432–442.

Riskind, J. H., & Maddux, J. E. (1993). Loomingness, helplessness, and fearfulness: An integration of harm-looming and self-efficacy models of fear and anxiety. *Journal of Social and Clinical Psychology, 12*, 73–89.

Riskind, J. H., & Mizrahi, J. (2000). *Mediating cognitive processes in musical performance anxiety: The role of looming vulnerability.* Unpublished manuscript.

Riskind, J. H., Moore, R., & Bowley, L. (1995). The looming of spiders: The fearful perceptual distortion of movement and menace. *Behaviour Research and Therapy, 33*, 171–178.

Riskind, J. H., & Wahl, O. (1992). Moving makes it worse: The role of rapid movement in fear of psychiatric patients. *Journal of Social and Clinical Psychology, 11*, 349–364.

Riskind, J. H., & Williams, N. L. (1999a). Cognitive case conceptualization and the treatment of anxiety disorders: Implications of the looming vulnerability model. *Journal of Cognitive Psychotherapy, 13*(4), 295–316.

Riskind, J. H., & Williams, N. L. (1999b). Specific cognitive content of anxiety and catastrophizing: Looming vulnerability and the looming maladaptive style. *Journal of Cognitive Psychotherapy, 13*(1), 41–54.

Riskind, J. H., & Williams, N. L. (2005). The Looming Cognitive Style and generalized anxiety disorder: Distinctive danger schemas and cognitive phenomenology. *Cognitive Therapy and Research, 29,* 7–27.

Riskind, J. H., Williams, N. L., Altman, A., Black, D. O., Balaban, M. S., & Gessner, T. L. (2004). Developmental antecedents of the looming maladaptive style: Parental bonding and parental attachment insecurity. *Journal of Cognitive Psychotherapy, 18,* 43–52.

Riskind, J. H., Williams, N. L., Gessner, T., Chrosniak, L., & Cortina, J. (2000). A pattern of mental organization and danger schema related to anxiety: The looming maladaptive style. *Journal of Personality and Social Psychology, 79*(5), 837–852.

Riskind, J. H., Williams, N. L., & Kyrios, M. (2002). Experimental methods for studying cognition. In R. O. Frost & G. Steketee (Eds.), *Cognitive approaches to obsessions and compulsions: Theory, assessment, and treatment* (pp. 139–164). Amsterdam, Netherlands: Pergamon/Elsevier Science.

Roy-Byrne, P. P., & Katon, W. (2000). Anxiety management in the medical setting: Rationale, barriers to diagnosis and treatment, and proposed solutions. In D. I. Mostofsky & D. H. Barlow (Eds.), *The management of stress and anxiety in medical disorders* (pp. 1–14). Boston: Allyn & Bacon.

Salkovskis, P. M., Shafran, R., Rachman, S., & Freeston, M. H. (1999). Multiple pathways to inflated responsibility beliefs in obsessional problems: Possible origins and implications for therapy and research. *Behaviour Research and Therapy, 37,* 1055–1072.

Shneidman, E. S. (1989). Approaches and commonalities of suicide. In R. F. W. Diekstra & R. Maris (Eds.), *Suicide and its prevention: The role of attitude and imitation* (pp. 14–36). Netherlands: E. J. Brill.

Tweed, J., Schoenbach, V., & George, L. K. (1989). The effects of childhood parental death and divorce on six-month history of anxiety disorders. *British Journal of Psychiatry, 154,* 823–828.

Vasey, M. W., & Borkovec, T. D. (1992). A catastrophizing assessment of worrisome thoughts. *Cognitive Therapy and Research, 16,* 505–520.

Wegner, D. M. (1994). Ironic processes of mental control. *Psychological Review, 101,* 34–52.

Wells, A. (1995). Meta-cognition and worry: A cognitive model of generalized anxiety disorder. *Behavioural and Cognitive Psychotherapy, 23,* 301–320.

Williams, N. L. (2002). *The cognitive interactional model of appraisal and coping: Implications for anxiety and depression.* Unpublished doctoral dissertation, George Mason University, Fairfax.

Williams, N. L., & Elwood, L. S. (2004). *Cognitive vulnerabilities to anxiety and depression in female victims of sexual assault.* Manuscript in preparation.

Williams, N. L., McDonald, T., & Riskind, J. H. (2004). *Mentation sampling during instructed anticipation and worry: The LCS is associated with a predominance of imagery-based mentation.* Manuscript in preparation.

Williams, N. L., & Reardon, J. (2004). *A comparison of vulnerabilities to anxiety: The looming cognitive style and anxiety sensitivity.* Manuscript submitted for publication.

Williams, N. L., & Riskind, J. H. (2004a). Adult romantic attachment and cognitive vulnerabilities to anxiety and depression: Examining the interpersonal basis of vulnerability models. *Journal of Cognitive Psychotherapy, 18,* 7–24.

Williams, N. L., & Riskind, J. H. (2004b). *The cognitive interactional model of appraisal and coping: Coping styles and coping flexibility.* Manuscript in preparation.

Williams, N. L., & Riskind, J. H. (2004c). *A prospective investigation of cognitive vulnerability to anxiety.* Manuscript in preparation.

Williams, N. L., Riskind, J. H., Olatunji, B. O., & Elwood, L. S. (2004). *Cognitive vulnerability to anxiety and information processing: Implications of the looming maladaptive style.* Manuscript in preparation.

Williams, N. L., & Riskind, J. H., Olatunji, B. O., & Tolin, D. (2004). *Cognitive vulnerabilities to contamination fears and obsessional thoughts.* Manuscript submitted for publication.

Williams, N. L., Shahar, G., Riskind, J. H., & Joiner, T. E. (2004). The looming cognitive style has a general effect on an anxiety disorder symptoms factor: Further support for a cognitive model of vulnerability to anxiety. *Journal of Anxiety Disorders, 19,* 157–175.

Zuckerman, M. (1999). *Vulnerability to psychopathology: A biosocial model.* Washington, DC: American Psychological Association.

8

Cognitive Vulnerability to Panic Disorder

Norman B. Schmidt
Florida State University

Kelly Woolaway-Bickel
The Ohio State University

In the mid-1980s, several cognitive theories were advanced that dramatically influenced research on the nature and treatment of panic disorder (Barlow, 1988; Clark, 1986; Reiss & McNally, 1985). Since that time, results from a number of studies of cognitive aspects of panic disorder have greatly extended our understanding such that there is compelling evidence for several cognitive parameters that appear to play a role in the pathogenesis of this condition. This chapter focuses on knowledge of cognitive vulnerability factors that has evolved from cognitive theories of panic disorder. After providing background about panic disorder and various cognitive models of panic, a summary model is presented that integrates a variety of cognitive factors. Then the empirical support for the pathways delineated in this model are described. Finally, comments are made concerning future directions and implications of this research.

THE PHENOMENOLOGY AND EPIDEMIOLOGY
OF PANIC DISORDER

Anxiety is an innate, adaptive mechanism that readies human beings for action and protects them from anticipated threat. Unfortunately, this "alarm system" can become maladaptive when it is triggered for excessive lengths of time, in situations known to be harmless, or for no apparent cause (Hoehn-Saric & McLeod, 1988). A *panic attack* is described as a discrete period of intense fear or discomfort accompanied by four or more somatic and/or cognitive symptoms (e.g., sweating, fear of dying) (APA, 1994). These symptoms develop abruptly and reach a peak within a 10-minute period. Panic attacks are seen across the spectrum of anxiety disorders, but a formal diagnosis of panic disorder is warranted when an individual experiences recurrent, unexpected panic attacks followed by at least 1 month of persistent concern about having additional attacks, worry about the implications of additional panic attacks, and/or a significant change in behavior related to the attacks. The additional diagnosis of agoraphobia (i.e., panic disorder with agoraphobia) is considered when an individual exhibits significant avoidance of or distress associated with places or situations from which escape might be difficult or embarrassing, or in which help may not be available in the event of a panic attack (APA, 1994).

Data from epidemiological studies such as the Epidemiological Catchment Area (ECA) study suggest that, over a lifetime, as many as 30%–40% of all individuals will experience clinically significant anxiety (Shepherd, Cooper, Brown, & Kalton, 1996), approximately 28%–34% will experience isolated panic attacks (Norton, Harrison, Hauch, & Rhodes, 1985), and 1.5%–6% will meet diagnostic criteria for panic disorder with and without agoraphobia (APA, 1994; Eaton & Keyl, 1990). At any given time, 3% of the adult population in the United States report recurrent panic attacks and 10% report occasional or isolated attacks (Jacobi et al., 2004; Weissman, 1988; Wittchen, 1986).

COGNITIVE THEORIES OF PANIC
AND PANIC DISORDER

Cognitive models of panic and panic disorder generally focus on the relation between fear and cognitive appraisal and parameters that affect the appraisal process. The three most influential cognitive models of panic disorder are Barlow's (1988) emotion-based model, Clark's (1986) cognitive model, and Reiss' (1991) expectancy model.

Barlow's Model

Barlow's (1988, 2002) model of panic and panic disorder describes panic primarily from an emotion theory perspective, but also incorporates cognitive, learning, and biological aspects. According to Barlow, the etiology of panic begins with a biological vulnerability that disposes the individual toward being neurobiologically overreactive to stress. In addition to possessing a biological vulnerability, Barlow proposed that certain individuals possess an additional psychological vulnerability to developing panic disorder, which consists of a sense that events and emotions are uncontrollable and unpredictable. This vulnerability results in an inward shift in attention during arousal, which contributes to a process of developing anxious apprehension regarding additional attacks. Individuals with anxious apprehension about future attacks have a propensity to associate interoceptive cues with the original false alarm through classical conditioning (i.e., "learned alarms"; Barlow, 1988). Learned alarms may then be triggered by specific bodily sensations, and with anxiety focused on future panic, "additional somatic and cognitive cues become available to trigger the panic attacks, resulting in the development of panic disorder" (Antony & Barlow, 1996, p. 60). Conscious appraisal of sensations is not a necessary factor in the development or occurrence of panic attacks, although Barlow's (1988) model acknowledges that some attacks may be preceded by the appraisal of danger regarding bodily sensations.

Clark's Model

Whereas Clark's (1986) cognitive model of panic is similar to Barlow's in that it implicates bodily sensations as an important factor in panic disorder architecture, Clark's model proposes that all panic is triggered by bodily sensations that are catastrophically misinterpreted as threatening. Catastrophic misinterpretation involves interpreting sensations as much more threatening than they really are. For example, an individual might perceive slight breathlessness as evidence of respiratory failure and consequent impending death (Clark, 1986). This perceived threat leads to more bodily sensations, greater perceived threat, and the cycle is repeated until the apprehension rises to panic. The misinterpreted bodily sensations may come from a variety of events, both emotional (e.g., anxiety-related palpitations) and nonemotional (e.g., ingestion of caffeine). These panic-triggering sensations may also change across time depending on which bodily sensations are noticed and the fears that the individual has been able to discount (Clark, 1986).

Clark (1986) noted that biological factors may play a role in panic and may increase an individual's vulnerability to panic in various ways. For instance, biological factors may contribute to the triggering of an attack if they cause the individual to experience more symptoms or more intense symptom fluctuations. For example, a diabetic may be prone to panic due to somatic perturbations associated with fluctuations in blood sugar. In addition, biological factors may influence the extent to which a perceived threat produces an increase in bodily sensations. For example, a deficiency in the alpha-2-adrenergic autoreceptor would cause an individual to experience larger than normal surges in sympathetic nervous system activity in response to a perceived threat.

Expectancy Theory

Expectancy theory predicts that panic attacks, phobias, and other fear reactions arise from three fundamental fears: fear of negative evaluation, injury/illness sensitivity, and anxiety sensitivity (Reiss, 2004; Reiss & McNally, 1985). Fear of negative evaluation refers to apprehension and distress about receiving negative evaluations from others, expectations that others will provide negative evaluations, and avoidance of evaluative situations. Injury/illness sensitivity is characterized by fears of injury, illness, and death (Reiss, 1991; Taylor, 1993). Finally, anxiety sensitivity is the fear of anxiety symptoms arising from beliefs regarding the consequences of experiencing anxiety (Reiss, 1991). In the case of panic disorder, anxiety sensitivity is the only aspect of expectancy theory that has been extensively investigated. Future work evaluating the other fundamental fear domains may also provide useful information about cognitive vulnerability for panic.

Bodily sensations do not invariably provoke panic, and in fact can prompt a wide variety of affective responses (McNally, 1994; Schmidt, Richey, & Fitzpatrick, in press). Reiss and McNally (1985) and Reiss (1991) proposed that preexisting beliefs regarding the harmfulness of symptoms determine whether or not someone will panic in response to bodily sensations. They asserted that a trait known as anxiety sensitivity embodies such beliefs. The construct of anxiety sensitivity refers to the extent to which an individual believes that autonomic arousal can have harmful consequences (Reiss & McNally, 1985). For example, individuals with high anxiety sensitivity may believe that shortness of breath signals suffocation or that heart palpitations indicate a heart attack, whereas those with low anxiety sensitivity experience these sensations as unpleasant but nonthreatening.

Consistent with most cognitive theories of anxiety, the anxiety sensitivity conceptualization posits that cognitive misappraisal is critical for the generation of anxiety. However, the anxiety sensitivity hypothesis is distinct from other psychological theories. For example, anxiety sensitivity is similar to Clark's (1986) "enduring tendency" to catastrophically misinterpret bodily sensations, but a difference in conceptualizations is evident. Like Clark's panic patient, an individual with high anxiety sensitivity is especially prone to catastrophic ideation. However, people high in anxiety sensitivity would not necessarily misinterpret sensations like rapid heartbeat as being a heart attack. Rather, a high anxiety sensitivity individual could become fearful because of a belief that rapid heartbeat may lead to a future heart attack. McNally (1994) explained that "the anxiety-sensitivity hypothesis does not require that patients misconstrue anxiety as something else (e.g., impending heart attack) for panic to be highly aversive" (p. 116).

Anxiety sensitivity is believed to be a relatively stable belief system that may precede the development of panic attacks. Individual differences in anxiety sensitivity are hypothesized to emerge from a variety of experiences that ultimately lead to the acquisition of beliefs about the potentially aversive consequences of arousal. Such experiences may include hearing others express fear of such sensations, receiving misinformation about the harmfulness of certain sensations, witnessing a catastrophic event such as the fatal heart attack of a loved one, and so forth. Thus, there are likely to be a variety of paths that lead to the acquisition of beliefs that constitute anxiety sensitivity. Importantly, anxiety sensitivity constitutes a disposition to developing anxiety and does not necessarily require the actual experience of anxiety or panic in its own development.

INTEGRATED COGNITIVE VULNERABILITY MODEL OF PANIC DISORDER

This section borrows from the earlier cognitive models of panic disorder to describe a model that stresses cognitive processes that are likely to make an individual vulnerable to the development of panic disorder (see Fig. 8.1). It highlights three distal cognitive vulnerability factors that have received empirical support. These factors include anxiety sensitivity beliefs, predictability and control beliefs, and information-processing biases. In addition, it also includes a factor termed *catastrophic cognition*, which appears to operate as a specific, proximal cognitive vulnerability for panic disorder. Before turning to a more detailed description of this model, it is important to clarify the nature of risk factors versus vulnerability factors and their relation to panic disorder.

Ingram, Miranda, and Segal (1998, pp. 80–83) noted a useful distinction between risk and vulnerability. Although these terms are often used interchangeably, *risk* can be used to refer to factors that are associated with an increased likelihood of experiencing the disorder without a clear sense of the causal status of these factors. Thus, risk refers to a statistical level of analysis rather than a causal one. On the other hand, *vulnerability* factors imply something about the underlying processes that are important in pathogenesis. A vulnerability factor informs us about the mechanisms believed to exist that are responsible for the development of the condition. According to this distinction, all vulnerability factors must be risk factors, but not vice versa. Moreover, risk factors might be considered to interact

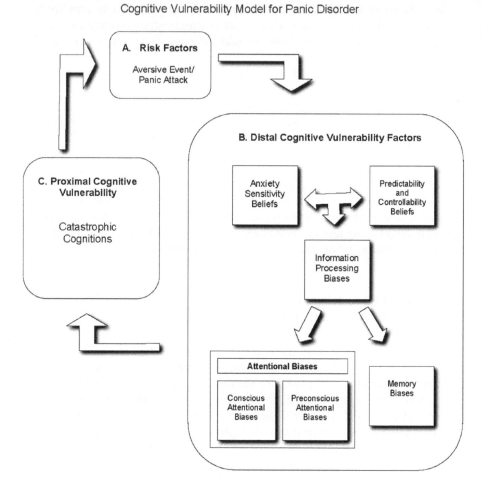

FIG. 8.1.   A model of panic disorder integrating cognitive risk and cognitive vulnerability factors.

with vulnerability factors in the development of the condition. A stressful life event (risk factor) may generally increase the likelihood of the development of panic attacks, but only because it contributes to changes in a cognitive diathesis (vulnerability factor). For example, the stressor increases anxiety sensitivity, which in turn increases the likelihood of panic. The proposed model (Fig. 8.1) distinguishes between risk factors for panic disorder, cognitive vulnerability factors for panic, and the interrelations among these factors.

The integrated cognitive vulnerability model of panic disorder is characterized by a number of interrelated cognitive processes. It is notable that the processes are described within a "vicious cycle" model whereby it is postulated that certain processes serve to maintain themselves. This model is divided into three main domains indicated by the three large boxes entitled Aversive Event/Panic Attack, Distal Cognitive Vulnerability Factors, and Proximal Cognitive Vulnerability. A reasonable starting point in describing the model is the box labeled Aversive Event/Panic Attack. This particular aspect is the postulated entry point for the inception of the cognitive vulnerability factors. Distal cognitive vulnerability factors are typically hypothesized to evolve out of a specific type of learning history that often involves aversive events. The model also included the experience of a panic attack as a specific instance of an aversive event, but obviously panic attacks are an important outcome of the cycle to be described. In the case of such an attack, a tautology is avoided because panic attacks per se are necessary but not sufficient for a diagnosis of panic disorder.

In terms of this entry point, it is also worth noting that risk factors for panic are also likely to impact both the likelihood of certain types of aversive events (e.g., strange cardiac sensations that result from having MVP), as well as the likelihood that these events will lead to the type of pernicious cognitive changes characterized by the cognitive vulnerability factors. The best established risk factors for panic disorder include gender, age, medical conditions, and negative life events. Epidemiological data suggest that gender is a risk factor for panic disorder (Katerndahl & Realini, 1993; Robins et al., 1984). Females have approximately twice the lifetime risk for panic disorder than males after adjusting for race, marital status, and socioeconomic status. The median age of onset for panic disorder is 24 years, and young adults appear to be at the highest risk for the development of panic disorder (Barlow, 1988; Eaton & Keyl, 1995). In addition, medical conditions such as a history of migraines appear to increase risk for the development of anxiety pathology (Breslau & Davis, 1993). Finally, the experience of negative life events, such as loss (e.g., death), has been associated with the development of panic (Faravelli & Pallanti, 1989). Two controlled studies found that patients with panic disorder experienced more negative life events during the year prior to panic than a matched group of nonclinical controls during the same period (Faravelli & Pallanti, 1989; Roy-Byrne, Geraci, & Uhde, 1986).

Exactly how these risk factors operate in panic disorder is open to some speculation. For example, these risks may be related to an underlying pathophysiologic factor. In the context of a cognitive vulnerability model, however, it would be hypothesized that these risk factors convey a specific risk for the production of change to the cognitive processes involved in the model. For example, individuals with certain medical conditions that produce unpleasant bodily sensations are likely to be at increased risk for heightened anxiety sensitivity. Similarly, females or individuals at a certain age may also be more prone toward change in certain types of cognitive processes relevant to the model.

The general idea is that certain types of aversive experiences are likely to be involved in the initial development of cognitive vulnerability factors. Within the box identified as distal cognitive vulnerability factors in the proposed model, there are three interrelated domains: anxiety sensitivity beliefs, predictability and control beliefs, and information-processing biases. Information-processing biases are further subdivided into attentional processes (both conscious and preconscious) and explicit memory biases. These are believed to represent the core cognitive processes that are likely to result in the generation and maintenance of panic disorder. A reciprocal relation among these processes is suggested because general cognitive changes are likely to be related and to exert some influence on other types of related cognitive processes. For example, seeing a loved one unexpectedly die from a heart attack (aversive event) is likely to create cardiac fears (heighten anxiety sensitivity), as well as beliefs about the predictability and control over aversive events. These changes in beliefs should also likely affect information processing for threat-relevant (e.g., cardiac) cues. The proposed interrelations among these cognitive risk factors is one of the more speculative aspects of the model as there are relatively few studies that have specifically examined these relations. However, some degree of independence or even complete independence is not problematic for this particular model because all of these factors are proposed to have a common outcome.

According to our model, individuals develop a number of related cognitive vulnerability factors but they are distinguished from the final factor, which has been labeled proximal cognitive vulnerability. In this case, the cognitive vulnerability is the production of catastrophic cognition. Catastrophic cognition involves thoughts about threat or danger (e.g., "I'm having a heart attack," "This anxiety will lead me to lose control of my car," "I'm going to make a fool of myself"). Consistent with cognitive models of fear, threat-related cognition is necessary for the production of a fear response such as a panic attack.

There are a number of reasons to distinguish catastrophic cognition from the other cognitive processes already described. As the labels would imply, a distinction is made between one factor that is believed to be more directly or proximally involved in pathogenesis (i.e., catastrophic cognition) and other factors believed to increase the risk for pathogenesis (i.e., anxiety sensitivity, predictability and control beliefs, and information-processing biases). Therefore, higher levels of distal cognitive vulnerability factors will increase the likelihood for the specific cognitive vulnerability factor (e.g., high anxiety sensitivity increases the likelihood that the individual will experience catastrophic cognition resulting in a panic attack, information-processing biases directed toward threat increase the likelihood that the individual will perceive the "threat" that can be catastrophically appraised).

It is also useful to distinguish between the cognitive vulnerability factors in terms of necessity versus sufficiency, and proximity or state versus trait qualities. In relation to necessity, each of the cognitive theories of panic posits that catastrophic ideation of some sort (conscious or preconscious) is necessary and sufficient for the production of a fear response. The model where this is clearest is Clark's description of catastrophic misinterpretation. In the case of Reiss' model, catastrophic ideation results from the interaction between the set of predisposing beliefs that constitute anxiety sensitivity and the experience of arousal (e.g., "These cardiac symptoms I'm experiencing mean I'm probably going to have a heart attack").

The role of catastrophic cognition is least apparent in Barlow's model. His model has an implicit appraisal of threat connected with perceptions regarding loss of control. Thus, an implicit or explicit and conscious or "preconscious" threat appraisal appears to be central to the main cognitive theories of panic. The term *catastrophic cognition* may be used to distinguish this element from catastrophic misinterpretation (Cox, 1996). Catastrophic cognition implies a state characterized by the active perception of threat, but it does not imply a "misinterpretation of arousal," which is potentially problematic for Clark (see McNally, 1994).

The rationale for a distinction between cognitive vulnerability factors rests with the assumption that certain cognitive factors may less immediately influence the pathogenesis of panic. Whereas distal cognitive vulnerability factors may exist in an individual, and they are believed to be necessary in the development of panic disorder, factors such as anxiety sensitivity are not sufficient for the production of acute fear responses. For example, there are many individuals with high anxiety sensitivity that do not have a history of panic attacks or clinical anxiety disorders (Schmidt & Bates, 2003). On the other hand, an individual who has a catastrophic thought ("I'm dying") should have a fear response regardless of the presence or severity of the distal cognitive vulnerability factors.

Catastrophic cognition can be separated from other cognitive vulnerability factors to convey a proximal distinction from catastrophic ideation, which can be viewed as one of the most proximal components of the fear response. In other words, catastrophic ideation is believed to immediately precede the generation of a fear response. Cognitive vulnerability factors, such as anxiety sensitivity or information-processing biases, might be viewed as more distal factors that do not necessarily or immediately trigger a fear response but simply increase the risk for catastrophic ideation.

Another way of considering this process is that catastrophic cognition can be considered to be more of a state variable that is required for the creation of a fear response, whereas cognitive risk variables are trait characteristics of the individual.

What makes the integrated model somewhat distinct from previous models is the separation that is being made between a set of distal cognitive factors and a more proximal cognitive vulnerability factor. Recalling the various models of panic, Clark emphasized the proximal vulnerability component (i.e., catastrophic cognition), whereas the Barlow and Reiss models underscore distal factors (i.e., anxiety sensitivity, predictability and control). McNally (1994) highlighted this distinction in terms of cognitive risk factors being dispositional constructs and catastrophic cognition being an occurrent (i.e., episodic) concept.

This so-called integrated cognitive model proposed herein is certainly not an entirely novel concept. Indeed, a similar model has been proposed by Cox (1996). Cox speculated that panic disorder arises from a multidimensional trait that interacts with a trait congruent trigger to produce catastrophic ideation. In this model, the multidimensional trait is basically an expanded version of anxiety sensitivity. In the presence of an appropriate cue such as somatic perturbations, this trait predisposes the individual to have catastrophic thoughts. The primary difference between our integrated cognitive model and that proposed by Cox is that Cox's model does not incorporate other cognitive risk factors such as perceptions of predictability and control (Plaks et al., 2005) or information-processing biases. These factors that are explicitly delineated in the present model, however, appear to be compatible with the Cox model.

EVIDENCE SUPPORTING THE COGNITIVE VULNERABILITY MODEL OF PANIC DISORDER

Now that an integrated cognitive model of panic disorder has been described, the following sections review evidence supporting these cognitive factors, their interrelations, and their links with panic.

Origins of Distal Cognitive Vulnerability Factors

The initial section of the model (Aversive Event/Panic Attack) represents a composite element that may contain factors that influence cognitive vulnerability factors as well as outcomes of cognitive vulnerability for panic. It represents a potential starting point for consideration of the development or influences on cognitive vulnerability factors (e.g., an aversive event leads to a change in cognitive beliefs relevant to anxiety sensitivity).

This section is also a termination point for the cascade of cognitive and emotional processes that occur during a fear response (e.g., panic attack). Thus, the vicious cycle highlights the idea that these events will also maintain and exacerbate existing maladaptive cognitive processes.

First consider the data supporting this link. Specifically, the "Where do these cognitive vulnerability factors come from?" aspect of the model deserves attention because relatively little is known about the etiology of these cognitive vulnerability factors. In terms of anxiety sensitivity, there are few studies that have investigated factors that contribute to its development. Watt, Stewart, and Cox (1998) retrospectively examined the impact of learning history on anxiety sensitivity and found that a childhood history of frequent experiences with anxiety and parentally reinforced sick-role behavior were significant predictors of adult levels of anxiety sensitivity. Watt et al. (1998) hypothesized that the pathway to the development of anxiety sensitivity is by learning to fear general body sensations rather than anxiety-specific symptoms.

Watt and Stewart (2000) supported and extended this finding through an investigation of how instrumental and vicarious learning were influenced by parental responses to both a child's and a parent's own nonanxiety-related (i.e., pain, lumps, stomach problems, and tiredness) and anxiety-related symptoms (Watt & Stewart, 2000). Instrumental and vicarious childhood learning experiences that displayed parental reinforcement and modeling of both general-anxiety-related and nonanxiety-related symptoms were found to be related to higher levels of anxiety sensitivity (Watt & Stewart, 2000). Stewart et al. (2001) subsequently developed a model explaining the relations between childhood learning history, anxiety sensitivity, and the development of panic attacks using retrospective self-reports of college students. Stewart and colleagues proposed that childhood learning history directly influences the development of panic attacks; childhood learning experiences directly influence anxiety sensitivity levels; and heightened anxiety sensitivity levels directly influence panic attacks. These hypotheses were confirmed in the study and are in agreement with prior research investigations (Stewart et al., 2001). These proposals, in turn, led to some additional work suggesting that heightened anxiety sensitivity acts as a mediating factor between childhood learning experiences and panic attacks in adulthood (Stewart et al., 2001).

Research on the etiology of anxiety sensitivity was extended through a prospective test of whether or not the experience of stressors like a panic attack may be partially responsible for increases in anxiety sensitivity. This hypothesis fits with data showing higher levels of anxiety sensitivity in nonclinical and clinical samples reporting panic attacks. In terms of a specific mechanism, it is likely that the experience of intense arousal (panic) provides an opportunity for the development of erroneous beliefs about arousal symptoms. We were particularly interested in evaluating the relation between anxiety sensitivity and the experience of one specific experience (i.e., spontaneous panic) that creates high levels of arousal as well as the experience of more general emotional experiences (e.g., anxiety and depression) also associated with unpleasant bodily sensations. In our study, levels of anxiety sensitivity were evaluated prior to and following basic training in a large military sample. Data indicated that the specific stressor of experiencing a panic attack as well as general stressors creating significant anxiety symptoms uniquely contributed to increased levels of anxiety sensitivity over time regardless of prior history of panic (Schmidt, Lerew, & Joiner, 2000). It was concluded that anxiety-related stressors appear to have the potential to "scar" individuals in regard to this cognitive vulnerability factor.

Studies of adults suffering from anxiety disorders have consistently found evidence that anxiety is associated with information-processing biases such as attention and memory biases toward threatening or negative information (for a review see Mogg & Bradley, 1998; Coles & Heimberg, 2002; Lang & Sarmiento, 2004). But how do these information-processing biases develop? Despite a fairly extensive literature on information processing, relatively few studies reveal anything about development of these information-processing biases. The relevant few suggest that information-processing biases can be learned and, similar to the case with anxiety sensitivity, conditioning in the context of aversive events may play an important role in their development (Merckelbach, van Hout, de Jong, & van den Hout, 1990). An extensive review of evidence by Coles and Heimberg (2002) regarding the involvement of memory biases in anxiety disorders discusses three theories of information processing in anxiety disorders: Beck's theory of cognitive schemata, Bower's theory of associative networks, and a model proposed by Williams, Watts, MacLeod, and Mathews (1988, 1997). Although Beck's theory of cognitive schemata and Bower's theory of associative networks both failed to make a distinction between explicit and implicit memory in information processing regarding anxiety, Williams et al. (1988) incorporated these memory processes along with reasons for a cognitive bias in anxiety versus depression into an integrative model explaining how information processes might develop (Coles & Heimberg, 2002). Williams et al. (1988) interpreted the results of previous studies to infer a vigilance–avoidance pattern for information processing with anxiety disorders suggesting that there is an initial increase in automatic attention to threat (vigilance) followed by strategic efforts to distance from it (avoidance). This pattern is believed to maintain anxiety by preventing habituation to threatening material. Coles and Heimberg (2002) pointed out inconsistencies in findings regarding the vigilance–avoidance model in anxiety disorders and indicated that much more research is needed in order to investigate the development and patterns of memory biases in the anxiety disorders.

In terms of attentional bias involved in information processing, MacLeod, Ebsworthy, and Rutherford (2002) manipulated information-processing biases and demonstrated that an attentional bias can be trained. In this study, attentional bias toward threat was produced following training in which participants' attention was consistently directed toward threat versus neutral words during a probe detection task. This study suggests that when individuals learn to direct their attention toward threatening information, the attentional processing can become an automatic information-processing bias.

The literature on early influences on controllability and predictability is much more extensive. A thorough summary is beyond the scope of this chapter because the support for these vulnerability factors is extensive and has been thoroughly reviewed elsewhere (Chorpita & Barlow, 1998). In general, this literature suggests that a variety of developmental, physiological, and biological factors influence a person's subsequent perception of control and the predictability of anxiety-related events (although much of this research is inferential). Thus, experiencing the world as uncontrollable and unpredictable during childhood and adolescence is implicated in subsequent deficits in control-related cognitions (Chorpita & Barlow, 1998).

Distal Cognitive Vulnerability Factors

Anxiety Sensitivity

Although anxiety sensitivity is elevated in panic disorder and other anxiety disorders (Taylor, Koch, & McNally, 1992), an important prediction of the anxiety sensitivity conceptualization is that anxiety sensitivity should act as a vulnerability factor for the development of panic attacks and related anxiety disorders. Taken together, laboratory and prospective studies provide converging evidence for anxiety sensitivity as a vulnerability factor in the development of anxiety pathology.

Challenge studies using nonclinical subjects with no history of spontaneous panic have demonstrated that anxiety sensitivity is predictive of fearful responding to hyperventilation, caffeine, and 35% carbon dioxide inhalation (Donnell & McNally, 1989; Harrington, Schmidt, & Telch, 1996; Rapee & Medoro, 1994; Schmidt & Telch, 1994; Telch, Silverman, & Schmidt, 1996). For example, Schmidt and Telch (1994) investigated the singular and joint effects of anxiety sensitivity and perceived safety of hypocapnia-induced bodily cues on nonclinical subjects' subjective and psychophysiological response to a 2-minute hyperventilation challenge. Subjects with no history of spontaneous panic were randomly assigned to one of two informational conditions (Safety Information vs. No Safety Information). When anticipating hyperventilation, High Anxiety Sensitivity–Safety Information subjects reported higher subjective anxiety compared to Low Anxiety Sensitivity–Safety Information subjects. During hyperventilation, anxiety and safety information exerted independent effects on subjective responding. High anxiety sensitivity subjects reported higher levels of subjective fear and physical symptoms compared to low anxiety sensitivity subjects; subjects who received safety information reported lower levels of anxiety and physical symptoms as compared to those who did not receive safety information.

Whereas longitudinal studies of clinical populations allow for the examination of the role of anxiety sensitivity in the long-term course of anxiety pathology, prospective studies of anxiety sensitivity in nonclinical samples permit the evaluation of the initial incidence of anxiety pathology. Such studies are important in evaluating the effects of anxiety sensitivity because in nonclinical and symptom-free individuals with no history of anxiety disorder, anxiety sensitivity cannot be attributed to preexisting anxiety pathology (Schmidt, 1999). In general, longitudinal studies suggest that individuals with elevated anxiety sensitivity are at increased risk for the development of anxiety pathology (Ehlers, 1995; Maller & Reiss, 1992).

Our lab was responsible for two large prospective studies using a military sample (Schmidt, Lerew, & Jackson, 1997, 1999). These data were collected at the U.S. Air Force Academy (USAFA) during Basic Cadet Training (BCT). The context of basic training is ideal for evaluating individuals under a great amount of stress and is therefore appropriate for evaluating diathesis–stress relations. In each study, more than 1,000 cadets were evaluated over the course of their first 5 weeks of training.

Both studies (Schmidt et al., 1997, 1999) revealed that approximately 6% of the sample reported experiencing at least one spontaneous panic attack during BCT. In most of these cases, there was no prior history of panic. As predicted, anxiety sensitivity was significantly associated with the development of spontaneous panic. This is true both for new cases of panic as well as for those cadets with a history of panic attacks. Although the Schmidt et al. studies did not utilize diagnostic interviews, we did assess for additional anxiety symptoms that allow for tentative conclusions about the development of anxiety disorder diagnoses. In the first study, of those reporting spontaneous panic attacks during BCT, 22% reported three or more such attacks and 28% reported significant worry about having additional attacks or the consequences of panic. Many of these individuals also endorsed symptoms on the Beck Anxiety Inventory (BAI) and Beck Depression Inventory (BDI) in the clinically significant range. In addition, those experiencing multiple panic attacks or panic-related worry generally reported that anxiety had created moderate levels of impairment in their ability to function during BCT. In this regard, we may tentatively conclude that higher levels of anxiety sensitivity are not only predictive of the incidence of spontaneous panic but are associated with the development of a broader range of clinically significant anxiety symptoms and possibly formal anxiety disorders.

In addition, Plehn and Peterson (2002) conducted another study investigating the relation between anxiety sensitivity and the development of panic attacks and panic disorder. A sample consisting of 505 undergraduate subjects attending an urban university was recruited between 1986 and 1988. In 1999, 178 of these subjects were contacted for a follow-up inquiry. The researchers found that anxiety sensitivity was a significant predictor of later panic attacks (Plehn & Peterson, 2002). Unexpectedly, anxiety sensitivity did not predict panic disorder. In a large prospective study, Weems, Hayward, Killen, and Taylor (2002) followed over 2,000 high school students for 4 years. High anxiety sensitivity, as well as unstable anxiety sensitivity, was predictive of panic attacks. In concordance with Schmidt et al. (1997, 1999), anxiety sensitivity appears to be a predispositional variable that plays a role in the development of later anxiety symptoms and panic attacks but evidence for full-blown clinical syndromes is not compelling as yet.

In terms of assessing anxiety sensitivity, the Anxiety Sensitivity Index (ASI) is the most widely employed assessment tool. Evidence suggest that the ASI is really a hierarchical model consisting of three group factors (AS–Physical Concerns, AS–Mental Incapacitation Concerns, and AS–Social Concerns) and one general factor (global anxiety sensitivity) (Zinbarg & Schmidt, 2002). Due to the hierarchical nature of the ASI, some questions have been raised concerning which factors of the ASI are measuring anxiety sensitivity and which elements of the ASI factor into particular anxiety disorders. Zvolensky and Forsyth (2002) investigated the relation between the three lower order factors of ASI and bodily sensations in a nonclinical population. They found that the AS–Physical Concerns was the best predictor of body vigilance, whereas the AS–Mental Incapacitation Concerns subscale had predictive validity concerning emotional avoidance (Zvolensky & Forsyth, 2002). Also, Zinbarg, Brown, Barlow, and Rapee (2001) found evidence suggesting that the AS–Physical Concerns factor is the most critical in accounting for panic attacks (Zinbarg et al., 2001). Zinbarg and colleagues did note that it would be premature to dismiss the role of all three group factors in the etiology and maintenance of other anxiety disorders. Clearly, this is an area that merits further investigation.

Predictability and Control Beliefs

Predictability and controllability of aversive events are believed to be important parameters that affect the generation of anxiety and panic (Barlow, 1988). Specifically, unpredictable and uncontrollable threatening events are believed to produce greater anxiety relative to predictable and controllable events (Mineka & Kihlstrom, 1978). Although predictability and control are likely to have relevance to a number of anxiety conditions, these constructs appear to be particularly relevant for panic attacks and panic disorder (Chorpita & Barlow, 1998). For example, predictability is likely to be crucial in terms of the spontaneous panic attacks that are the hallmark feature of panic disorder (Barlow, Chorpita, & Turovsky, 1996). However, the construct of controllability has received greater attention and has resulted in a number of theoretical models that postulate uncontrollability as a vulnerability factor for anxiety (Alloy, Kelly, Mineka, & Clements, 1990; Chorpita & Barlow, 1998).

There is also reasonable empirical support for the relation between predictability and control and the development of anxiety. In terms of predictability, the majority of evidence is based on animal studies (Minor, Dess, & Overmier, 1991). However, Schmidt and Lerew (2002), using a nonclinical sample, found some evidence that predictability interacts with anxiety sensitivity to predict anxiety. Furthermore, evidence from clinical samples is consistent with the notion that unpredictability of aversive events such as panic attacks is likely to engender greater concern and anxiety symptoms (Craske, Glover, & DeCola, 1995). Finally, laboratory studies suggest that humans prefer predictable aversive stimuli to unpredictable aversive stimuli (Lejuez, Eifert, Zvolensky, & Richards, 2000).

In terms of control, studies of clinical and nonclinical samples indicate that lower levels of perceived control are related to anxiety (Chorpita, Brown, & Barlow, 1998; Roy-Byrne, Mellman, & Uhde, 1986). More specifically, patients with panic disorder report that they have low control regarding regulation of their emotional experiences (Clum & Knowels, 1991) as well as little ability to control or cope with panic attacks (Telch, Brouillard, Telch, Agras, & Taylor, 1989). Sanderson, Rapee, and Barlow (1989) demonstrated the importance of perceived control in the genesis of panic. Using a CO_2 challenge, Sanderson et al. instructed patients with panic disorder that a dial placed nearby would allow them to control the flow of CO_2 (i.e., the intensity of sensations) during the test if a light was illuminated. The light was illuminated for half of the subjects (illusion of control group), but in reality the dial was inoperative for all subjects. The illusion of control group, in line with the cognitive mediation hypothesis, was significantly less likely to panic and reported fewer catastrophic cognitions than the control group. More recent research indicates that control exerts a similar influence on high anxious nonclinical subjects in the context of biological challenges (Telch et al., 1996; Zvolensky, Eifert, Lejuez, & McNeil, 1999). For example, subjects were randomly assigned to either a perceived control (PC) or a no perceived control (NPC) instructional set during a caffeine (450 mcg) challenge (Telch et al., 1996). Perceived control over caffeine-induced arousal was manipulated by providing half of the subjects an ostensible "caffeine antidote" with instructions that they could ingest the antidote and counteract the caffeine should its effects become too uncomfortable (perceived control). The other half of the subjects were told that the effects of the caffeine, however unpleasant, would persist for several hours (no perceived control). As expected, those in the perceived control condition reported lower subjective anxiety in the context of the challenge. Another study has suggested that lack of control over external events might be associated with a greater interpretive bias toward threat (Zvolensky et al., 2001). Zvolensky et al. tested a nonclinical sample and found that a lower level of perceived control was associated with greater interpretive bias for threat (Zvolensky et al., 2001). These findings suggest that the response to ambiguous situations might be influenced by a person's perceived lack of control in regard to anxiety-related events.

Information-Processing Biases

Conscious Attentional Biases. The process of monitoring internal states has broad relevance for many theories of emotion and has been described by terms such as visceral perception, autonomic perception, symptom perception, and interoception (McLeod & Hoehn-Saric, 1993; Pennebaker, 1982). There are individual differences in monitoring and evaluation of internal sensations. Some individuals fail to seek medical care despite symptoms or report no awareness of significant physiological events such as myocardial infarction (Beunderman, van Dis, & Duyvis, 1987). Others closely monitor internal sensations and repeatedly present for medical evaluation when there is no evidence to suggest organic etiology. In the case of panic disorder, individuals appear to excessively monitor internal sensations because they report very high levels of symptoms and repeatedly seek out medical evaluations despite reassurances from health care providers (Weissman, 1991). In a related study, Schmidt, Lerew, and Trakowski (1997) investigated the role of conscious attentional vigilance in panic disorder. In particular, *body vigilance* refers to conscious attention focused on internal bodily sensations and perturbations. Excessive body vigilance is elevated in panic disorder relative to other anxiety disorders and appears to be a natural consequence of learning to fear bodily sensations and, therefore, is likely to play a role in the development of panic disorder (Schmidt, Lerew, & Trakowski, 1997). The vigilance concept is distinguished from previous work in that it focuses on changes in conscious attention regardless of accuracy. Accordingly, the act of perception, independent of its accuracy, is a process that may contribute to maintaining panic disorder.

According to Richards, Cooper, and Winkelman (2003), nonclinical panickers more often and more accurately predicted change in the sympathetic nervous system than control nonpanickers indicating an association between body vigilance and panic. Stewart, Buffett-Jerrott, and Kokaram (2001) tested heart rate reactivity, perceived heart rate, and anxiety sensitivity in a group of nonclinical college students. Findings indicated that there was no difference in heart rate reactivity to an arousal-induced challenge and there were no significant differences between groups in terms of physiological reactivity to stressors (Stewart, Buffett-Jerrott, & Kokaram, 2001). They did reveal that subjects with high anxiety sensitivity levels were more accurate in estimating heart rate regardless of arousal level (Stewart, Buffett-Jerrott, & Kokaram, 2001). This research is in line with other findings, which indicate interoceptive acuity or body vigilance might be characteristic of high anxiety sensitivity (Stewart, Buffett-Jerrott, & Kokaram, 2001).

The model of body vigilance described by Schmidt, Lerew, and Trakowski (1997) suggests that panic-related worry (i.e., worry about autonomic arousal or anxiety sensitivity) should lead to vigilance for related interoceptive threat cues. This hypothesis was tested experimentally, and consistent with this model, body vigilance was significantly associated with anxiety sensitivity in both the nonclinical and panic disorder samples. Thus, there is some evidence for an association between the vulnerability factors posited in Fig. 8.1. There was actually a higher level of association in the clinical sample, suggesting that the development of a formal panic disorder syndrome may produce a closer connection between panic-related worry and body vigilance. Interestingly, posttreatment findings indicated that treated patients showed less body vigilance than nonclinical samples suggesting that vigilance is readily malleable when it becomes the focus of treatment intervention.

Preconscious Attentional Biases. Anxiety disordered patients, in general, and panic disordered patients, in particular, show a preconscious attentional bias to threat-related words (Burgess, Jones, Robertson, Radcliffe, & Emerson, 1981). For example, McNally, Riemann, and Kim (1990) compared attentional biases for threat words in patients with panic disorder and controls using a modified Stroop color naming task. During the Stroop task, patients showed longer response latencies relative to controls. This line of research is strengthened by evidence that patients have an attentional bias for disorder-relevant cues. Keogh, Dillon, Georgiou, and

Hunt (2001) tested subjects with high and low anxiety sensitivity using a visual dot-probe paradigm in order to evaluate attentional bias toward physical threatening, socially threatening, and positive words. Individuals with high physical anxiety sensitivity selectively attended to physically threatening words and selectively avoided positive words in relation to those low in anxiety sensitivity (Keogh et al., 2001). Those low in anxiety sensitivity selectively avoided physically threatening stimuli and attended to positive stimuli (Keogh et al., 2001). Socially threatening words elicited no processing differences from either group (Keogh et al., 2001). It appears that biased attentional processes toward physical threat may result from greater body vigilance in high anxiety individuals (Keogh et al., 2001). Hope, Rapee, Heimberg, and Dombeck (1990) compared panickers and social phobics on attentional bias for physical, neutral, or social threat words using a modified Stroop task. Findings indicated that patients with panic disorder had relatively longer latencies in terms of responding to physical threat words, whereas patients with social phobia had relatively greater attentional biases to social threat cues. There are also prospective studies indicating that attentional biases predict the development of anxiety reactions (MacLeod & Hagan, 1992).

Memory Biases. In addition to attentional biases, patients with panic disorder show a memory bias for threat-related cues. It has been suggested that cognitive representations of threat may be in a somewhat primed state in memory that allows them to be more readily accessed by patients that are cued into threat (McNally, 1994). In general, patients with panic disorder can recall more anxiety than nonanxiety words, whereas nonclinical controls show the reverse pattern (McNally, Foa, & Donnell, 1989). However, the memory bias in panic disorder appears to be primarily explicit. Explicit memory is indicated by conscious recollection of previous experiences, but implicit memory is assessed using tasks that do not require deliberate recollection of these experiences. Coles and Heimberg (2002) reviewed all previous work on explicit and implicit memory noting that 15 studies have investigated explicit memory biases in panic disorder but only 5 have addressed implicit memory biases. Explicit memory is typically assessed using free recall and cued recall tasks; implicit memory is usually assessed using word stem completion tasks. For example, Lundh, Czyzykow, and Ost (1997) compared patients with panic disorder to nonclinical controls on explicit (cued recall) and implicit (word stem completion) memory tasks for physical and social threat words, as well as neutral cues. Results showed that patients had an explicit memory bias but not an implicit memory bias for physical threat words. Overall, of the studies evaluated by Coles and Heimberg (2002), 9 of 15 studies have shown evidence of an explicit memory bias for threat. The remaining 6 studies that have shown little or no support for explicit memory bias, in general, did not encourage depth of processing while presenting "a large number of stimuli" (Coles & Heimberg, 2002). Out of the 5 studies that examined implicit memory bias in panic disorder, only 2 have shown a bias for threat (Coles & Heimberg, 2002). This led these authors to suggest that it would be premature to draw any conclusions from the current studies because of the lack of research on implicit memory bias in panic disorder. Harrison and Turpin (2003) studied implicit memory in individuals who were not clinically anxious but who were ranked as either high or low in trait anxiety (Harrison & Turpin, 2003). The study was unusual in that it implemented implicit memory, heart rate, and electrodermal responses. The findings indicated, for all subjects, an implicit memory bias toward nonthreat words, as measured by performance and psychophysiological indices, on an implicit memory paradigm (Harrison & Turpin, 2003). Clearly, more research is needed to better understand the effects of memory biases on panic disorder.

Proximal Cognitive Vulnerability

Laboratory studies have yielded considerable support for a cognitive vulnerability for panic. Consistent with cognitive models (most notably Clark, 1986), patients with panic disorder report that thoughts of danger typically accompany their panic attacks (Beck, Laude, & Bohnert, 1974; Hibbert, 1984; Ottavani & Beck, 1987), and such thoughts tend to occur after the detection of a bodily sensation (Hibbert, 1984; Ley, 1985). Clark (1986) predicted that panic in response to a challenge procedure will occur only when the sensations associated with the procedure are catastrophically interpreted. Evidence tends to support this idea because patients with panic disorder who panic in response to challenge procedures report catastrophic cognition such as thoughts of going crazy or losing control, whereas those who do not panic when challenged report no such thoughts (Yeragani, Balon, & Pohl, 1989).

Additional evidence in support of the hypothesis that catastrophic cognition influences whether an individual panics during biological challenge is provided by studies that manipulate the tendency to catastrophize during challenges. It has been demonstrated that manipulation of danger expectancies can influence the degree of anxiety experienced during CO_2 inhalation (van den Hout & Griez, 1982) and lactate infusion (van der Molen, van den Hout, Vroeman, Lousberg, & Griez, 1986). For example, Rapee (1986) manipulated the pre CO_2 challenge instructions given to two groups of patients. One group was provided instructions that described the sensations induced by an inhalation of 50% CO_2 gas. All possible sensations were detailed, and their cause was attributed to the CO_2. A second group was provided with no explanation of the procedure. As predicted, the no explanation group reported significantly more catastrophic cognitions and significantly more panic in response to the inhalation than the detailed information group. Similarly, Clark et al. (1992) tested the cognitive mediation hypothesis by manipulating pre-challenge instructions using a lactate challenge. Patients were randomized to one of two pre-infusion instructional sets, both of which emphasized that lactate is harmless and the patient could stop the infusion at any time. In the experimental group however, the instructions also stressed that lactate is a normal substance, that it is normal to experience sensations during infusion, and such sensations do not indicate bodily harm or danger. During the infusion, patients given the experimental instructions reported significantly less anxiety, less panic, and had smaller physiological arousal.

It is also worth noting that several prominent researchers have argued that catastrophic misinterpretation is not a necessary or sufficient ingredient for panic (D. F. Klein & H. M. Klein, 1989; Teasdale, 1988). Empirical studies have also questioned the necessity of catastrophic cognition. Some challenge studies have found that some patients will panic without reporting catastrophic cognitions (Aronson, Whitaker-Azmitia, & Caraseti, 1989). In addition, Rachman (1988) found that some patients with panic disorder report catastrophic ideation without actually panicking, whereas other patients will report panic without catastrophic ideation (Rachman, Lopatka, & Levitt, 1988). Barlow's (1988) model would explain the absence of apparent catastrophic cognition though interoceptive conditioning, but Clark (1986) maintained that catastrophic misinterpretation may occur preconsciously. Unfortunately, this aspect of Clark's (1986) theory appears to render it unfalsifiable. As McNally (1994) pointed out, "If misinterpretations can be either conscious or unconscious, it is difficult to imagine what would count as evidence against the hypothesis that misinterpretations necessarily precede panics" (p. 115). Despite some conceptual problems, as well as some empirical evidence regarding the necessity of catastrophic cognition, evidence suggests that catastrophic ideation is likely to play a role in some panic attacks and in the development of some (perhaps most) cases of panic disorder.

Cognitive vulnerability to panic disorder has received considerable attention. A review of this literature clearly indicates that cognitive factors play an important role in its development. In the past decade, a number of such factors have been delineated, including anxiety sensitivity beliefs, predictability and control beliefs, and several types of information-processing bias. Evidence also suggests that catastrophic cognition, often directed at aversive somatic cues, is likely to be a proximal cognitive vulnerability factor for panic disorder. But what is the overall association between any specific cognitive factor and outcomes such as panic disorder? In most studies, the association between cognitive vulnerability factors and outcome variables such panic attack occurrence, psychological distress, and physical and functional impairment, although significant, accounts for only a limited amount of variance. In terms of panic attack frequency, for example, the unique variance accounted for by anxiety sensitivity in our prospective studies was only about 5% (Schmidt et al., 1999). These data indicate that focus on one or two specific cognitive factors is not likely to be sufficient.

Furthermore, a limitation of this literature is that most studies examine the effects of a single cognitive factor. In part, this is likely due to the fact that considerable effort is needed to simply establish the role of these factors as vulnerability variables. Now that we are in a position to more clearly state that factors such as anxiety sensitivity are established vulnerability factors, it may be useful to approach future studies with a constellation of vulnerability factors in mind. Schmidt and Lerew (2002) investigated the interactions and independent effects of control, predictability, anxiety sensitivity, and the pathogenesis of panic in the context of basic training. There was no evidence that perceived control or predictability exerted an independent effect on the development of panic or anxiety, but there was some evidence of an interaction between anxiety sensitivity and perceived predictability to predict anxiety and between anxiety sensitivity and perceived control to predict panic (Schmidt & Lerew, 2002). The investigators noted that much more work is needed to identify other interactions between factors in the pathogenesis of anxiety and panic disorder (Schmidt & Lerew, 2002). To facilitate future investigations, a composite measure of risk/vulnerability could be constructed that borrows measures from several domains (e.g., bodily hypervigilance, controllability, and anxiety sensitivity). For example, it would be potentially interesting to examine the influence of more proximal perceptions of predictability and control beliefs, more distal beliefs about predictability/control beliefs, as well as the relation between these beliefs and anxiety sensitivity. Evaluation of multiple measures will allow us not only to determine both additive and interactive vulnerability factor effects. The evaluation of the combinations of vulnerability factor variables may substantially increase our capacity to predict outcomes.

Thus, although there is strong evidence to support the role of cognitive variables in panic disorder, considerable additional work is needed to identify other psychological parameters as well as the interaction between psychological, physiological, and even genetic factors in the pathogenesis of anxiety. In a somewhat larger context, it is important to consider cognitive parameters in light of the considerable biological research on panic disorder. In a twin study, Stein and colleagues reported evidence for the heritability of anxiety sensitivity (Stein, Jang, & Livesley, 1999). Another study investigated the levels of anxiety sensitivity in first-degree relatives of patients with panic disorder and indicated that in comparison with healthy controls, first-degree relatives of panic disorder patients were found to have higher anxiety sensitivity levels (Van Beek & Griez, 2003). This is evidence for the involvement of possible genetic factors regarding a cognitive vulnerability factor for panic disorder. Significant advances have been made in the identification of genetic risk factors for anxiety pathology (Gershon & Cloninger, 1994). Converging lines of evidence suggest that anxiety disorders in adulthood may represent manifestations of an underlying constitutional vulnerability or diathesis for anxiety that is partly genetic and variably expressed over the life cycle. An individual's overall risk for pathology is believed to be a function of personal genetic and nongenetic resiliency and vulnerability factors, environmental risk and protective factors, and an interaction among these factors.

We have been very interested in developing an etiological model that integrates well-established biobehavioral models of anxiety (see Schmidt, Storey, et al., 2000). Similar to the model described in this chapter, this theoretical model proposes that there are two necessary processes involved in the pathogenesis of fear, including sets of biological and cognitive processes. These processes essentially include the generation of physiological arousal and the misappraisal of arousal. Whereas deterministic genetic and biological conceptualizations have typically focused on the sufficiency of genetic factors in the pathogenesis of fear, while describing perceptual or attributional processes as epiphenomenal and noncausal, psychobiological conceptualizations of anxiety propose that the generation and perception of arousal are necessary precursors to catastrophic appraisal, which is the final essential element for the development of fear (e.g., Barlow, 1988).

A critical step toward understanding the assumed nature of anxiety pathology should integrate genetic and environmental factors. Advances in molecular genetics now offer the opportunity to incorporate genetic strategies in studies of experimental psychopathology. In accord with the literature, although there is now evidence to support the role of specific cognitive factors in the potentiation of anxiety disorders, considerable additional work is needed to identify other genetic and psychological parameters and to assess their interactive effects on the pathogenesis of panic.

ACKNOWLEDGMENTS

This research was supported by National Institute of Mental Health Grant (MH62056), Ohio Department of Mental Health Grant 00.1136, and an Ameritech Faculty Research Grant.

REFERENCES

Alloy, L. B., Kelly, K. A., Mineka, S., & Clements, C. M. (1990). Comorbidity of anxiety and depressive disorders: A helplessness-hopelessness perspective. In J. D. Maser & C. R. Cloninger (Eds.), *Comorbidity of mood and anxiety disorders* (pp. 499–543). Washington, DC: American Psychiatric Press.

American Psychiatric Association. (1994). *Diagnostic and statistical manual of mental disorders* (4th ed.). Washington, DC: Author.

Antony, M. M., & Barlow, D. H. (1996). Emotion theory as a framework for explaining panic attacks and panic disorder. In R. M. Rapee (Ed.), *Current controversies in the anxiety disorders* (pp. 55–76). New York: Guilford.

Aronson, T. A., Whitaker-Azmitia, P., & Caraseti, I. (1989). Differential reactivity to lactate infusions: The relative role of biological, psychological, and conditioning variables. *Biological Psychiatry, 25*, 469–481.

Barlow, D. H. (1988). *Anxiety and its disorders*. New York: Guilford.

Barlow, D. H. (2002). *Anxiety and its disorders* (2nd ed.). New York: Guilford.

Barlow, D. H., Chorpita, B. F., & Turovsky, J. (1996). Fear, panic, anxiety, and disorders of emotion. In D. Hope (Ed.), *Nebraska symposium on motivation* (pp. 251–328). Lincoln: University of Nebraska Press.

Beck, A. T., Laude, R., & Bohnert, M. (1974). Ideational components of anxiety neurosis. *Archives of General Psychiatry, 31*, 319–325.

Beunderman, R., van Dis, H., & Duyvis, D. (1987). Eine Vergleichsstudie somatischer und psychologischer Symptome bei Patienten mit nicht kardial bedingtem Brustschmerz und solchen mit Myokardinfarkt [A comparison study of somatic and psychological symptoms between patients with noncardiac chest pain and those with myocardial infarction]. In D. O. Nutzinger, D. Pfersmann, T. Welan, & H. G. Zapotoczky (Eds.), *Herzphobie* (pp. 56–65). Stuttgart: Enke.

Breslau, N., & Davis, G. C. (1993). Migraine, physical health and psychiatric disorder: A prospective epidemiologic study in young adults. *Journal of Psychiatric Research, 27*, 211–221.

Burgess, I. S., Jones, L. M., Robertson, S. A., Radcliffe, W. N., & Emerson, E. (1981). The degree of control exerted by phobic and non-phobic verbal stimuli over the recognition behaviour of phobic and non-phobic subjects. *Behaviour Research and Therapy, 19*, 233–243.

Chorpita, B. F., & Barlow, D. H. (1998). The development of anxiety: The role of control in the early environment. *Psychological Bulletin, 124*, 3–21.

Chorpita, B. F., Brown, T. A., & Barlow, D. H. (1998). The development of anxiety: The role of control in the early environment. *Psychological Bulletin, 124*, 3–21.

Clark, D. M. (1986). A cognitive approach to panic. *Behaviour Research and Therapy, 24*, 461–470.

Clark, D. M., Salkovskis, P. M., Middleton, H., Anastasiades, P., Hackmann, A., & Gelder, M. G. (1992). [Cognitive mediation of lactate induced panic]. Unpublished raw data.

Clum, G. A., & Knowels, S. L. (1991). Why do some people with panic disorders become avoidant?: A review. *Clinical Psychology Review, 11*, 295–313.

Coles, M. E., & Heimberg, R. G. (2002). Memory biases in the anxiety disorders: Current status. *Clinical Psychology Review, 22*, 587–627.

Cox, B. J. (1996). The nature and assessment of catastrophic thoughts in panic disorder. *Behaviour Research and Therapy, 34*(4), 363–374.

Craske, M. G., Glover, D., & De Cola, J. (1995). Predicted versus unpredicted panic attacks: Acute versus general distress. *Journal of Abnormal Psychology, 104*, 214–223.

Donnell, C. D., & McNally, R. J. (1989). Anxiety sensitivity and history of panic as predictors of response to hyperventilation. *Behaviour Research and Therapy, 27*, 325–332.

Eaton, W. W., & Keyl, P. M. (1990). Risk factors for the onset of Diagnostic Interview Schedule/*DSM–III* agoraphobia in a prospective, population-based study. *Archives of General Psychiatry, 47*, 819–824.

Ehlers, A. (1995). A 1-year prospective study of panic attacks: Clinical course and factors associated with maintenance. *Journal of Abnormal Psychology, 104,* 164–172.

Faravelli, C., & Pallanti, S. (1989). Recent life events and panic disorder. *American Journal of Psychiatry, 146,* 622–626.

Gershon, E. S., & Cloninger, C. R. (1994). *Genetic approaches to mental disorders.* Washington, DC: American Psychiatric Press.

Harrington, P. H., Schmidt, N. B., & Telch, M. J. (1996). Prospective evaluation of panic potentiation following 35% CO_2 challenge in a nonclinical sample. *American Journal of Psychiatry, 153,* 823–825.

Harrison, L. K., & Turpin, G. (2003). Implicit memory bias and trait anxiety: A psychophysiological analysis. *Biological Psychology, 62,* 97–114.

Hibbert, G. A. (1984). Ideational components of anxiety: Their origin and content. *British Journal of Psychiatry, 144,* 618–624.

Hoehn-Saric, R., & McLeod, D. (1988). Panic and generalized anxiety disorders. In C. G. Last & M. Hersen (Eds.), *Handbook of anxiety disorders* (pp. 109–126). Elmsford, NY: Pergamon.

Hope, D. A., Rapee, R. M., Heimberg, R. G., & Dombeck, M. J. (1990). Representations of the self in social phobia: Vulnerability to social threat. *Cognitive Therapy and Research, 14,* 177–189.

Ingram, R. E., Miranda, J., & Segal, Z. V. (1998). *Cognitive vulnerability to depression.* New York: Guilford.

Jacobi, F., Wittchen, H. U., Holting, C., Hofler, M., Pfister, H., Muller, N., & Lieb, R. (2004). Prevalence, co-morbidity and correlates of mental disorders in the general population: Results from the German Health Interview and Examination Survey (GHS). *Psychological Medicine, 34,* 597–611.

Katerndahl, D. A., & Realini, J. P. (1993). Lifetime prevalence of panic states. *American Journal of Psychiatry, 150,* 246–249.

Keogh, E., Dillon, C., Georgiou, G., & Hunt, C. (2001). Selective attentional biases for physical threat in physical anxiety sensitivity. *Anxiety Disorders, 15,* 299–315.

Klein, D. F., & Klein, H. M. (1989). The substantive effect of variations in panic measurement and agoraphobia definition. *Journal of Anxiety Disorders, 3,* 45–56.

Lang, A. J., & Sarmiento, J. (2004). Relationship of attentional bias to anxiety sensitivity and panic. *Depression and Anxiety, 20,* 190–194.

Lejuez, C. W., Eifert, G. H., Zvolensky, M. J., & Richards, J. B. (2000). Preference between onset predictable and unpredictable administrations of 20% carbon dioxide-enriched air: Implications for better understanding the etiology and treatment of panic disorder. *Journal of Experimental Psychology: Applied, 6,* 349–359.

Ley, R. (1985). Agoraphobia, the panic attack, and the hyperventilation syndrome. *Behaviour Research and Therapy, 23,* 79–81.

Lundh, L.-G., Czyzykow, S., & Ost, L.-G. (1997). Explicit and implicit memory bias in panic disorder with agoraphobia. *Behaviour Research and Therapy, 35,* 1003–1014.

MacLeod, C., Ebsworthy, G., & Rutherford, E. M. (2002). Selective attention and emotional vulnerability: Assessing the causal basis of their association through the experimental induction of attentional bias. *Journal of Abnormal Psychology, 111,* 107–123.

MacLeod, C., & Hagan, R. (1992). Individual differences in the selective processing of threatening information, and emotional responses to a stressful life event. *Behaviour Research and Therapy, 30,* 151–161.

Maller, R. G., & Reiss, S. (1992). Anxiety sensitivity in 1984 and panic attacks in 1987. *Journal of Anxiety Disorders, 6,* 241–247.

McLeod, D. R., & Hoehn-Saric, R. (1993). Perception of physiological changes in normal and pathological anxiety. In R. Hoehn-Saric & D. R. McLeod (Eds.), *Biology of anxiety disorders* (pp. 223–243). Washington, DC: American Psychiatric Press.

McNally, R. J. (1994). *Panic disorder: A critical analysis.* New York: Guilford.

McNally, R. J., & Foa, E. B. (1987). Cognition and agoraphobia: Bias in the interpretation of threat. *Cognitive Therapy and Research, 11,* 567–581.

McNally, R. J., Foa, E. B., & Donnell, C. D. (1989). Memory bias for anxiety information in patients with panic disorder. *Cognition and Emotion, 3,* 27–44.

McNally, R. J., Riemann, B. C., & Kim, E. (1990). Selective processing of threat cues in panic disorder. *Behaviour Research and Therapy, 28,* 407–412.

Merckelbach, H., van Hout, W., de Jong, P., & van den Hout, M. A. (1990). Classical conditioning and attentional bias. *Journal of Behavior Therapy and Experimental Psychiatry, 21,* 185–191.

Mineka, S., & Kihlstrom, J. F. (1978). Unpredictable and uncontrollable events: A new perspective on experimental neurosis. *Journal of Abnormal Psychology, 87,* 256–271.

Minor, T. R., Dess, N. K., & Overmier, J. B. (1991). Inverting the traditional view of "learned helplessness." In M. R. Denny (Ed.), *Fear, avoidance, and phobias: A fundamental analysis* (pp. 87–134). Hillsdale, NJ: Lawrence Erlbaum Associates.

Mogg, K., & Bradley, B. P. (1998). A cognitive-motivational analysis of anxiety. *Behaviour Research and Therapy, 36,* 809–848.

Norton, G. R., Harrison, B., Hauch, J., & Rhodes, L. (1985). Characteristics of people with infrequent panic attacks. *Journal of Abnormal Psychology, 94,* 216–221.

Ottavani, R., & Beck, A. T. (1987). Cognitive aspects of panic disorders. *Journal of Anxiety Disorders, 1,* 15–28.

Pennebaker, J. W. (1982). *The psychology of physical symptoms.* New York: Springer-Verlag.

Plaks, J. E., Grant, H., & Dweck, C. S. (2005). Violations of implicit theories and the sense of prediction and control: Implications for motivated person perception. *Journal of Personality and Social Psychology, 88,* 245–262.

Plehn, K., & Peterson, R. A. (2002). Anxiety sensitivity as a predictor of the development of panic symptoms, panic attacks, and panic disorder: A prospective study. *Anxiety Disorders, 16,* 455–474.

Rachman, S. (1988). Panics and their consequences: A review and prospect. In S. Rachman & J. D. Maser (Eds.), *Panic: Psychological perspectives* (pp. 259–303). Hillsdale, NJ: Lawrence Erlbaum Associates.

Rachman, S., Lopatka, C., & Levitt, K. (1988). Experimental analyses of panic: II. Panic patients. *Behaviour Research and Therapy, 26,* 33–40.

Rapee, R. M. (1986). Differential response to hyperventilation in panic disorder and generalized anxiety disorder. *Journal of Abnormal Psychology, 95,* 24–28.

Rapee, R. M., & Medoro, L. (1994). Fear of physical sensations and trait anxiety as mediators of the response to hyperventilation in nonclinical subjects. *Journal of Abnormal Psychology, 103,* 693–699.

Reiss, S. (1991). Expectancy model of fear, anxiety, and panic. *Clinical Psychology Review, 11,* 141–153.

Reiss, S. (2004). Multifaceted nature of intrinsic motivation: The theory of 16 basic desires. *Review of General Psychology, 8,* 179–193.

Reiss, S., & McNally, R. J. (1985). Expectancy model of fear. In S. Reiss & R. R. Bootzin (Eds.), *Theoretical issues in behavior therapy* (pp. 107–121). San Diego, CA: Academic Press.

Richards, J. C., Cooper, A. J., & Winkelman, J. H. (2003). Interoceptive accuracy in nonclinical panic. *Cognitive Therapy and Research, 27,* 447–461.

Robins, L. N., Heizer, J. E., Weissman, M. M., Orvaschel, H., Gruenberg, E., Burke, J. D., Jr., & Regier, D. A. (1984). Lifetime prevalence of specific psychiatric disorders in three sites. *Archives of General Psychiatry, 41,* 949–958.

Roy-Byrne, P. B., Geraci, M., & Uhde, T. W. (1986). Life events and the onset of panic disorder. *American Journal of Psychiatry, 143,* 1424–1427.

Roy-Byrne, P., Mellman, T., & Uhde, T. (1986). Effects of one night's sleep deprivation on mood and behavior in panic disorder. *Archives of General Psychiatry, 43,* 895–899.

Sanderson, W. C., Rapee, R. M., & Barlow, D. H. (1989). The influence of an illusion of control on panic attacks induced via inhalation of 5.5% carbon dioxide-enriched air. *Archives of General Psychiatry, 46,* 157–162.

Schmidt, N. B. (1999). Prospective evaluations of anxiety sensitivity. In S. Taylor (Ed.), *Anxiety sensitivity: Theory, research and treatment of the fear of anxiety* (pp. 217–235). Mahwah, NJ: Lawrence Erlbaum Associates.

Schmidt, N. B., & Bates, M. J. (2003). Evaluation of a pathoplastic relationship between anxiety sensitivity and panic disorder. *Anxiety, Stress & Coping: An International Journal, 16,* 17–30.

Schmidt, N. B., & Lerew, D. R. (2002). Prospective evaluation of perceived control, predictability, and anxiety sensitivity in the pathogenesis of panic. *Journal of Psychopathology and Behavioral Assessment, 24,* 207–214.

Schmidt, N. B., Lerew, D. R., & Jackson, R. J. (1997). The role of anxiety sensitivity in the pathogenesis of panic: Prospective evaluation of spontaneous panic attacks during acute stress. *Journal of Abnormal Psychology, 106,* 355–364.

Schmidt, N. B., Lerew, D. R., & Jackson, R. J. (1999). Prospective evaluation of anxiety sensitivity in the pathogenesis of panic: Replication and extension. *Journal of Abnormal Psychology, 108,* 532–537.

Schmidt, N. B., Lerew, D. R., & Joiner, T. E., Jr. (2000). Prospective evaluation of the etiology of anxiety sensitivity: Test of a scar model. *Behaviour Research and Therapy, 38,* 1083–1095.

Schmidt, N. B., Lerew, D. R., & Trakowski, J. H. (1997). Body vigilance in panic disorder: Evaluating attention to bodily perturbations. *Journal of Consulting & Clinical Psychology, 65,* 214–220.

Schmidt, N. B., Richey, J. A., & Fitzpatrick, K. K. (in press). Discomfort intolerance: Development of a construct and measure relevant to panic disorder. *Journal of Anxiety Disorders.*

Schmidt, N. B., Storey, J., Greenberg, B. D., Santiago, H. T., Li, Q., & Murphy, D. L. (2000). Evaluating gene x psychological risk factor effects in the pathogenesis of anxiety: A new model approach. *Journal of Abnormal Psychology, 109,* 308–320.

Schmidt, N. B., & Telch, M. J. (1994). The role of safety information and fear of bodily sensations in moderating responses to a hyperventilation challenge. *Behavior Therapy, 25,* 197–208.

Shepherd, M., Cooper, B., Brown, A., & Kalton, C. W. (1996). *Psychiatric illness in general practice.* London: Oxford University Press.

Stein, M. B., Jang, K. L., & Livesley, W. J. (1999). Heritability of anxiety sensitivity: A twin study. *American Journal of Psychiatry, 156,* 246–251.

Stewart, S. H., Buffett-Jerrott, S. E., & Kokaram, R. (2001). Heartbeat awareness and heart rate reactivity in anxiety sensitivity: A further investigation. *Anxiety Disorders, 15,* 535–553.

Stewart, S. H., Taylor, S., Lang, K. L., Cox, B. J., Watt, M. C., Fedoroff, I. C., & Borger, S. C. (2001). Causal modeling of relations among learning history, anxiety sensitivity, and panic attacks. *Behaviour Research and Therapy, 39,* 443–456.

Taylor, S. (1993). The structure of fundamental fears. *Journal of Behavior Therapy and Experimental Psychiatry, 24,* 289–299.

Taylor, S., Koch, W. J., & McNally, R. J. (1992). How does anxiety sensitivity vary across the anxiety disorders? *Journal of Anxiety Disorders, 6,* 249–259.

Teasdale, J. (1988). Cognitive models and treatments for panic: A critical evaluation. In S. Rachman & J. D. Maser (Eds.), *Panic: Psychological perspectives* (pp. 189–203). Hillsdale, NJ: Lawrence Erlbaum Associates.

Telch, M. J., Brouillard, M., Telch, C. F., Agras, W. S., & Taylor, C. B. (1989). Role of cognitive appraisal in panic-related avoidance. *Behaviour Research and Therapy, 27,* 373–383.

Telch, M. J., Silverman, A., & Schmidt, N. B. (1996). Effects of anxiety sensitivity and perceived control on emotional responding to caffeine challenge. *Journal of Anxiety Disorders, 10*(1), 21–35.

Van Beek, N., & Griez, E. (2003). Anxiety sensitivity in first degree relatives of patients with panic disorder. *Behaviour Research and Therapy, 41,* 949–957.

van den Hout, M. A., & Griez, E. (1982). Cognitive factors in carbon dioxide therapy. *Journal of Psychosomatic Research, 26,* 209–214.

van der Molen, G. M., van den Hout, M. A., Vroeman, J., Lousberg, H., & Griez, E. (1986). Cognitive determinants of lactate-induced anxiety. *Behaviour Research and Therapy, 24,* 677–680.

Watt, M. C., & Stewart, S. H. (2000). Anxiety sensitivity mediates the relationship between childhood learning experiences and elevated hypochondriacal concerns in young adulthood. *Journal of Psychosomatic Research, 49,* 107–118.

Watt, M. C., Stewart, S. II., & Cox, B. J. (1998). A retrospective study of the learning history origins of anxiety sensitivity. *Behaviour Research and Therapy, 36,* 505–525.

Weems, C. F., Hayward, C., Killen, J., & Taylor, C. B. (2002). A longitudinal investigation of anxiety sensitivity in adolescence. *Journal of Abnormal Psychology, 111,* 471–477.

Weissman, M. M. (1988). The epidemiology of panic disorder and agoraphobia. In R. E. Hales & A. Frances (Eds.), *Review of psychiatry* (Vol. 7, pp. 54–66). Washington, DC: American Psychiatric Press.

Weissman, M. M. (1991). Panic disorder: Impact on quality of life. *Journal of Clinical Psychiatry, 52,* 6–8.

Williams, J. M. G., Watts, F. N., MacLeod, C., & Mathews, A. (1988). *Cognitive psychology and emotional disorders.* Chichester, England: Wiley.

Williams, J. M. G., Watts, F. N., MacLeod, C., & Mathews, A. (1997). *Cognitive psychology and emotional disorders* (2nd ed.). Chichester, England: Wiley.

Wittchen, H. U. (1986). Epidemiology of panic attacks and panic disorders. In I. Hand & H. U. Wittchen (Eds.), *Panic and phobias: Empirical evidence of theoretical models and long-term effects of psychological treatments* (pp. 18–27). New York: Springer-Verlag.

Yeragani, V., Balon, R., & Pohl, R. (1989). Lactate infusions in panic disorder patients and normal controls: Autonomic measures and subjective anxiety. *Acta Psychiatrica Scandinavica, 79,* 32–40.

Zinbarg, R. E., Brown, T. A., Barlow, D. H., & Rapee, R. M. (2001). Anxiety sensitivity, panic and depressed mood: A reanalysis teasing apart the contributions of the two levels in the hierarchical structure of the Anxiety Sensitivity Index. *Journal of Abnormal Psychology, 110,* 372–377.

Zinbarg, R. E., & Schmidt, N. B. (2002). Evaluating the invariance of the structure of anxiety sensitivity over five weeks of basic cadet training in a large sample of Air Force cadets. *Personality and Individual Differences, 33,* 815–832.

Zvolensky, M. J., Eifert, G. H., Lejuez, C. W., & McNeil, D. W. (1999). The effects of offset control over 20% carbon dioxide-enriched air on anxious responding. *Journal of Abnormal Psychology, 108,* 624–632.

Zvolensky, M. J., & Forsyth, J. P. (2002). Anxiety sensitivity dimensions in the prediction of body vigilance and emotional avoidance. *Cognitive Therapy and Research, 26,* 449–460.

Zvolensky, M. J., Heffner, M., Eifert G. H., Spira, A. P., Feldner, M. T., & Brown, R. A. (2001). Incremental validity of perceived control dimensions in the differential prediction of interpretative biases for threat. *Journal of Psychopathology and Behavioral Assessment, 23,* 75–83.

9

Cognitive Vulnerability to Obsessive-Compulsive Disorders

Stanley J. Rachman
University of British Columbia

Roselyn Shafran
Oxford University

John H. Riskind
George Mason University

Studies have shown that patients diagnosed with obsessive-compulsive disorder (OCD), and nonclinical participants who score highly on OCD measures, show evidence of significant cognitive biases. They also tend to endorse a number of extreme beliefs that may well promote OCD, especially a significantly elevated sense of personal responsibility. The significance of these findings is examined in detail.

Ideally, the search for factors that increase vulnerability to a psychological disorder should be guided by our construal of the nature and causes of the particular disorder. In the absence of any firm theoretical starting point, this search can decline into a more or less random selection of tests given to diagnosed cases in the hope that statistical analyses will reveal some enlightening results. In addition to the need for a firm theoretical basis on which to construct the search into vulnerability factors, there is an unavoidable need to carry out prospective studies to confirm or disconfirm the hypotheses, but these studies are of course laborious, demanding, and expensive.

Distal vulnerability factors are risk factors that were present long before the development of disorder, and increase the probability that the given disorder will occur in the future. Such distal cognitive factors can be distinguished from proximal cognitive features (e.g., "online" appraisals or memory biases) that are present only when the disorder itself is present. Preexisting vulnerabilities that put persons at risk for disorder must be examined with prospective, longitudinal designs. Such prospective designs can also be used to examine possible exacerbating factors (e.g., the role of stress, depression, or other aversive factors that occur after onset of the disorder), as well as protective factors (e.g., social support, or coping skills), that mitigate the effects of cognitive vulnerabilities or stress. The search for these factors is guided by the possession of a theory.

The goal of identifying the cognitive vulnerability factors for OCD the requirement of a theoretical starting point is partly met. But there is a lack of prospective data in the current literature against which to test the prevailing hypotheses. However, before turning to the role of cognitive factors and possible vulnerabilities, the common view that depression/anxiety are predisposing factors must be recognized. It has repeatedly been shown that OCD correlates positively with depression and with elevated levels of anxiety (Rachman & Hodgson, 1980; Swinson, Antony, Rachman, & Richter, 1998). Moreover, after the successful treatment of cases of OCD, the emergence or reemergence of anxiety/depression is considered to place the person at risk for the recurrence of OCD (Rachman & Hodgson, 1980; Swinson et al., 1998). Before the publication of statistical evidence of positive correlations of depression and OCD (see Clark, 2002, for a review), and anxiety and OCD, clinicians consistently described the connection between depression and OCD and, to a lesser degree, between anxiety and OCD (see, e.g., the classic writings of Lewis, 1936, 1957, 1965). Many rich descriptions were clinicians' unsystematized accounts of the "natural history" of OCD as they observed it in their patients, many of whom were followed over long periods of time—there were no dependably effective methods of treatment available and OCD was oftentimes truly chronic. These reports were "pre-scientific" prospective studies, but nevertheless valuable sources of information, and Ricciardi and McNally (1995) reported interesting observations in the relation between depression and compulsions, and depression and obsessions (depression is most closely associated with obsessions).

Regrettably, attempts to detect OCD vulnerability factors in the data collected in the unique Dunedin prospective study (comprising extremely detailed information on all of the children born in that city between April 1, 1972, and March 31, 1973) proved fruitless (Poulton, personal communication, 1998). This database contains a usable number of cases of OCD occurring in childhood and early adulthood, but numerous directed searches failed to uncover possible early predictors of the disorder. These searches included investigating elevated psychopathology in the families of people who met diagnostic criteria for OCD, but little information was found, although studies of clinical samples have demonstrated elevated parental psychopathology in children with the disorder (Lenane et al., 1990; Riddle et al., 1990). The Dunedin study also differed from the clinical studies in finding that only 10% of children who had obsessive-compulsive symptoms at 11 years met diagnostic criteria for OCD at age 21. This suggests a reassuringly less chronic form of the disorder than has been noted in previous clinical samples. It should be remembered that searching to discover the cognitive predictors of the disorder was limited in the Dunedin study due to the lack of inclusion of cognitive measures. This is because the study was designed and introduced in 1972–1973 when psychology had not yet turned so determinedly cognitive. Recent research on OCD has yielded promising evidence of a significant contribution to the disorder made by cognitive factors.

COGNITIVE FACTORS

Patients with OCD, and high scoring research participants, show evidence of significant cognitive biases (they tend to endorse extreme beliefs and also express an elevated sense of responsibility). There is also some evidence that these two groups, patients with OCD and the high scorers on OCD measures, display memory biases and selected perceptions (see Amir & Kozak, 2002, for a review). These examples of skewed information processing, however, are not specific to OCD. They may well be part of the anxiety disorders spectrum itself rather than vulnerability factors, and there is no suggestion that these types of processing variations are particular to OCD. Without the necessary prospective designs, there is no persuasive evidence at present that skewed information processing acts as a vulnerability factor in OCD, or increases the probability of the first episode of the disorder.

In order to appreciate the relevance of the cognitive distortions referred to in the previous paragraph, it is necessary first to place them in context. In recent decades, there have been important changes in the construal of OCD, most particularly by the infusion of cognitive analyses and explanations in approaching this disorder. Indeed, important advances have been made in the cognitive analysis of various types of anxiety disorder, notably panic, and Salkovskis applied this approach in his stimulating, fresh analysis of obsessional disorders (Salkovskis, 1985; Salkovskis & Forrester, 2002; Salkovskis & Kirk, 1997). In a similar manner to other cognitive theorists, Salkovskis argued that to make sense of OCD it is necessary to gain an understanding of the person's thinking on the subject, their interpretations and understanding of potential threats to their well-being, and the meaning of the actions that they undertake—or avoid—in their attempts to reduce threat and ensure safety. Salkovskis placed particular emphasis on the role of elevated feelings of responsibility, with responsibility defined as "the belief that one has power which is pivotal to bring about, or prevent, subjectively crucial negatively outcomes" (Salkovskis, Rachman, Ladouceur, & Freeston, 1992).

An exaggerated sense of responsibility can take various forms: It can be too extensive, too intense, too personal, too exclusive, or all of these. The sense of responsibility can take extraordinary extremes in which the affected individuals "confess" to the police that they have been responsible for crimes or accidents of which they in fact have little or no knowledge. A sense of excessive responsibility typically is manifested at home or at work, but can spread to any situation in which people may come to work—if the affected person feels some belongingness in the place. They also have a tendency to experience guilt, not only for their own actions but also for those of other people. People who harbor feelings of excessive responsibility may well include in this range of responsibilities their intrusive thoughts, as well as any action or omission that may form the basis of compulsive checking for safety. The exaggerated sense of responsibility is also at play in obsessional thinking so that when the individuals experience an unwanted obsessional thought they feel unduly responsible for the "consequences" of the thought and its potential significance.

The range of psychometric and experimental evidence is consistent with Salkovskis' cognitive-behavioral analysis emphasizing the role of responsibility appraisal (e.g., Freeston, Ladouceur, Thibodeau, & Gagnon, 1992; Lopatka & Rachman, 1995; Salkovskis & Forrester, 2002; Shafran, 1997). Lopatka and Rachman (1995) conducted an experimental study suggesting that changes in perceived responsibility will be followed by corresponding changes in the urge to check compulsively. The study directly manipulated perceived responsibility by experimental instructions with 30 subjects who were diagnosed with OCD. The therapist induced high responsibility in OCD participants by stating: "I want you to know that you will have to take complete responsibility if anything bad happens or anything is not perfect." In contrast, the therapist induced low responsibility by stating: "I want you to know that I will take complete responsibility if anything bad happens or anything is not perfect. You are *not* responsible." The experimental manipulation succeeded in increasing or decreasing the participant's perceived responsibility, as intended. Decreased responsibility was followed by significant declines in discomfort and the urge to carry out compulsive checking. Likewise, increased responsibility was followed by increases in discomfort and urges, but these failed to reach a statistically significant level. In other studies, responsibility has been manipulated in a variety of other direct or indirect ways (e.g., Ladouceur et al., 1995; Shafran, 1997). Shafran (1997) obtained similar results when indirectly manipulating perceived responsibility by means of the presence or absence of the therapist during a behavioral task.

ORIGINS OF ELEVATED RESPONSIBILITY

There are few data addressing the possible origins of an inflated sense of responsibility, despite its important place in the cognitive theory of OCD. It has been suggested (Salkovskis, Shafran, Rachman, & Freeston, 1998) that there are multiple pathways to inflated responsibility beliefs in obsessional problems. These include an early developed sense of responsibility that is encouraged during childhood, for example, a first-born child caring for younger siblings. Second, responsibility can be inflated as a result of rigid and extreme codes of conduct and duty such as those inculcated by educational and religious instruction. Third, children who are overly protected from responsibility may be overly sensitive to ideas of responsibility as adults, or unable to cope with the responsibilities of adult life. In these cases, the children may have anxious parents who convey a sense that danger is imminent and they will be unable to cope with it. Fourth, an incident in which individuals' actions or inaction actually contributed to a serious misfortune affecting themselves or others may predispose to the development of exaggerated responsibility, as could an incident in which it appeared that their thoughts and/or actions or inaction contributed to a misfortune. Although there are reasons to believe that some general patterns can be identified, it is suggested that the origins of obsessional problems are best understood in terms of complex interactions specific to each individual.

In some instances, rather imaginary formative incidents may contribute to inflated responsibility. For example, a 24-year-old young woman felt guilty about not spending time with her father on the night before his unexpected death. This distorted perception of responsibility was elaborated into fantastic forms that only she found credible. She believed she had to avoid a certain spot in a nearby city park at all costs because of a demonic sign that would cause her to go back in time and blurt out hurtful things to her father.

Given the evidence that inflated responsibility is implicated in OCD, there is the possibility that people who believe they have extreme and personal responsibility for avoiding harm and ensuring safety will be at risk for developing OCD. However, remember that the presence of elevated responsibility is not always associated with OCD; there is far more elevated responsibility than there is OCD. In addition, whereas the presence of elevated feelings of responsibility might make a contribution to the development of the disorder, one must think in terms of vulnerability–stress models in which the presence of elevated levels of personal responsibility might interact with other cognitive vulnerabilities, to produce disorder. A study by Bouchard, Rheaume, and Ladoucer (1999) provides an example. Their results suggest that, as compared to less perfectionistic individuals, highly perfectionist individuals showed greater increases in perceived responsibility after a responsibility induction.

COGNITIVE THEORY OF OBSESSIONS

In addition to Salkovskis' broad reanalysis of the nature of obsessional disorders, a theory specifically designed to account for obsessional problems has been advanced and a concise description is necessary in order to place within context the cognitive biases' standing as risk factors. It has been proposed that obsessions are caused by catastrophic misinterpretations of the significance of one's intrusive thoughts (images and impulses) (Rachman, 1997, 1998). The parallel is to the role that catastrophic misinterpretations of ordinary bodily sensations can play in the etiology and treatment of panic disorder (see chap. 8, this vol.). By a similar deduction, it has been argued that obsessions will persist for as long as the misinterpretations continue, and the obsessions will diminish or disappear as a functioning of the weakening or elimination of the misinterpretations. In addition, two testable deductions were drawn from the theory. It was predicted that people who experience these obsessions (recurrent, unwanted, repugnant thoughts) are far more likely than people who do not experience them to attach important and personal significance to their intrusive thoughts. Among those who experience obsessions, those intrusive thoughts that are interpreted by them as being highly significant will feature in the content of their obsessions, and those thoughts interpreted as being of minimal significance will not feature in the content of their obsessions. One of the starting points for this theory was the demonstration that almost everybody experiences unwanted intrusive thoughts. But, among OCD patients, these thoughts are more intense, longer lasting, more insistent, more repugnant and distressing, and more adhesive than other varieties of intrusive thoughts (Rachman & de Silva, 1978).

This summary of the cognitive theory of obsessions affirms that the core of the theory is indeed cognitive, resting on the affected person's interpretation of meaning in particular experiences. The evidence and arguments for and against the theory are provided in Rachman (1997). But, for present purposes, a separate question is whether the maladaptive cognitions were present prior to the emergence of the disorder, or whether they emerge only after the disorder is established. Ultimately, the predisposing role of maladaptive cognitions in OCD remains to be tested by conducting the appropriate research. However, the accumulating evidence about the prominence of particular forms of cognitive distortions in OCD encourages the hope that the path may eventually lead to unearthing of specific risk factors.

COGNITIVE DISTORTIONS

Thought–action fusion (TAF) is a cognitive distortion that appears in two forms: *Probability TAF*, in which the intrusive thought is believed to increase the probability that a specific negative event is going to occur, and *Moral TAF*, in which experiencing the intrusive thought is interpreted as almost morally equivalent to carrying out a prohibited action. This distortion is especially prominent in obsessions, is closely related to guilt, and is associated with subsequent attempts at neutralization. The TAF scale (Shafran, Thordarson, & Rachman, 1996) is designed to tap both forms of the distortion, with 7 items for Probability TAF (e.g., "If I think of a relative/friend being in a car accident, this increases the risk that he/she will have a car accident") and 12 items for Moral TAF (e.g., "If I wish harm on someone, it is almost as bad as doing harm").

The cognitive distortions described as thought–action fusion was first encountered in the work on pure obsessions. "Fusion refers to the psychological phenomenon in which the patient appears to regard the obsessional activity and the forbidden action as being morally equivalent" (Rachman, 1993, p. 152). The concept arose from the theoretical proposition that patients with OCD were inclined to assume that "a thought is like an action" (Salkovskis, 1985, p. 574) and from clinical observations. It soon became apparent, however, that there is an additional or third form of thought–action fusion, which is just as common and perhaps equally or more important than the first (Rachman & Shafran, 1999).

An early example of TAF was encountered during the treatment of a 33-year-old patient who was oppressed by compulsive checking and a group of obsessions on the theme of death. Each night he dreaded going to bed because he feared that he might die in his sleep. He rated the probability of such an untimely death as 10%–20%. However, he rated the probability of a therapist or relative or friend dying in the same manner as less than one in a million. When asked to explain this bias—why he, in particular, was at such a high risk—he replied that he was more likely to die in this way precisely because he had the thought that he might do so. He believed that the probability of his death was significantly increased by his intrusive thoughts. In effect, he felt that thoughts of dying in one's sleep are dangerous and potentially harmful. In contrast, he reasoned that people who do not share these thoughts have a negligible probability of dying in their sleep. In another example, a young student was plagued by obsessional images of his family, who lived 250 miles away, being injured or killed in a vehicle accident. He was certain that the probability of his relatives being harmed in an accident was significantly increased by his recurrent thoughts and images. Unsurprisingly, the obsessions made him feel wretched, anxious, and extremely guilty for putting his family at serious risk.

There is also a second form of TAF in which the obsessional thoughts were interpreted by the patient as being morally equivalent to carrying out the prohibited actions. A conscientious and devout young woman who was devoted to her work as a nursing assistant caring for elderly patients experienced a period of stress unrelated to her work and then began to experience intrusive thoughts about attacking or even killing her patients. Naturally these obsessions caused great distress, guilt, and serious loss of self-esteem. She concluded that she had turned into a true monster and a hypocrite. In her view and experience, the intrusive thoughts of harming the patients were morally equivalent to causing actual harm; she felt compromised and described herself as "a bad person, no better than a vicious criminal."

The connection between the type of thought–action fusion, probability and moral equivalence, requires explanation because they are related but not identical. In some cases, the two forms of TAF become intertwined, as illustrated by a man who had a recurrent unwanted intrusive impulse to abuse his baby son while changing his diapers. He interpreted the impulse as showing that he was highly immoral and dangerous. In addition, he believed that the frequency of the impulse increased the probability that he would lose control and eventually harm his son.

Of course, it is easy and most common to believe that bad thoughts are immoral without also believing that the thoughts can cause such bad events to happen. In psychometric studies of people with obsessive-compulsive problems, the correlation between the two types of TAF was moderate ($r = .44$) and the relation between TAF and obsessional problems was confirmed (Shafran, Teachman, Kerry, & Rachman, 1996).

Rassin, Muris, Schmidt, and Merckelbach (2000) used structural equation modeling to examine the relations and covariances between scores on TAF, thought suppression (Wegner et al.'s White Bear Suppression Inventory, Wegner & Zanakos, 1994), and obsessive-compulsive symptoms. Rassin et al. provided evidence that TAF triggers thought suppression, and thought suppression, in turn, promotes obsessive-compulsive symptoms. These findings give added weight to the importance of the TAF construct and lend support to the assumption that it is an antecedent of thought suppression and symptoms.

Although there is supportive evidence on TAF, recent research indicates a continuing need for study. Shafran and Rachman (2004) reviewed the literature on TAF and concluded that the moral form of TAF is less robust than the likelihood form. Indeed, several recent studies have given rise to questions about whether likelihood TAF is more closely related to OCD than moral OCD (Lee, Cougle, & Telch, 2005; Rassin, Muris, Schmidt, & Merckelback, 2000). For example, Amir, Freshman, Ramsey, Neary, and Brigidi (2001) found that OCD participants and nonanxious controls did not differ on ratings of TAF moral. Moreover, Abramowitz, Whiteside, Lynam, and Kalsy (2002) found evidence that moral TAF was actually related to depression (or general distress), although Lee et al. (2005) did not find this. Shafran and Rachman suggested that both scales may be best used as a starting point in identifying beliefs and conducting experimental investigations.

A second question that has emerged from recent research is whether TAF is a general feature common to anxiety disorders not specific to OCD. Hazlett-Stevens, Zucker, and Craske (2002) found that TAF likelihood was elevated in GAD. Similarly, Abramowitz et al. (2002) found significant associations between TAF likelihood and anxiety. In a study on children (ages 7 to 13), Barrett and Healy (2003) found no difference in thought–action fusion between those with OCD and other anxious children. Thus there is a possibility that the associations between likelihood TAF and OCD are mediated by anxiety (depression) symptoms.

In combination with this evidence of the nonspecificity of TAF to OCD, other evidence suggests it may reflect a more general propensity to magical thinking (e.g., Einstein & Menzies, 2004a, 2004b). Einstein et al. examined the associations between measures of magical thinking, TAF, and obsessive-compulsive symptoms. They found that magical ideation (on MI scales) had large and significant relationships to measures of OCD even when TAF was held constant. But TAF no longer had significant relationships to measures of OCD when magical ideation was held constant. Results suggested that magical thinking is the central construct that underlies the relationship between TAF and OC symptoms. Likelihood (but not moral) TAF has also been found to be related to schizotypal traits, which are thought to involve magical thinking (Lee et al., 2005). Thus, there is a need for further research to explore whether a general magical thinking tendency underpin links between TAF, and OC symptom severity.

TAF AND RESPONSIBILITY

Another type of cognitive bias (originally described by Lopatka & Rachman, 1995) incorporates elements of TAF and excessive responsibility. In the Lopatka and Rachman study, patients with OCD rated the probability of an aversive event occurring as substantially increased if they felt personally responsible for ensuring safety. For example, one patient said that the probability of the family home catching fire was .001% when other members of the family were the last to close up the house before leaving, but the chance rose to as high as 30% when she was the last person to leave the home. Hence, she felt totally responsible for ensuring the safety of the home.

Clinical observation of this kind and the psychometric research created interest in the connections between these two types of cognitions. As a start, it was felt necessary to determine the relative frequency with which thought–action fusion is reported in order to ascertain the relation between TAF and elevated responsibility, and to establish whether or not there is a particular and exclusive connection between thought–action fusion and OCD. In order to examine the possible connection between the two types of cognition, we carried out two interconnected psychometric studies on large groups of students (Rachman, Thordarson, Shafran, & Woody, 1995). TAF emerged as one of four factors, in addition to factors for responsibility for harm, positive responsibility, and responsibility in a social context. The TAF subscale correlated significantly with measures of obsessionality and guilt and the correlations remained significant even after measures of depression were controlled.

The relation between TAF and responsibility has also been examined by an international working group that was established in 1995 to formulate and measure the beliefs and appraisals associated with OCD (OCCWG, or Obsessive-Compulsive Cognitions Working Group, 1997, 2003). General beliefs and specific interpretations concerning personal responsibility and the importance of thoughts (including TAF) were assessed. An interim report of these measures is based on a sample of 426 people, including those with OCD, community controls, student controls, and a small sample (n = 35) of people with anxiety disorders other than OCD (OCCWG, 1997, 2003). Initial examination of reliability and validity indicated excellent internal consistency, stability, and encouraging evidence of validity. The OCD group scored significantly higher than all other groups on both responsibility and importance of thoughts subscales of these measures. The high correlations between beliefs about responsibility and the importance of thoughts (r = .6), and between the interpretation of intrusions in these domains (r = .85), indicates a close link between these cognitive distortions.

It is not argued that these cognitive distortions in the form of TAF and elevated responsibility are confined to people who have OCD. This would be an overgeneralization and the extant psychometric and clinical data argue against this. Rather, it is being proposed that these cognitive distortions are particularly pronounced in people diagnosed with OCD or who score highly on OCD measures and, given the prevailing cognitive theory of obsessions summarized earlier, that the operation of these cognitive distortions may well promote OCD.

OTHER COGNITIVE FACTORS

Additional cognitive factors other than responsibility and TAF that are thought to be associated with OCD have been examined by the international Obsessive-Compulsive Cognitions Working Group (OCCWG,

1997). Such beliefs include perfectionism, the intolerance of uncertainty, beliefs about the importance of controlling thoughts, and the overestimation of threat estimation. Although these beliefs are not suggested to be specific to OCD, they overlap significantly with beliefs concerning responsibility and the importance of thoughts (all $r > .6$) and may also function to promote OCD in certain individuals (OCCWG, 2003).

A different type of cognitive bias has been suggested to function as an antecedent vulnerability factor for anxiety. Riskind and his colleagues propose a bias called the sense of looming vulnerability, which refers to the internal generation mental scenarios and expectations of repeatedly increasing danger and rapidly intensifying risk (see chap. 7, this vol.; Riskind, Williams, Gessner, Chrosniak, & Cortina, 2000). By their view, different symptom-specific forms of looming vulnerability are specific to different particular subtypes of OCD. For example, fears of contamination seem to be related to a tendency to construct mental scenarios of rapidly spreading contamination (Riskind, Abreu, Strauss, & Holt, 1997; Riskind, Wheeler, & Picerno, 1997), whereas fears of harming others may be related to mental scenarios of rapidly overwhelming urges to harm others. Besides this, a more global and trait-like sense of looming vulnerability, referred to as the "looming cognitive (or maladaptive) style" may operate as a cognitive vulnerability that cuts across anxiety disorders (see chap. 7, this vol.). Thus, this looming cognitive style may be OCD relevant but not OCD specific (Williams, Shahar, Riskind, & Joiner, 2005). In a recent unpublished study, Black (2004) used a retrospective behavioral high-risk design (see chap. 1, this vol.) and found with college students that the looming maladaptive style predicts past history of OCD. This was true even when current symptoms were controlled and individuals with current OCD were excluded from study.

COMPARABLE COGNITIVE BIASES
IN OTHER DISORDERS

It is of interest that a comparable form of cognitive bias to TAF has been found operating in people with eating disorders. *Thought–shape fusion* occurs when merely thinking about eating a forbidden food increases the person's estimate of their shape or weight, elicits a perception of moral wrongdoing, and/or makes the person feel fat. Thought–shape fusion was found to be significantly associated with eating disorder psychopathology in 119 undergraduate students ($r = .61$). In addition, an experimental study based on the method of Rachman, Shafran, Mitchell, Trant, and Teachman (1996) indicated that eliciting this distortion produced negative emotional reactions and prompted the urge to engage in behavior such as neutralizing. Moreover, engaging in neutralizing behavior reduced the negative reactions elicited by activating the distortion. These findings were recently replicated in a sample of 20 patients with anorexia nervosa (Radomsky, de Silva, Todd, Treasure, & Murphy, 2002).

FUTURE RESEARCH

As already mentioned, the attempts in the Dunedin prospective study to detect OCD vulnerability factors bore no fruits. Regrettably, the Dunedin study lacked suitable cognitive vulnerability measures. Future studies of this type that include measures of possible cognitive vulnerabilities such as TAF could help increase understanding of these predictors. Suitable modification of measures for use in childhood would, of course, be required.

Coupled with this, it would be desirable to include suitable measures of protective factors such as positive parental relationships or social support. The Dunedin study found a lower rate of a chronic form of the disorder than clinical studies have reported before. It is possible that these findings would be clarified by considering possible protective factors (e.g., strong attachment relationships or bonds with parents) that might mitigate the risk of chronic disorder.

Another issue to explore emerges from growing evidence that OCD symptoms correspond to several symptom subgroups. Moreover, it currently appears that cognitive biases such as inflated responsibility and TAF play different roles in obsessions related to compulsive checking, but not in those related to nonchecking symptom patterns. For example, Foa, Sachs, Tolin, Prezworski, and Amir (2002) found that, as compared to noncheckers and nonanxious controls, OC checkers had an inflated perception of responsibility for harm, and this perception may lead to undue needs to rectify potentially harmful situations. Thus, the cognitive vulnerability factors or biases that put individuals at risk for other nonchecking OCD symptom subgroups, such as contamination obsessions, still remains largely an open question.

Thus far, evidence has accumulated to show that the particular cognitive distortions described here are especially common and pronounced in people with OCD and in participants who score highly on OCD measures, and this gives rise to the clear possibility that these cognitive biases, extreme beliefs, and misappraisals are also vulnerability factors. Yet, at the same time, a limitation of the findings is that they are primarily cross-sectional, and do not provide a clear basis for causal inferences about cognitive vulnerability. Factors such as TAF or responsibility could be correlates of the disorder, but do not play a vulnerability role that increases the probability of developing the disorder.

Ultimately, the demonstration that the preexistence of these cognitive distortions increases the risk of developing OCD can only be confirmed or disconfirmed by conducting the appropriate prospective studies. Implementing such studies would involve assessing theoretically specified cognitive vulnerability factors such as TAF or responsibility at a time before the first appearance of any symptoms of disorder. Also, it would entail eliminating people with the vulnerability factors who already have symptoms. Pending such studies, further experimental analyses and psychometric studies of these intriguing cognitive distortions should be on the table in the hope of illuminating their character and their role in obsessional-compulsive disorders.

REFERENCES

Abramowitz, J. S., Whiteside, S., Lynam, D., & Kalsy, S. (2003). Is thought–action specific to obsessive-compulsive disorder?: A mediating role of negative affect. *Behaviour Research and Therapy, 41,* 1069–1079.

Amir, N., Freshman, M., Ramsey, B., Neary, E., & Brigidi, B. (2001). Thought–action fusion in individuals with OCD symptoms. *Behaviour Research and Therapy, 39,* 765–776.

Amir, N., & Kozak, M. J. (2002). Information processing in obsessive compulsive disorder. In R. O. Frost & G. Steketee (Eds.), *Cognitive approaches to obsessions and compulsions: Theory, assessment, and treatment* (pp. 165–182). Boston: Elsevier.

Barrett, P. M., & Healy, L. J. (2003). An examination of a cognitive processes involved in childhood obsessive compulsive disorder. *Behaviour Research and Therapy, 41,* 285–299.

Black, D. O. (2004). *Lifetime history of anxiety and mood disorders predicted by cognitive vulnerability to anxiety.* Unpublished dissertation, George Mason University.

Bouchard, C., Rheaume, J., & Ladouceur, R. (1999). Responsibility and perfectionism in OCD: An experimental study. *Behaviour Research and Therapy, 37,* 239–248.

Clark, D. A. (2002). A cognitive perspective on obsessive compulsive disorder and depression: Distinct and related features. In G. R. Frost & G. Steketee (Eds.), *Cognitive approaches to obsessions and compulsions: Theory, assessment, and treatment* (pp. 107–116). New York: Elsevier Science.

Einstein, D. A., & Menzies, R. G. (2004a). The presence of magical thinking in obsessive compulsive disorder. *Behaviour Research and Therapy, 42,* 539–549.

Einstein, D. A., & Menzies, R. G. (2004b). Role of magical thinking in obsessive-compulsive symptoms in an undergraduate sample. *Depression and Anxiety, 19,* 174–179.

Foa, E. B., Sachs, M. B., Tolin, D. F., Prezworski, A., & Amir, N. (2002). Inflated perceptions of responsibility for harm in OCD patients with and without checking compulsions: A replication and extension. *Journal of Anxiety Disorders, 16,* 443–457.

Freeston, M. H., Ladouceur, R., Thibodeau, N., & Gagnon, F. (1992). Cognitive intrusions in a non-clinical population: II. Associations with depressive, anxious, and compulsive symptoms. *Behaviour Research and Therapy, 30,* 263–271.

Hazlett-Stevens, H., Zucker, B. G., & Craske, M. G. (2002). The relationship of thought–action fusion to pathological worry and generalized anxiety disorder. *Behaviour Research and Therapy, 41,* 285–299.

Ladouceur, R., Rheaume, J., Freeston, M. H., Aublet, F., Jean, K., Lachance, S., et al. (1995). Experimental manipulations of responsibility: An analogue test for models of obsessive-compulsive disorder. *Behaviour Research and Therapy, 33,* 937–946.

Lee, H.-J., Cougle, J. R., & Telch, M. J. (2005). Thought–action fusion and its relationship to schizotype and OCD symptoms. *Behaviour Research and Therapy, 43,* 29–41.

Lenane, M. C., Swedo, S. E., Leonard, H., Pauls, D. L., Sceery, W., & Rapoport, J. L. (1990). Psychiatric disorders in first degree relatives of children and adolescents with obsessive compulsive disorder. *Journal of the American Academy of Child and Adolescent Psychiatry, 29,* 407–412.

Lewis, A. (1936). Problems of obsessional illness. *Proceedings of the Royal Society of Medicine, 29,* 325 336.

Lewis, A. (1957). Obsessional illness. RMPA Lecture, *Acta Neurosiq., Argentina, 3,* 323.

Lewis, A. (1965). A note on personality and obsessional illness. *Psychiatria et Neurologia, 150,* 299–305.

Lopatka, C., & Rachman, S. (1995). Perceived responsibility and compulsive checking: An experimental analysis. *Behaviour Research and Therapy, 33,* 673–684.

Obsessive Compulsive Cognitions Working Group. (1997). Cognitive assessment of obsessive-compulsive disorder. *Behaviour Research and Therapy, 35,* 667–681.

Obsessive Compulsive Cognitions Working Group. (2003). Psychometric validation of the Obsessive Beliefs Questionnaire and the Interpretation of Intrusions Inventory: Part I. *Behaviour Research and Therapy, 41,* 863–878.

Rachman, S. (1993). Obsessions, responsibility and guilt. *Behaviour Research and Therapy, 31,* 149–154.

Rachman, S. (1997). A cognitive theory of obsessions. *Behaviour Research and Therapy, 35,* 793–802.

Rachman, S. (1998). A cognitive theory of obsessions: Elaborations. *Behaviour Research and Therapy, 36,* 385–401.

Rachman, S., & de Silva, P. (1978). Abnormal and normal obsessions. *Behaviour Research and Therapy, 16,* 233–238.

Rachman, S., & Hodgson, R. (1980). *Obsessions and compulsions.* Englewood Cliffs, NJ: Prentice-Hall.

Rachman, S., & Shafran, R. (1999). Cognitive distortions: Thought–action fusion. *Journal of Clinical Psychology and Psychotherapy, 6,* 80–85.

Rachman, S., Shafran, R., Mitchell, D., Trant, J., & Teachman, B. (1996). How to remain neutral: An experimental analysis of neutralization. *Behaviour Research and Therapy, 34,* 889–898.

Rachman, S., Thordarson, D. S., Shafran, R., & Woody, S. R. (1995). Perceived responsibility: Structure and significance. *Behaviour Research and Therapy, 33,* 779–784.

Radomsky, A. S., De Silva, P., Todd, G., Treasure, J., & Murphy, T. (2002). Thought–shape fusion in anorexia nervosa: An experimental investigation. *Behaviour Research and Therapy, 40,* 1169–1177.

Rassin, E., Muris, P., Schmidt, H., & Merckelbach, H. (2000). Relationships between thought–action fusion, thought suppression and obsessive-compulsive symptoms: A structural equation modelling approach. *Behaviour Research and Therapy, 38,* 889–897.

Ricciardi, J. N., & McNally, R. J. (1995). Depressed mood is related to obsessions, but not to compulsions, in obsessive-compulsive disorder. *Journal of Anxiety Disorders, 9,* 249–256.

Riddle, M. A., Scahill, L., King, R. A., Hardin, M. T., Towbin, K. E., Ort, S. I., Leckman, J. F., & Cohen, D. J. (1990). Obsessive compulsive disorder in children and adolescents: Phenomenology and family history. *Journal of the American Academy of Child and Adolescent Psychiatry, 29,* 766–772.

Riskind, J. H., Abreu, K., Strauss, M., & Holt, R. (1997). Looming vulnerability to spreading contamination in subclinical OCD. *Behaviour Research and Therapy, 35,* 405–414.

Riskind, J. H., Wheeler, D. J., & Picerno, M. R. (1997). Using mental imagery with subclinical OCD to "freeze" contamination in its place: Evidence for looming vulnerability theory. *Behaviour Research and Therapy, 35,* 757–768.

Riskind, J. H., Williams, N. L., Gessner, T. L., Chrosniak, L. D., & Cortina, J. M. (2000). The looming maladaptive style: Anxiety, danger, and schematic processing. *Journal of Personality and Social Psychology, 79,* 837–952.

Salkovskis, P. M. (1985). Obsessional-compulsive problems: A cognitive-behavioural analysis. *Behaviour Research and Therapy, 23,* 571–583.

Salkovskis, P. M., & Forrester, E. (2002). Responsibility. In G. R. Frost & G. Steketee (Eds.), *Cognitive approaches to obsessions and compulsions: Theory, assessment, and treatment* (pp. 45–62). Oxford: Elsevier Science.

Salkovskis, P. M., & Kirk, J. (1997). Obsessive-compulsive disorder. In D. M. Clark & C. G. Fairburn (Eds.), *Science and practice of cognitive behaviour therapy* (pp. 179–208). Oxford, England: Oxford University Press.

Salkovskis, P. M., Rachman, S. R., Ladouceur, R., & Freeston, M. H. (1992). *Proceedings of the Toronto Cafeteria.* Association for Advancement of Behavior Therapy.

Shafran, R. (1997). The manipulation of responsibility in obsessive-compulsive disorder. *British Journal of Clinical Psychology, 36*(3), 397–408.

Shafran, R., & Rachman, S. (2004). Thought–action fusion: A review. *Journal of Behavior Therapy and Experimental Psychiatry, 35,* 87–107.

Shafran, R., Teachman, B. A., Kerry, S., & Rachman, S. (1999). A cognitive distortion associated with eating disorders: Thought–shape fusion. *British Journal of Clinical Psychology, 38,* 167–179.

Shafran, R., Thordarson, D. S., & Rachman, S. (1996). Thought–action fusion in obsessive compulsive disorder. *Journal of Anxiety Disorders, 10,* 379–391.

Swinson, R. P., Antony, M. M., Rachman, S., & Richter, M. A. (Eds.). (1998). *Obsessive-compulsive disorder: Theory, research, and treatment.* New York: Guilford.

Wegner, D. M., & Zanakos, S. (1994). Chronic thought suppression. *Journal of Personality, 62,* 615–640.

Williams, N. L., Shahar, G., Riskind, J. H., & Joiner, T. E. (2005). The looming maladaptive style predicts shared variance in anxiety disorder symptoms: Further support for a cognitive model of vulnerability to anxiety. *Journal of Anxiety Disorders, 19,* 157–175.

10

Cognitive Vulnerability to Social Anxiety Disorder

Deborah Roth Ledley
University of Pennsylvania

David M. Fresco
Kent State University

Richard G. Heimberg
Temple University

Historically, the notion of cognitive vulnerability to psychopathology has most often been associated with the study of depression, and particularly with the study of hopelessness depression, a subtype of the disorder proposed by Abramson, Metalsky, and Alloy (1989). The hopelessness theory of depression distinguishes between distal and proximal factors that contribute to the disorder. Distal factors occur at the beginning of the chain of events that eventually leads to the expression of the symptoms of hopelessness depression. According to Abramson and her colleagues, a major distal influence is attributional style. Specifically, people who end up depressed tend to make stable and global attributions for negative events in their lives. Yet, simply having this attributional style does not cause depression. Rather, people must also experience negative events in their lives. Abramson et al. (1989) proposed that a diathesis–stress approach can be used to understand these contributory factors, such that a depressogenic attributional style (the diathesis) and negative life events (the stress) interact to increase the likelihood that a person will experience the symptoms of depression in the future.

In their hopelessness theory of depression, Abramson et al. (1989) also discussed a specific proximal cause of the disorder—hopelessness. Hopelessness occurs close in proximity to the onset of depressive symptoms, and according to these authors, is a "sufficient" cause, in other words, the presence of hopelessness guarantees the occurrence of depressive symptoms. They suggested that when people expect negative outcomes of events in their lives and believe that they are helpless to change these outcomes, they will experience the symptoms of hopelessness depression. Other proximal contributory causes, such as lack of social support, might also play a role in the onset of depressive symptoms. Abramson et al.'s (1989) hopelessness theory of depression is premised on the idea that there is a specific and identifiable chain of events leading from distal and contributory proximal causes to an eventual culmination in hopelessness (the proximal sufficient cause), which then elicits the symptoms of hopelessness depression; research has provided ample support for this notion (see Abramson et al., 1989).

This chapter discusses cognitive vulnerability for social anxiety disorder. The concept of cognitive vulnerability is not as well developed in social anxiety disorder as it is in depression. Yet, the literature provides information on possible distal and proximal risk factors that may contribute to the development of social anxiety disorder or the occurrence of episodes of social anxiety. This discussion first looks at possible distal risk factors—those that occur relatively early in the chain of events that culminates in the symptoms of social anxiety disorder. Specifically, events that may occur in the family and within the context of peer relations are reviewed. Early experiences with either family or peers may contribute to the development of thinking styles associated with social anxiety disorder. Later, possible proximal risk factors, those that seem to occur in closer relation to the onset of symptoms, are explored. Specifically, the cognitive styles of adults with social anxiety disorder are investigated, focusing on attentional biases, memory biases, and judgment-interpretation biases that might play a role in the onset and maintenance of the disorder.

EARLY RISK FACTORS FOR COGNITIVE
VULNERABILITY TO SOCIAL ANXIETY DISORDER

Social anxiety disorder, the most prevalent of the anxiety disorders, is characterized by intense fear and discomfort in social and/or performance situations (American Psychiatric Association, APA, 1994). Commonly feared situations include public speaking; initiating and maintaining conversations; asserting oneself; and eating, drinking, and writing in front of others (Holt, Heimberg, Hope, & Liebowitz, 1992). These fears often lead to significant impairment in social, educational, and occupational functioning (e.g., Schneier et al., 1994). In the National Comorbidity Survey (NCS; Kessler et al., 1994), the lifetime prevalence rate of social anxiety disorder, defined by the criteria specified in the *Diagnostic and Statistical Manual of Mental Disorders, Third Edition, Revised* (*DSM–III–R*; APA, 1987), was 13.3%.

Various cognitive models of social anxiety disorder have been proposed (e.g., Clark & Wells, 1995; Rapee & Heimberg, 1997). Rapee and Heimberg's (1997) model posits that individuals with social anxiety disorder come to view the world as a harsh and critical place and thus conduct their lives as though they are constantly under the scrutiny of others. Specifically, socially anxious people come to view themselves from the perspective of the audience (most often perceived as critical). However, this mental representation is unlikely to be veridical, but instead is a compilation of the individuals' concerns about how they may come across to others, feedback from internal and external cues, and memories for (mostly negative) events. They then compare this mental representation of self as seen by the audience to the standards that they perceive the audience holds for them. The more the mental representation of the self as seen by the audience falls short of the perception of the audience's standards for them, the greater the likelihood that the individuals with social anxiety disorder will expect to be negatively evaluated. The judgment of likely negative evaluation initiates behavioral, cognitive, and physiological symptoms of anxiety, which serve to confirm the socially anxious individuals' beliefs that they have been or will be negatively evaluated by others, and a vicious cycle ensues. Rapee and Heimberg (1997) also pointed out that when attention is shifted to the representation of the self as seen by the audience, external indicators of negative evaluation (e.g., a person yawning in the audience during a public speaking experience or a single piece of criticism in an otherwise positive job evaluation) become highly salient.

It is important to the Rapee and Heimberg model that the person believes that others are likely to be critical and that negative evaluation is a probable outcome in social situations. One way to elucidate the origins of these beliefs is to look to early experiences with parents and peers.

Factors Related to the Family Environment and Parenting

Attachment.   Beginning in early infancy, people develop schemas for understanding their social world via the parent–infant relationship. Bowlby (1982) and others (see Greenberg, 1999) posited that the early parent–infant relationship has a major impact on personality development and can be predictive of later psychopathology. Attachment theorists have distinguished between secure and insecure attachment relationships (see Dozier, Stovall, & Albus, 1999). Securely attached children have parents who are attentive and responsive. These children, who develop the beliefs that they are loved and that their caregivers are loving people, come to possess strong self-esteem and perceptions of competence. Insecurely attached children, on the other hand, have parents who are rejecting and undependable. These children develop the beliefs that they are unloved and that their caregivers are unloving, leading to feelings of anger, mistrust, and anxiety. Indeed, Bowlby proposed that anxiety is "the fundamental condition underlying insecure attachment" (Greenberg, 1999, p. 488).

Researchers have not yet explored the relation between parent–child attachment patterns and the later development of social anxiety disorder. Rather, patterns of *adult* attachment have been studied in individuals with social anxiety disorder based on the assumption that the way people relate to one another as adults has its roots in the early parent–child relationship. Mickelson, Kessler, and Shaver (1997) explored adult attachment styles in the NCS and found that social anxiety disorder was negatively related to having a secure attachment style and positively related to having an avoidant or anxious attachment style. Another study (Eng, Heimberg, Hart, Schneier, & Liebowitz, 2001) also found social anxiety disorder to be associated with insecure attachment styles. Eng et al. (2001) found that individuals with social anxiety disorder were more likely than nonclinical controls to be classified as insecurely attached, and insecure attachment was associated with greater severity of social anxiety disorder symptoms. Although some people with social anxiety disorder do exhibit secure attachment styles, it is interesting to note that those with insecure attachment styles were also more likely to become depressed.

Behavioral Inhibition. Another issue to consider with regard to infant–parent interaction patterns is infant temperament. Temperament refers to behavioral tendencies that are present in infancy and are presumed to be inherited, given their very early presentation. Interaction patterns are undoubtedly influenced by parental factors (e.g., parental mental illness, marital discord, etc.) but can also be influenced by these early tendencies exhibited by the infant. Particularly relevant to the anxiety disorders is the temperamental style referred to as behavioral inhibition to the unfamiliar. Approximately 15% of infants can be described as behaviorally inhibited. These infants react to novel stimuli (including unfamiliar people) in a fearful way, evidenced by both behavior (e.g., crying) and physiological reactivity (e.g., increased heart rate). According to Kagan, Reznick, and Snidman (1988), three quarters of children who were identified as either behaviorally inhibited or uninhibited at age 2 are similarly classified when reassessed at age 8.

It is interesting to consider how behavioral inhibition can influence interactions very early in life. People might be less likely to approach infants who cry and appear fearful than infants who have a more outgoing disposition. This aversion might carry into childhood when peers and adults realize that these children might "do better" when left to their own devices.

In other words, children who are behaviorally inhibited might have less experience interacting with others and also find that when they do interact with others, the feedback that they get is less than positive.

Research has suggested that behavioral inhibition bears some relation to social anxiety disorder. Parents of behaviorally inhibited children have higher rates of social anxiety disorder than do the parents of uninhibited children (Rosenbaum, Biederman, Hirshfeld, Bolduc, & Chaloff, 1991). Furthermore, a number of studies have demonstrated a relationship between behavioral inhibition in childhood and social anxiety disorder (Biederman et al., 2001; Hayward, Killen, Kraemer, & Taylor, 1998; Mick & Telch, 1998).

Other Family Factors. Children might also learn about social relations from the way that their parents relate to others. Two major themes emerge in the research literature. First, people who develop social anxiety disorder seem to grow up in families where a great deal of importance is placed on making a good impression on others. Caster, Inderbitzen, and Hope (1999) found that adolescents who described themselves as socially anxious were more likely than less socially anxious adolescents to report that their parents were concerned with the opinions of others. Similarly, Bruch, Heimberg, Berger, and Collins (1989) reported that people with social anxiety disorder were more likely than people with agoraphobia to recall that their parents overemphasized the opinions of others. In Caster et al.'s (1999) study, socially anxious adolescents were also more likely to report that their parents were ashamed of their children's shyness and difficulties in social performance.

How may parental emphasis on the opinions of others be related to the development of cognitive vulnerability to social anxiety disorder? When parents have strong social evaluative concerns, it makes sense that they will correct their children, constantly telling them how to act and what to say (see Rapee & Spence, 2004). This scenario may lead children to come to expect threat in social situations and may also lead them to believe that making a good impression on others is a difficult, if not impossible, goal to accomplish (Bruch et al., 1989; Buss, 1980; Cloitre & Shear, 1995).

The second major theme that has emerged in the literature is that children can learn about social relations by watching their parents' behavior in the social arena. This can apply not only to parents' relations with their own peers, but also to parents' abilities to help their children navigate the social world. Whereas some parents who have socially reticent children may purposefully set up social interactions for their children, parents who themselves are socially anxious may be more than happy to facilitate avoidance for their children (which, in turn, serves their own desire to avoid). Bruch et al. (1989) found that people with social anxiety disorder were more likely than people with agoraphobia to report that their parents isolated them from social experiences when they were children. In that same study, people with social anxiety disorder were also more likely to report that their families rarely socialized as a unit. Similarly, in Caster et al.'s (1999) study, socially anxious adolescents were more likely than nonanxious adolescents to perceive their parents as socially isolated.

Two points are important to consider here. Parents who fail to provide their children with the opportunity to learn to interact with others also prevent their children from learning that such interactions can be rewarding and pleasurable. From a young age, then, some people may get caught in a vicious cycle of social avoidance and distress. Furthermore, parents may also communicate to their children that social situations are dangerous and should be feared. Thus, children may become more likely to notice threat in the environment and, furthermore, may be more likely to respond to such threat in a negative and maladaptive way.

Factors Related to Peer Relationships

As children grow older, they spend less time in the company of family and more time in the company of peers. As such, their beliefs about their abilities in the social world are undoubtedly influenced by peer relationships. The relation between social anxiety and peer relationships is a difficult one to disentangle. The research seems to suggest the existence of a reciprocal relationship such that socially anxious children are more likely than nonanxious children to experience negative peer relationships, most notably peer neglect (La Greca, Dandes, Wick, Shaw, & Stone, 1988; Strauss, Lahey, Frick, Frame, & Hynd, 1988), and these experiences lead to the exacerbation and maintenance of social anxiety.

Two studies have examined this complex relation. Rubin and Mills (1988) assessed different types of social isolation in a group of schoolchildren during the second, fourth, and fifth grades. Children who were classified as behaving in a passive, solitary way while at school were rated by their peers as more anxious, withdrawn, and asocial than other children and were also more likely to be rejected (and less likely to be accepted) by their peers. This relation between passive withdrawal and peer rejection got stronger as children got older. The authors also reported that the best predictor of loneliness during the fifth grade was low self-perceived social competence during the second grade. This study suggests that repeated peer rejection directed at passive, withdrawn children might contribute to the cognitive style associated with social anxiety disorder. Such children, based on repeated social failure, may develop a belief that they cannot succeed in social situations, leading them to then avoid social interactions with their peers and, in turn, leading to increasing loneliness as they get older.

Vernberg, Abwender, Ewell, and Beery (1992) looked at the relation between social anxiety and peer relationships in a sample of adolescents whose families had recently moved to a new community. Studying the adolescents over the course of their first year in the new community, Vernberg et al. (1992) found that social anxiety was associated with less frequent peer interactions in the first few months of school (for both boys and girls) and to less intimate friendships (for girls only) in the later part of the year. Peer exclusion was associated with increased social anxiety as the year progressed. In light of Vernberg et al.'s study, it is interesting to note that in an epidemiological study, moving more than three times as a child was positively related to a diagnosis of social anxiety disorder among children (Chartier, Walker, & Stein, 2001). However, these data do not permit an examination of cause and effect; as in Vernberg et al.'s study, it might be the case that socially anxious children have a more difficult time with making new friends after moving and these difficulties lead to an exacerbation of social anxiety over time.

One interesting study on the relation between social anxiety and peer relationships in a clinical sample also deserves comment. In line with research in nonclinical samples of socially anxious children, Spence, Donovan, and Brechman-Toussaint (1999) found that children with social anxiety disorder experienced more negative social interactions than did control children. Based on school observations, children with social anxiety disorder were found to have fewer positive interactions with their peers than were control children (the groups did not differ on negative or "ignore" interactions). Furthermore, children with social anxiety disorder initiated interactions with peers less frequently than control children and also had fewer peer interactions, suggesting that other children tended not to initiate interactions with them either. Spence et al. (1999) also reported on the impact that these experiences seemed to have in terms of cognitive style. When children in their study were presented with negative and positive social events and asked about the likelihood of these events occurring, children with social anxiety disorder were less likely than control children to expect positive social situations to occur and tended to be more likely than control children to expect negative social situations to occur. It is interesting to note that this pattern is in line with findings in the literature in adults with social anxiety disorder (e.g., Amir, Foa, & Coles, 1998a), suggesting that cognitive biases with regard to social experiences may develop very early.

In line with the findings on difficulties with peer relationships in socially anxious children, two studies have explored retrospective memories of childhood peer relationships in socially anxious adults. Roth, Coles, and Heimberg (2002) found that college students' high scores on a measure of social anxiety were related to reports of frequent teasing during childhood (see also Storch et al., 2004). A recent study by McCabe, Antony, Summerfeldt, Liss, and Swinson (2003) indicated that 92% of participants with social anxiety disorder recalled having been teased or bullied during childhood. Patients with social anxiety disorder were more likely to recall having been teased or bullied than were patients with obsessivecompulsive disorder or panic disorder. These studies suggest that difficulties with peer relationships during childhood can continue to have an impact into adulthood.

Other Life Events

Other life events may also contribute to cognitive vulnerability for social anxiety disorder. For example, marital conflict, including early parental separation or divorce (Chartier et al., 2001; Davidson, Hughes, George, & Blazer, 1993), lack of a close relationship with an adult during childhood (Chartier et al., 2001), and long-lasting separation from either parent during childhood (Wittchen, Stein, & Kessler, 1999) have all been associated with the development of social anxiety disorder.

Magee (1999) explored the influence of traumatic life events on the development of social anxiety disorder using data from the NCS. The onset of social anxiety disorder before age 12 in females was associated with rape and/or molestation by a relative. Chartier et al. (2001) also found a relation between childhood sexual and physical abuse and incidence of social anxiety disorder. Magee (1999) suggested that because some perpetrators of rape or molestation blame their victims, people who have this type of experience might develop a more generalized fear of being criticized by others. Although Magee did not find that parental divorce increased the odds of an individual developing social anxiety disorder (in contrast to the findings of Davidson et al., 1993), the onset of social anxiety disorder was strongly associated with verbal aggression between respondents' parents. Magee pointed out that observing verbal aggression between parents can also be related to the development of generalized fears of being criticized by others. Watching one's own parents be verbally aggressive toward one another might suggest to a child that social relationships, even between people who are supposed to love one another, can be characterized by intense criticism and instability.

Various studies have also reported a link between the presence of psychopathology in parents and the development of social anxiety disorder in offspring (Chartier et al., 2001; Davidson et al., 1993; Wittchen et al., 1999). Lieb et al. (2000) explored this issue in greater detail, using data that was collected from over 1,000 community adolescents. As suggested by research reviewed earlier, children of parents with social anxiety disorder were significantly more likely to also have social anxiety disorder than were children whose parents did not have the disorder. The presence of social anxiety disorder in the parent was the best predictor of social anxiety disorder in the adolescent, but other anxiety disorders, depressive disorders, and alcohol use disorders in parents were also associated with social anxiety disorder in their children.

Lieb et al. (2000) also reported that respondents who met criteria for social anxiety disorder were more likely than those who did not meet criteria to describe their parents as overprotective and rejecting. It is interesting to note that the association between parental rejection and adolescents' social anxiety disorder was significantly greater when parents were affected by psychopathology of any kind.

The common thread in these studies seems to be that people who develop social anxiety disorder may be more likely than others to have parents who were unavailable (because of poor mental health or because they actually left the home). In such situations, children may come to blame themselves and may come to see themselves as unable to establish and maintain positive social relationships. Furthermore, such experiences may lead children to develop the belief that social relationships are tenuous and that any "mis-step" could lead to their dissolution.

COGNITIVE FACTORS ASSOCIATED WITH SOCIAL ANXIETY DISORDER

Much of the chapter thus far has offered an account of factors that may contribute to the development of cognitive styles characteristic of social anxiety disorder. This section reviews the available evidence that cognitive factors may play a role in the onset and maintenance of social anxiety disorder. Much of the evidence concerns the study of biased information processing. In particular, three kinds of biased information processing—attentional biases, memory biases, and judgment biases—have been extensively studied in these disorders, and the literature relevant to these areas is reviewed.

Attentional Biases in Social Anxiety Disorder

Definitions and Methodology.   The various cognitive models of psychopathology share the premise that affected individuals have a "sensitivity to and preoccupation with stimuli in their environment that represent their concern" (Williams, Mathews, & MacLeod, 1996, p. 3). Whereas it is generally adaptive to be vigilant to threat in the world (people are likely to live longer that way!), persons with social anxiety disorder are *hyper*vigilant, looking for potential social catastrophe (and finding it) around every corner. Biased attention of this nature may be the result of disorder, but it is also possible that these attentional biases play more of a causal or mediational role in the development of social anxiety disorder, as well as in its maintenance.

Two primary tasks have been used to explore attentional biases in the anxiety disorders and in other forms of psychopathology. The most common is the Stroop (1935) color naming task. In the original Stroop task, individuals were required to name the color in which a word was printed rather than reading the particular word aloud. Performance on the task was measured by the speed and accuracy in which words were color named, and the greatest degree of interference with performance was observed when the participant was required to name the color of ink in which the name of a color was printed (e.g., responding with "green" when the word "red" appeared in green ink rather than reading the word "red" aloud).

In a very influential study, Mathews and MacLeod (1985) developed a modified Stroop task in which threat words, rather than color names, were used as stimuli. In this study, anxious patients were slower at color naming during the modified Stroop task than were nonanxious controls. More importantly, anxious individuals were found to be particularly slow at color naming words related to threat. Since that time, researchers have developed Stroop tasks that involve disorder-relevant threat cues. In studies of individuals with social anxiety disorder, threatening stimuli are generally of a social or evaluative nature (e.g., boring, foolish, inferior; see Mattia, Heimberg, & Hope, 1993). The general assumption underlying the "emotional Stroop" is that individuals will take longer to color name words that represent threat (or current concern) to them because the content of the word diverts their attention from the color in which the word is printed.

Another task used to assess attentional bias in psychopathology is the visual dot-probe paradigm (MacLeod, Mathews, & Tata, 1986). In this paradigm, participants are presented with a pair of words on a computer screen. The words, generally oriented one above the other, are presented briefly (typically for about 500 ms) and then disappear. Afterward, a dot (.) is presented in the position previously occupied by one of the words. Participants are to respond as quickly as possible (usually by pressing a key) when the dot first appears on the screen. When a participant's attention is drawn to a word in the top position and the dot is presented in the top position, there may be facilitation of responding. Conversely, when the dot appears in the alternate position, responding may be slowed.

Studies of Stroop Response in Social Anxiety Disorder. As noted earlier, cognitive theories of anxiety posit that individuals with a specific disorder are highly vigilant to threat in their environment that is related to their specific concerns. In the case of individuals with social anxiety disorder, this "selective attention" should be directed to social threat. A study by Hope, Rapee, Heimberg, and Dombeck (1990) offers support for this hypothesis. In their study, patients with social anxiety disorder and patients with panic disorder were presented with neutral words, social threat-related words (e.g., stupid, embarrassed, boring), and physical threat-related words (e.g., fatal, illness, doctor) using a modified Stroop task. Individuals with social anxiety disorder demonstrated greater response latencies for social threat words than neutral words. However, their response latencies for physical threat words and neutral words did not differ. As would be expected, patients with panic disorder exhibited longer latencies for physical threat words but not social threat words. Two additional studies comparing patients with social anxiety disorder to matched community controls also provide support for the selective attention hypothesis (Lundh & Öst, 1996b; Mattia et al., 1993). In these studies, patients with social anxiety disorder exhibited longer latencies than did control participants on all word types (social threat, physical threat, and matched neutral words), but were particularly slow to respond to social threat words.

Maidenberg, Chen, Craske, Bohn, and Bystritsky (1996) addressed the question of whether selective attention was related specifically to threat or whether attention was drawn to words with a more generally negative valence. Patients with social anxiety disorder, panic disorder, and normal controls completed a modified Stroop task with word stimuli drawn from seven categories: social-threat (e.g., inferior), social-positive (e.g., respected), panic-threat (e.g., gasping), panic-positive (e.g., healthy), general-threat (cancer), general positive (e.g., happy), and neutral (e.g., identical). Among the patients with social anxiety disorder, latencies to color name the various types of threat words (social, panic, general) did not differ. However, when latencies to color name threat words were compared to latencies to color name neutral words, differences emerged only for the social-threat words, with social anxiety disorder patients taking longer to color name the social threat words than neutral words. In contrast, panic disorder patients demonstrated longer latencies for all threat-related words (as compared to neutral words), leading the authors to conclude that social anxiety disorder is characterized by a more specifically focused fear network than that of panic disorder (Maidenberg et al., 1996).

Recently, DiPino and Riskind (2000) tried to determine the specific nature of social-threat words most relevant to shy people and people with social anxiety disorder. In their study, participants with social anxiety disorder, participants who had been classified as shy (but who did not meet criteria for social anxiety disorder) and nonclinical control participants completed a Stroop task that included neutral words and four kinds of affect words (i.e., words related to shame, guilt, evaluation, and shyness). Although significant group differences did not emerge on the shyness, guilt, or evaluation words, participants with social anxiety disorder and participants who were shy showed more interference on shame words (e.g., ashamed, exposed, embarrass, humiliate) than did nonclinical control participants. This is the first study to examine shame and its potential relation to social anxiety; further study is warranted.

Finally, it is interesting to note that successful treatment for social anxiety disorder can reduce the interference produced by social threat words in the Stroop color naming task. In the Mattia et al. (1993) study, patients with social anxiety disorder who responded to a variety of treatments demonstrated a significant reduction in response latency for social threat words following treatment and patients classified as treatment non-responders did not. The groups did not differ in their responses to physical threat words or color names. Similar findings were reported by Lundh and Öst (2001). Whereas nonresponders to CBT continued to show Stroop interference, patients who were deemed treatment responders showed a significant reduction in attentional bias for social threat words.

Studies of Dot-Probe Response in Social Anxiety Disorder. Only one study has employed the classic dot-probe paradigm in the study of social anxiety disorder. Asmundson and Stein (1994) employed the dot-probe task to compare patients with social anxiety disorder to nonanxious control participants by presenting pairs of words that were either both neutral, one neutral/one physical threat, or one neutral/one social threat. In addition to viewing the words, participants were asked to read aloud the top word and then to quickly press the space bar for trials in which a dot appeared in the position of either word. Consistent with the selective attention hypothesis, patients with social anxiety disorder responded more rapidly to the presentation of the dot when social threat words were presented in the top position. Patients with social anxiety disorder did not show differences in response rates when physical threat or neutral words appeared in the top position. Furthermore, nonanxious control participants did not differ in their response rates for any pairings of words and dot probes.

Three studies have used a creative variation on the dot-probe paradigm to study attentional biases toward (or away from) different facial expressions. Facial expressions have been used in studies exploring attention and memory biases in social anxiety disorder because these stimuli are viewed as more externally valid than mere words. By definition, people with this disorder are exquisitely sensitive to the feedback that they receive from others and facial expressions are an important way in which that feedback is communicated.

Bradley et al. (1997, Exp. 1) explored attentional biases for facial expressions using a modified dot-probe task in a nonclinical sample of participants who had been divided into high and low socially anxious groups according to their scores on the Fear of Negative Evaluation Scale (FNE; Watson & Friend, 1969). Bradley et al. (1997) did not find evidence for a social anxiety related attentional bias for angry faces. Yet, in a study by Yuen (1994) in which participants were told that they would have to give a speech after completing the dot-probe task, those who scored high on the FNE scale responded more slowly to probes that were presented after negative faces than to probes presented after neutral faces. This bias was not exhibited by participants who scored low on the FNE scale.

In a follow-up, Mansell, Clark, Ehlers, and Chen (1999) had participants—half of whom had been told that they would have to make a speech after they had finished the task—complete the modified dot-probe task. Whereas Yuen (1994) only presented participants with negative and neutral faces, Mansell et al. (1999) also included happy faces. In line with Yuen's (1994) findings, highly socially anxious participants reacted more slowly to probes presented after they had seen negative faces than to probes that were presented after they had seen neutral faces, but only in the social threat condition (i.e., when they expected they would soon be giving a speech). In the social threat condition, highly socially anxious participants also reacted more slowly to probes presented after they had seen positive faces than to probes that were presented after they had seen neutral faces.

Mansell and colleagues advanced some interesting suggestions concerning why the attentional bias was demonstrated in reaction to both positive and negative faces. It is possible that *any* emotionally valenced expression could remind socially anxious individuals that they are being evaluated, leading them to direct their attention elsewhere. They may also misinterpret positive expressions, thinking instead that they are being laughed at, for example. These findings are interesting to interpret in light of findings by Wallace and Alden (1997). These authors found that social success can actually lead to negative emotional states in people with social anxiety disorder because they perceive that others will expect even more of them following success, increasing the likelihood that they will not be able to live up to others' expectations during future interactions.

It is important to mention that the findings of the dot-probe studies that used faces as stimuli seem incongruent with the findings from Stroop tasks and from dot-probe studies that used words as stimuli. Stroop studies, as well as the study using the classical dot-probe paradigm, suggest that attention is directed toward threat words. Studies using the modified dot-probe paradigm suggest that attention is directed away from emotional faces (as compared to neutral faces). On closer consideration, these patterns need not necessarily be seen as discrepant. In the modified dot-probe studies of facial stimuli, differences in reaction time did emerge between neutral and emotional faces. In order for this difference to emerge, participants must have initially attended to the faces. Once the facial expressions were perceived as being emotionally laden, participants may have subsequently diverted their attention. This pattern of findings fits well with what Mogg, Mathews, and Weinman (1987) termed the vigilance–avoidance pattern of cognitive processing. People who are anxious are vigilant to threat in their environments, and they are motivated to avoid threat, reduce its impact, or to act as if it does not exist as well.

The vigilance–avoidance pattern of processing could have important implications for the maintenance of social anxiety disorder. At some stage in information processing, people with social anxiety disorder direct their attention away from the facial expressions of others. By not being attuned to the finer points of facial expressions (which is likely if they rapidly divert their attention), people with social anxiety disorder may miss out on positive feedback from others (in the forms of smiles, nods, etc.) or, at least, the opportunity to learn that these pleasant expressions are not harbingers of future negative outcomes. Their beliefs about their lack of ability in social situations might therefore be perpetuated. Furthermore, by turning away from facial expressions, people with social anxiety disorder might miss out on important social cues, making it more likely that they will come across as less socially skilled than others. This too can serve to perpetuate social anxiety over time, because individuals with the disorder might actually have negative social interactions with others, serving to confirm their beliefs that they lack the ability to successfully negotiate social situations.

Studies Using Alternative Methodologies to Explore Attentional Bias in Social Anxiety Disorder. Researchers using other paradigms have also recognized the importance of studying reactions to facial expressions among people with social anxiety disorder. Gilboa-Schechtman, Foa, and Amir (1999) made use of a "face-in-the-crowd" paradigm to explore attentional biases for faces in social anxiety disorder. In their study, participants with social anxiety disorder and nonclinical controls were shown arrays of faces. On some trials, all of the faces in the crowd shared the same expression (neutral, happy, or angry), and on other trials, one face in the crowd exhibited a different emotional expression (neutral, angry, happy, or disgust) than the rest of the group. Participants were asked to indicate if there was a discrepant face in each array that they were shown.

All participants were quicker at finding an angry face in a crowd of neutral faces than they were at finding a happy face in a crowd of neutral faces. However, this discrepancy was more pronounced in individuals with social anxiety disorder. This task took longer when participants with social anxiety disorder were exposed to happy or angry crowds than when they were exposed to neutral crowds. Explanations for this pattern of findings were similar to those advanced for the findings in Mansell et al. (1999). It is possible that people with social anxiety disorder are sensitive to emotional reactions of any type in others and it is also possible that people with the disorder view even positive faces in a negative way (e.g., a smile actually means that someone is laughing at you).

At a quick glance, the findings from Gilboa-Schechtman et al. (1999) seem to be in contrast to those of Mansell et al. (1999) in that the latter study indicated that socially anxious people diverted their attention away from emotional faces, whereas the former study found that people with social anxiety disorder directed their attention toward emotional faces. Yet, as already noted, in the Mansell et al. (1999) study, it seems that participants must have initially directed their attention toward the faces, identified the expressions, and subsequently diverted their attention when they saw that the faces were of an emotional nature. That Mansell et al. (1999) used more real-life stimuli than Gilboa-Schechtman et al. (1999) supports this argument.

In a study with better external validity than most, Veljaca and Rapee (1998) asked participants who had scored either high or low on a measure of social anxiety to give a speech to an audience of confederates who had been trained to engage in an equal number of positive (e.g., leaning forward) and negative (e.g., yawning) feedback behaviors, many of which included some sort of facial feedback. Whereas participants low in social anxiety detected more positive feedback behaviors than negative feedback behaviors from audience members, participants high in social anxiety showed the opposite effect.

Finally, in a unique study using words as stimuli, Amir, Foa, and Coles (1998b) used a homograph paradigm (a homograph is a word with multiple meanings) to study attentional bias in individuals with social anxiety disorder. In this paradigm, participants are presented with a sentence, which is then followed by a word. Participants must decide if this word is related to the sentence they have just seen. In Amir et al.'s study, the word that followed each sentence was presented either at a very short delay or at a longer delay in an effort to study the sequence of vigilance and avoidance hypothesized by Mogg et al. (1987).

Two types of sentences were used for the critical trials in their study. Half of the sentences ended in a nonhomograph and the word following the sentence was a social threat word (e.g., She cut off the string. ABANDON). The other half of the sentences ended in a homograph and the stimulus word following the sentence implied the socially threatening meaning of the homograph but did not fit the meaning of the sentence (e.g., She wrote down the mean. UNFRIENDLY). It was assumed that the threatening meaning of homograph had been activated if participants took longer to respond to social threat words following sentences ending in homographs than those ending in nonhomographs.

Significant results did in fact emerge for the sentences ending in socially relevant homographs. When words followed sentences at a short delay, people with social anxiety disorder showed more interference than they did after a long delay; nonclinical controls did not show this effect. Amir et al. (1998b) interpreted these findings in terms of Mogg et al.'s vigilance–avoidance notion. It might be that cues in the environment (like the socially relevant homographs) can immediately activate threat-relevant information in anxious people. Yet, given that this type of information is aversive, they may be motivated to shift their attention away from it. The longer delay between the sentence and the word in Amir et al.'s study might have permitted participants to do just that.

In summary, numerous tasks have been employed to explore the general hypothesis that people with social anxiety disorder selectively attend to social threat in their environments. Although the findings are often complex, they generally support this contention. It seems that people who are socially anxious have a natural tendency to attend to threat in their environments. However, once they have noticed threat (or what they perceive to be threatening), they may be motivated to divert attention away from it. This tendency to divert attention away from socially relevant information (be it truly threatening or just perceived as such) may be very important to understanding the etiology and maintenance of social anxiety disorder.

Memory Bias in Social Anxiety Disorder

Definitions and Methodology.   Researchers interested in memory biases distinguish between implicit memory and explicit memory. According to Schacter (1998), explicit memory is the form of memory demonstrated when someone attempts to learn new material and makes a specific effort to recall that material. Explicit memory requires conscious and effortful recollection of previous experiences. In contrast, implicit memory is the learning that takes place naturally in the course of everyday life. Individuals do not set out specifically to learn something, but their performance indicates that learning has indeed taken place.

Tests of implicit and explicit memory generally occur in two phases (see Roediger & McDermott, 1993). In the first phase, experimental participants are presented with test stimuli, generally words or pictures. In the second phase, task demands differ depending on the type of memory being assessed. Explicit memory tasks typically involve recall or recognition.

In recall tasks, for example, participants might be asked to list the words that they had previously rehearsed. In recognition tasks, they might simply indicate whether or not they had seen a particular word or picture during the first phase of the task—in other words, they must distinguish stimuli they had already seen from novel stimuli presented for the first time. Explicit memory biases would be said to have occurred if the person recalls more threatening words than words of other sorts, endorses more threat words than neutral words in a recognition test, or if this tendency was noted in patients but not in normal control participants.

In implicit memory tasks, participants are not instructed to rehearse material or led to believe that they will be tested on it later. Rather, they are led to believe that they are completing a task unrelated to the first phase of the study. For example, participants might be given word stems and be asked to complete the stems with the first word that comes to mind. The assumption is that participants will be more adept at completing stems of words that they had previously studied than words that were not on the original stimuli list; this facilitation is referred to as "priming" (see Schacter, 1998). Implicit memory biases would be demonstrated if more word stems were completed with previously seen threat words than with previously seen neutral words or if this tendency were noted in patients but not in normal control participants.

Studies of Memory Bias in Social Anxiety Disorder. It is clear that people who have difficulties with social anxiety selectively attend to social threat in their environments (although after having initially attended to threat, they might then direct their attention away from it). The literature on memory biases in social anxiety disorder is less clear-cut than the literature on attentional biases. Some studies have suggested that memory biases in social anxiety disorder do not exist. Rapee, McCallum, Melville, Ravenscroft, and Rodney (1994) ran four studies exploring both implicit and explicit memory biases in individuals with social anxiety disorder. Their studies involved both standard laboratory tasks (recall and recognition of social threat words as compared to physical threat words, positive words, and neutral words) and tasks with relevance to situations that are difficult for people with social anxiety disorder (memory for feedback on a public speaking task). None of the studies in Rapee et al.'s (1994) report showed any sort of memory bias. Lundh and Öst (1997) also failed to find evidence of implicit or explicit memory biases in people with social anxiety disorder.

Other studies have shown evidence of memory biases among patients with social anxiety disorder, with some demonstrating impaired memory and others enhanced memory for information relevant to social threat. Wenzel and Holt (2002) found evidence for memory impairments in a study in which patients with social anxiety disorder and nonclinical control participants were presented with prose passages, some relevant to evaluative threat and some neutral in content. Participants were asked to complete free recall tasks immediately after reading each passage. Patients with social anxiety disorder actually remembered less information from the passages pertaining to evaluative threat than did the nonclinical controls. The authors interpreted their findings in the context of vigilance–avoidance theory, proposing that patients with social anxiety disorder avoided content that was of a threatening nature to them. Other studies, however, have shown evidence of enhanced memory for social threat relevant information among patients with social anxiety disorder. Amir, Foa, and Coles (2000) found evidence for an implicit memory bias in the disorder using the white-noise judgment paradigm (Jacoby, Allan, Collins, & Larwill, 1988). This task was developed to reduce the influence of explicit memory processes on tasks meant to measure implicit memory. Participants were asked to listen to and then repeat neutral sentences and social threat related sentences. During the test phase, participants were presented with the sentences that they had heard before ("old") and with novel sentences ("new"), all of which were masked by white noise at variable volumes. Participants were then asked to rate the level of noise masking each sentence. Ratings of lower noise volume for old sentences than for new sentences have been taken as indicative of implicit memory (Jacoby et al., 1988), and, if this pattern were to occur specifically for socially threatening sentences among persons with social anxiety disorder, then an implicit memory bias would be demonstrated. Although nonclinical controls did not rate the noise volume of old and new sentences differently, people with social anxiety disorder did make lower noise ratings for old social threat sentences than for novel social threat sentences, providing support for an implicit memory bias.

In line with the research on attentional biases, some researchers have explored memory for faces in people with social anxiety disorder. In a study by Lundh and Öst (1996a; see also replication by Coles & Heimberg, 2005), participants with social anxiety disorder and nonclinical controls were presented with a series of faces and were asked to rate them as critical or accepting. Participants were subsequently presented with a larger set of faces (half of which they had rated and half of which they had never seen) and were asked to indicate if they recognized each face. Participants with social anxiety disorder and normal control participants did not differ in their judgments of faces as either critical or accepting, but participants with social anxiety disorder were better than normal control participants at recognizing the faces that they had rated as critical. In contrast, normal control participants showed a trend toward recognizing more of the faces that they had classified as accepting. It is interesting to note that this memory bias for critical faces seems to be unique to social anxiety disorder. In a study by Lundh, Thulin, Czyzykow, and Öst (1998), participants with panic disorder did not show a memory bias for faces that they had rated as critical, but rather showed a memory bias for faces that they had rated as safe (a more relevant concern for people with panic disorder).

In Foa, Gilboa-Schechtman, Amir, and Freshman (2000, Exp. 1), participants with social anxiety disorder were shown pictures of a series of people and were asked to learn each person's name. They were then presented with an encoding task in which they were asked to state the facial expression (happy, angry, or neutral) that each person exhibited. Subsequent to these learning and encoding tasks, participants performed a free recall task that involved listing the names of the people they had just seen and indicating the facial expression that each person had exhibited. People with social anxiety disorder performed better on the free recall task than did nonclinical controls. That is, individuals with social anxiety disorder were better than nonclinical controls at remembering the names of the persons they had seen earlier in the study and were better at correctly recalling the facial expression that each person had exhibited. This pattern supports the idea that socially anxious persons attend to others' facial expressions before diverting their attention.

Participants in Foa et al.'s (2000) Experiment 1 also performed a cued recall task in which they were given a list of names and asked to indicate which expression each person had exhibited during the second phase of the study. All participants showed better recall of happy faces than of neutral or angry faces, which did not support the hypothesis that people with social anxiety disorder would show enhanced memory for angry faces. On the cued recall task, people with social anxiety disorder again performed better than nonclinical controls, and as in the free recall task, all participants recalled happy faces better than angry or neutral faces. Yet, people with social anxiety disorder were found to recall angry expressions better than did nonclinical control participants.

In Foa et al.'s (2000) Experiment 2, individuals with social anxiety disorder and nonclinical controls were shown faces with neutral, happy, angry, or disgusted expressions. Later, these faces were interspersed with faces that the participants had not seen before, and they had to indicate if the faces were "new" or "old." In this study, participants with social anxiety disorder were better at recognizing old faces than were nonclinical controls and, furthermore, the clinical group was better at recognizing old negative facial expressions (anger and disgust) than they were at recognizing old nonnegative facial expressions.

In a similar task, Mansell et al. (1999) assessed recognition for faces that were used in the dot-probe task discussed earlier. After completing the dot-probe task, participants were presented with a number of faces (half of which had been used in the dot-probe task) and were asked to indicate which faces they had seen before. Low socially anxious participants did not show a recognition bias. High socially anxious participants did show a bias, which differed depending on the threat condition to which they were assigned. Participants who were under high threat were more likely to recognize any emotional face (positive or negative) as compared to neutral faces, but those who were not under threat were actually more likely to recognize neutral faces.

Data inconsistent with other studies of memory for facial expressions among individuals with social anxiety disorder were presented by Pérez-López and Woody (2001). Patients with social anxiety disorder and nonclinical controls were told that they would be giving a speech and were then shown photos of individuals who might be in the audience. In the photos, individuals exhibited threatening or reassuring facial expressions. After the encoding task, participants were given 3 minutes to prepare their speeches and were then presented with two side-by-side photos of each individual they had originally seen. In one photo, the person exhibited a threatening facial expression and, in the other, the person exhibited a reassuring facial expression; participants were asked to select which face they had seen during the encoding task. Contrary to expectations, patients with social anxiety disorder were less skilled than nonclinical control participants at recognizing previously seen faces and, although both groups showed a small bias in favor of remembering accepting faces, the bias index was only significant for patients with social anxiety disorder. These results were mediated by the level of state anxiety experienced by participants in anticipation of making their speeches. In other words, by focusing on the upcoming speech task, patients with social anxiety disorder might have been less able to encode information about the pictures that they had seen. This does not explain the bias in favor of remembering accepting faces; the authors pointed out, however, that this bias was quite small and was measured with an index that has limited utility.

In summary, the evidence for memory biases in social anxiety disorder is mixed. Whereas there is some evidence for enhanced memory for information relevant to social threat, other studies failed to find any evidence of memory bias and one study actually showed impaired memory for such information. The range of methodologies used to explore this issue might be a factor in these inconsistencies, suggesting that further research is required. It is quite likely that memory for social threat related information is at times enhanced and at times impaired; further research might be able to uncover the factors that lead to these divergent outcomes.

There is slightly stronger evidence to suggest that a bias might exist for memory of faces. The studies exploring this issue have shown, for the most part, that people with social anxiety disorder remember emotional faces (particularly when they are negative) better than neutral faces. This finding has important implications in terms of cognitive vulnerability for social anxiety disorder. If people come away from social situations remembering only the (real or perceived) critical people that they have encountered, then this might facilitate future avoidance and perpetuate the cycle of social avoidance and distress.

Although not specifically a memory bias, it is interesting to note that a number of studies show that memory for nonsocially threatening information may be disrupted in people with social anxiety disorder. Hope, Heimberg, and Klein (1990) asked female college students who had been classified as being high or low on social anxiety to interact with a male confederate. They were later asked to recall aspects of the interaction. Participants who scored high on the measure of social anxiety recalled less information (e.g., interests, appearance, background) about the male conversation partner and were more prone to make errors in their recall than were participants who scored low on the measure of social anxiety. In a subsequent study, Hope, Sigler, Penn, and Meier (1998) were not able to entirely replicate the earlier findings; however, socially anxious females did make more recall errors. Other studies with nonclinical samples show similar findings (e.g., Bond & Omar, 1990; Daly, Vangelisti, & Lawrence, 1989; Kimble & Zehr, 1982).

These findings fit very nicely with research on focus of attention in social anxiety disorder. When socially anxious individuals find themselves in stressful social situations, their attention is focused inward on themselves and on how they believe that they are coming across to others, rather than on the social situation at hand (e.g., Hackmann, Surawy, & Clark, 1998; Wells, Clark, & Ahmad, 1998; Wells & Papageorgiou, 1999). This shift in focus of attention has an impact on individuals with social anxiety disorder when they are in social situations, but also impacts on how they recall social situations once they are over. When imagining or remembering themselves in social situations, some people take an "observer perspective," seeing themselves as they imagine that others see them (almost as if viewing themselves on videotape); others take a "field perspective," recalling situations as viewed through their own eyes. Coles, Turk, Heimberg, and Fresco (2001) found that as the degree of anxiety associated with memories of social/performance situations increased, people with social anxiety disorder were more and more likely to take an observer perspective, whereas nonclinical controls were slightly more likely to take a field perspective. Furthermore, as the anxiety associated with these social memories increased, people with social anxiety disorder rated their behavior during the situations more negatively.

The excessive attention to how one is coming across to others (and to how one did come across to others, once social situations are over) has important implications for cognitive vulnerability to social anxiety disorder. By focusing attention on the self, rather than outward on the situation at hand, individuals with social anxiety disorder might come across to others as less socially skilled (e.g., not being able to follow the conversation, forgetting a person's name whom they have met many times, etc.), increasing the likelihood that they will receive negative feedback or be rejected by others. In addition, self-focused attention precludes socially anxious individuals from picking up on positive cues from others that might serve to disconfirm their beliefs. Because their focus is inward, they miss out on this important information and therefore judge the outcome of social situations on how they felt when they were in them, rather than on what actually occurred. This is clearly demonstrated in the Coles et al. (2001) study. When patients felt more anxious in social situations, they assumed that their performance was poorer. Coming away from social situations with biased data (overemphasis on the negative and missing out on the positive) could be important to both the onset and maintenance of social anxiety disorder. Furthermore, as already noted, being inwardly self-focused can actually lead to social impairments, which might also contribute to the onset and maintenance of the disorder.

Judgment and Interpretation Biases in Social Anxiety Disorder

A major factor implicated in the maintenance of social anxiety disorder is the fact that people with the disorder avoid social situations, often denying themselves the chance to learn that these situations are not as threatening as they perceive them to be. Studies of judgment and interpretation biases help in understanding the motivation behind this avoidance. First, socially anxious people tend to be harsh critics of their own social behavior. Following from this, it should come as no surprise that people who have difficulties with social anxiety expect negative outcomes in the social situations in which they find themselves. Further increasing the likelihood of avoidance, socially anxious people also perceive that they have little control over outcomes in their lives.

Judgments About the Self in Social Situations. Numerous studies have demonstrated that socially anxious people are their own worst critics. These studies typically place participants in a "mock" social situation and ask them to rate their own social behavior once the situation is over. Other participants in these mock social situations (usually experimental confederates) and/or objective observers are also asked to make similar ratings, allowing for a comparison between how socially anxious people judge themselves and how they are judged by others.

Stopa and Clark (1993) placed individuals with social anxiety disorder and nonanxious controls in a "get-acquainted" task with an experimental confederate. Participants were asked to rate their own social behavior, and tapes of the interaction were also rated at a later date by objective observers. As compared to nonclinical controls, participants with social anxiety disorder were rated higher on negative dimensions of social behavior (e.g., blushing, shaking, leaving gaps in the conversation) and lower on positive dimensions of social behavior (e.g., asking interesting questions, appearing socially competent, etc.) as assessed both by self-ratings and by ratings made by the observer. Of particular relevance, however, was the discrepancy between self-ratings and observer ratings. Participants in the social anxiety disorder group gave themselves significantly higher ratings on negative social behaviors and significantly lower ratings on positive social behaviors as compared to ratings made by the observer. In contrast, although nonclinical controls rated themselves somewhat lower on positive social behaviors than did the observer, self and observer ratings did not differ on negative social behaviors.

Alden and Wallace (1995) also used a "get-acquainted" task in which participants with social anxiety disorder and nonanxious controls interacted with a confederate who had been instructed to behave either positively or negatively toward the participant. Following the interaction, participants were asked to rate their own social behavior and were also rated by the confederate. As compared to ratings made by the confederate, people with social anxiety disorder rated themselves as less interesting and less likeable in both positive and negative interactions.

Other studies have made use of a speech task in which participants are asked to make a speech and are then rated by both themselves and objective observers. Rapee and Lim (1992) asked people with social anxiety disorder and nonclinical controls to make a speech in the presence of other study participants. Individuals rated their own performance and were also rated by the other participants. Whereas all participants (regardless of diagnosis) were more critical of themselves than others were of them, this was particularly true for people with social anxiety disorder. A similar finding was reported by Rapee and Hayman (1996).

People with social anxiety disorder also seem to differ from people without the disorder in terms of how they think that others interpret symptoms typically associated with anxiety such as blushing, shaking, or sweating. Roth, Antony, and Swinson (2001) reported that whereas nonclinical controls assume that others will interpret these symptoms as being indicative of some normal physical state like being hot or cold or tired, people with social anxiety disorder assume that others will interpret these symptoms as being indicative of an intense anxiety problem or some other psychiatric disorder. Going into social situations with this type of expectation most likely contributes to the tendency of people with social anxiety disorder to selectively attend to negative reactions from others. As already noted, this type of expectation precludes people with the disorder from noticing positive feedback in the environment and might also serve as a distraction, increasing the likelihood of real difficulties in the social arena.

It is interesting to reiterate at this point that people with social anxiety disorder take an observer perspective when viewing their own social behavior, that is, they tend to view themselves as if through the eyes of another person. This is a hallmark of cognitive models of social anxiety disorder and has also been demonstrated empirically in the literature (e.g., Hackmann et al., 1998). With this in mind, we can interpret the self-ratings made in these studies as measures of how people with social anxiety disorder assume they are viewed by others. Because they assume that they are viewed much worse than they really are and because they do little to gather discomfirmatory data, this tendency should perpetuate social avoidance and distress over time.

Judgments About the Social World. It has been established that people with social anxiety disorder tend to judge themselves quite harshly in social situations. It should then come as no surprise that people with the disorder tend to expect negative outcomes in social situations. Lucock and Salkovskis (1988) explored this issue, comparing patients with social anxiety disorder to matched control participants on the likelihoods they assigned to negative social and negative nonsocial events. Untreated patients with social anxiety disorder assigned a higher likelihood to a negative social event than did control participants. The two groups did not differ on the likelihood that negative nonsocial events would occur. Following treatment with cognitive behavior therapy, the patients with social anxiety disorder demonstrated significant improvement in their judgment bias for the likelihood of negative social events. Control participants did not repeat the assessment, however, leaving open the possibility that changes in the rated likelihood of negative social events were the result of repeated assessment rather than treatment.

Foa, Franklin, Perry, and Herbert (1996) replicated and extended the findings of Lucock and Salkovskis (1988) by comparing a sample of patients with social anxiety disorder to nonanxious controls. In this study, participants were also asked to assess the cost associated with negative events in addition to the likelihood of their occurrence. Nonanxious participants also repeated the task concurrent in time with the end of treatment for the patients with social anxiety disorder to control for repeated assessment and the passage of time. The findings of this study correspond favorably to those of Lucock and Salkovskis (1988). Untreated patients with social anxiety disorder were more likely than nonanxious participants to assign greater likelihoods to negative social events and to see their impact as being more costly. The groups did not differ in their likelihood and cost estimates for negative nonsocial events. Following cognitive behavioral treatment, estimates of likelihood and cost were attenuated for the patients with social anxiety disorder. In this case, drops in cost estimates were more related to improvement than changes in probability estimates, but this finding was not replicated by McManus, Clark, and Hackmann (2000).

Gilboa-Schechtman, Franklin, and Foa (2000) extended these findings by presenting patients with social anxiety disorder with both negative and positive social events. Participants were asked to rate the probability that each event would happen to them and were also presented with questions about their reactions to each event. As compared to nonclinical controls, patients with social anxiety disorder estimated that positive social events were less likely and negative social events were more likely. Furthermore, they associated a greater impact and more negative reactions to both positive and negative social events.

Participants in two studies were presented with ambiguous social situations (e.g., not obviously positively or negatively valenced) in an effort to identify a possible interpretation bias in social anxiety disorder. In Amir et al. (1998a), patients with social anxiety disorder, patients with obsessive-compulsive disorder (OCD), and nonanxious control participants were asked to consider a series of social and nonsocial scenarios. Participants were asked to rank order the likelihood that a positive, a neutral, and a negative outcome for each scenario would occur. As compared to patients with OCD and nonanxious controls, patients with social anxiety disorder were more likely to select the negative interpretation for social situations even when positive and neutral interpretations were available. The three groups did not differ in their interpretation of nonsocial events.

Stopa and Clark (2000) conducted a study similar to that of Amir et al. (1998a), comparing patients with social anxiety disorder to patients with any other anxiety disorder. In addition to rating ambiguous situations, participants were also asked to consider the meaning of mildly negative social events (e.g., "You've been talking to someone for a while and it becomes clear that they're not really interested in what you are saying."). Patients with social anxiety disorder were more likely than patients with other anxiety disorders to interpret ambiguous social situations as negative. They were also more likely than anxious controls to interpret the mildly negative social situations in catastrophic terms.

Not only do people with social anxiety disorder expect negative outcomes for themselves in social situations, but they also attribute outcomes in their lives to causes over which they have little control. Informed by research on attributional styles in depression (Abramson, Seligman, & Teasdale, 1978), Heimberg et al. (1989) gave a slightly modified version of the Attributional Styles Questionnaire (Peterson et al., 1982) to people with social anxiety disorder, other anxiety disorders, and depression. As compared to nonclinical controls, people with social anxiety disorder exhibited a more internal, global, and stable attributional style for negative events, quite similar to that exhibited by the depressed group. This attributional style suggests that people with social anxiety disorder attribute a great deal of responsibility for negative outcomes to unchangeable negative aspects of themselves. Two further studies (Cloitre, Heimberg, Liebowitz, & Gitow, 1992; Leung & Heimberg, 1996) shed additional light on the ways in which persons with social anxiety disorder explain the outcomes of events. In the study by Cloitre et al. (1992), patients with social anxiety disorder, patients with panic disorder, and normal controls completed a measure of locus of control. Both groups of anxiety disordered patients endorsed causes beyond their control more frequently than control participants. However, the patients differed in the nature of the causes of events in their lives. Panic patients attributed outcomes to chance, a finding that seems consistent with their concern about attacks of physiological symptoms that appear to come out of nowhere. Socially anxious patients, in contrast, viewed "powerful others" as controlling the outcomes of events. It seems that socially anxious persons do believe in an orderly and controllable world; they just believe someone else is at the switch!

These findings fit nicely with our knowledge about avoidance in persons with social anxiety disorder. Although these individuals avoid social situations because they want to avoid feeling "bad," their attributional style likely also plays an important role. Simply put, people with social anxiety disorder might avoid social situations because they see negative outcomes as inevitable regardless of their efforts to have an impact on the situation. Because of their avoidance, they never learn that they have more control over outcomes in their life than they think they do.

A definite strength of the research on social anxiety disorder has been the development of cognitive models for the disorder (e.g., Clark & Wells, 1995; Rapee & Heimberg, 1997). These models focus on factors that maintain the disorder, but they put less emphasis on the etiology or development of the disorder. Because cognitive models of social anxiety disorder have been informed by cognitive behavioral therapy for the disorder and have, in turn, helped to improve therapy for the disorder, etiology has not been emphasized. After all, cognitive behavioral therapy is effective regardless of whether or not patients have a clear understanding of the origins of their disorder. Yet, efforts to prevent the development of a psychological disorder develop from knowledge of its root causes.

As has been the case in research on depression, a diathesis–stress approach may be useful for organizing the distal factors that may contribute to the later development of social anxiety disorder. In terms of stressors, we have reviewed literature suggesting that certain negative events may contribute to the later onset of social anxiety disorder. Specifically, factors relating to parenting styles, family functioning, and peer relationships may influence the way that children come to see their social world and their ability to succeed therein. In terms of diatheses, the focus in social anxiety disorder has been different than it has been in research on mood disorders. Researchers in social anxiety disorder have focused most on the role that early temperament—specifically, behavioral inhibition to the unfamiliar—may play in the way that people come to experience their world. Although researchers have explored attributional style in people who currently have social anxiety disorder, this factor has yet to be explored downstream from the actual occurrence of social anxiety symptoms. It would be fruitful to employ longitudinal research methods to explore how specific negative life events and a negative attributional style eventually interact in the development of social anxiety disorder. It remains unclear whether attributional style develops first, influencing perceptions of negative life events, whether negative life events lead people to develop specific attributional styles, or whether other variables are involved as well. Understanding the nature of this effect seems important in terms of both treatment and prevention.

In terms of more proximal influences that might result in the expression of social anxiety disorder, we have focused here on biases in attention, memory, and interpretation of social stimuli. Again, these studies have examined individuals who currently have social anxiety disorder. People with social anxiety disorder are hypervigilant to social threat in their environments. They seem particularly likely to notice socially relevant information, to interpret it as threatening or dangerous, and in some situations, to then divert their attention away from it. This diversion of attention from socially relevant information may subserve the maintenance of social anxiety disorder by preventing people from attending to positive social cues that could serve to disconfirm their negative beliefs about their abilities in social situations. It may also lead to real impairments in social performance, serving to confirm and strengthen these negative beliefs. It comes as no surprise that people with social anxiety disorder expect negative outcomes in social situations and view their own social performance in a negative way, even though it is not always perceived that way by others.

When in the life of the socially anxious person do these biases become evident? Do they exist before a person actually develops problematic social anxiety? Or, are these biases actually symptoms of the disorder itself?

These questions require empirical investigation. Longitudinal studies are the essential next step in understanding the causal sequence of events that leads a person who experiences negative life events to actually develop a disorder.

A study by Schwartz, Snidman, and Kagan (1996) is an example of a "good start" in exploring some of these "links." As noted earlier in this chapter, there seems to be a connection between behavioral inhibition in infancy/childhood and the later development of social anxiety disorder. Schwartz et al. (1996) had adolescent participants who had been classified as behaviorally inhibited or uninhibited 11 years earlier complete a Stroop task that included physical threat words, social threat words, positive words, and neutral words. Although their results were quite complex, it appears that the responses of behaviorally inhibited adolescents (as classified 11 years earlier) included a greater proportion of words with threatening content than the responses of adolescents who had been classified as uninhibited. Although these inhibited teens had not yet been diagnosed with particular disorders, they exhibited response styles that one would expect to see in anxiety disordered adults. It would be interesting to look at this same sample again in a few years' time to see if these response styles were predictive of the later development of anxiety disorders. If so, there would be evidence showing a progression from an early temperamental style to later cognitive styles to still later anxiety disorder.

In conclusion, it will be worthwhile to establish causal models for the development and etiology of social anxiety disorder. In terms of distal factors, researchers should continue to explore negative life events that seem to be tied to the upstream development of social anxiety disorder, while also gaining a clearer understanding of the vulnerabilities (e.g., behavioral inhibition, attributional style) that might influence the way that we perceive these events. Further along the course of events, it will be important to see how cognitive styles change over time and whether, indeed, there is a culmination of sorts in that people who develop social anxiety disorder first develop an extreme concern about negative evaluation from others. Understanding these causal links will be very helpful in preventing or containing social anxiety disorder before it begins to have a negative impact on people's quality of life.

REFERENCES

Abramson, L. Y., Metalsky, G. I., & Alloy, L. B. (1989). Hopelessness depression: A theory-based subtype of depression. *Psychological Review, 96,* 358–372.

Abramson, L. Y., Seligman, M. E. P., & Teasdale, J. D. (1978). Learned helplessness in humans: Critique and reformulation. *Journal of Abnormal Psychology, 87,* 49–74.

Alden, L. E., & Wallace, S. T. (1995). Social phobia and social appraisal in successful and un-successful social interactions. *Behaviour Research and Therapy, 33,* 497–505.

American Psychiatric Association. (1987). *Diagnostic and statistical manual of mental disorders* (3rd ed., rev.). Washington, DC: Author.

American Psychiatric Association. (1994). *Diagnostic and statistical manual of mental disorders* (4th ed.). Washington, DC: Author.

Amir, N., Foa, E. B., & Coles, M. E. (1998a). Automatic activation and strategic avoidance of threat-relevant information in social phobia. *Journal of Abnormal Psychology, 107,* 285–290.

Amir, N., Foa, E. B., & Coles, M. E. (1998b). Negative interpretation bias in social phobia. *Behaviour Research and Therapy, 36,* 959–970.

Amir, N., Foa, E. B., & Coles, M. E. (2000). Implicit memory bias for threat-relevant information in generalized social phobia. *Journal of Abnormal Psychology, 109,* 713–720.

Asmundson, G. J. G., & Stein, M. B. (1994). Selective processing of social threat in patients with generalized social phobia: Evaluation using a dot-probe paradigm. *Journal of Anxiety Disorders, 8,* 107–117.

Biederman, J., Hirshfeld-Becker, D., Rosenbaum, J., Herot, C., Friedman, D., Snidman, N., Kagan, J., & Faraone, S. (2001). Further evidence of association between behavioral inhibition and social anxiety in children. *American Journal of Psychiatry, 158,* 1673–1679.

Bond, C. F., Jr., & Omar, A. S. (1990). Social anxiety, state dependence, and the next-in-line effect. *Journal of Experimental Social Psychology, 26,* 185–198.

Bowlby, J. (1982). Attachment and loss: Retrospect and prospect. *American Journal of Orthopsychiatry, 52,* 664–678.

Bradley, B. P., Mogg, K., Millar, N., Bonham-Carter, C., Fergusson, E., Jenkins, J., & Parr, M. (1997). Attentional biases for emotional faces. *Cognition and Emotion, 11,* 25–42.

Bruch, M. A., Heimberg, R. G., Berger, P., & Collins, T. M. (1989). Social phobia and perceptions of early parental and personal characteristics. *Anxiety Research, 2,* 57–65.

Buss, A. H. (1980). *Self-consciousness and social anxiety.* San Francisco: Freeman.

Caster, J. B., Inderbitzen, H. M., & Hope, D. (1999). Relationship between youth and parent perceptions of family environment and social anxiety. *Journal of Anxiety Disorders, 13,* 237–251.

Chartier, M. J., Walker, J. R., & Stein, M. B. (2001). Social phobia and potential childhood risk factors in a community sample. *Psychological Medicine, 31,* 307–315.

Clark, D. M., & Wells, A. (1995). A cognitive model of social phobia. In R. G. Heimberg, M. R. Liebowitz, D. A. Hope, & F. R. Schneier (Eds.), *Social phobia: Diagnosis, assessment, and treatment* (pp. 69–93). New York: Guilford.

Cloitre, M., Heimberg, R. G., Liebowitz, M. R., & Gitow, A. (1992). Perceptions of control in panic disorder and social phobia. *Cognitive Therapy and Research, 16,* 569–577.

Cloitre, M., & Shear, M. K. (1995). Psychodynamic perspectives. In M. B. Stein (Ed.), *Social phobia: Clinical and research perspectives* (pp. 163–187). Washington, DC: American Psychiatric Press.

Coles, M. E., & Heimberg, R. G. (2005). Recognition bias for critical faces in social phobia: A replication and extension. *Behaviour Research and Therapy, 43,* 109–120.

Coles, M. E., Turk, C. L., Heimberg, R. G., & Fresco, D. M. (2001). Effects of varying levels of anxiety within social situations: Relationship to memory perspective and attributions in social phobia. *Behaviour Research and Therapy, 39,* 651–665.

Daly, J. A., Vangelisti, A. L., & Lawrence, S. G. (1989). Self-focused attention and public speaking anxiety. *Personality and Individual Differences, 10,* 903–913.

Davidson, J. R., Hughes, D. L., George, L. K., & Blazer, D. G. (1993). The epidemiology of social phobia: Findings from the Duke Epidemiological Catchment Area Study. *Psychological Medicine, 23,* 709–718.

DiPino, R. K., & Riskind, J. H. (2000). *Shamed in social phobia: Shame proneness in social phobia and shyness.* Unpublished manuscript.

Dozier, M., Stovall, K. C., & Albus, K. E. (1999). Attachment and psychopathology in adulthood. In J. Cassidy & P. R. Shaver (Eds.), *Handbook of attachment: Theory, research, and clinical applications* (pp. 497–519). New York: Guilford.

Eng, W., Heimberg, R. G., Hart, T. A., Schneier, F. R., & Liebowitz, M. R. (2001). Attachment
in individuals with social anxiety disorder: The relationship among adult attachment
styles, social anxiety and depression. *Emotion, 1,* 365–380.

Foa, E. B., Franklin, M. E., Perry, K. J., & Herbert, J. D. (1996). Cognitive biases in generalized
social phobia. *Journal of Abnormal Psychology, 105,* 433–439.

Foa, E. B., Gilboa-Schechtman, E., Amir, N., & Freshman, M. (2000). Memory bias in generalized social phobia: Remembering negative emotional expressions. *Journal of Anxiety Disorders, 14,* 501–519.

Gilboa-Schechtman, E., Foa, E. B., & Amir, N. (1999). Attentional biases for facial expressions
in social phobia: The face-in-the-crowd paradigm. *Cognition and Emotion, 13,* 305–318.

Gilboa-Schechtman, E., Franklin, M. E., & Foa, E. B. (2000). Anticipated reactions to social
events: Differences among individuals with generalized social phobia, obsessive compulsive disorder, and nonanxious controls. *Cognitive Therapy and Research, 24,* 731–746.

Greenberg, M. T. (1999). Attachment and psychopathology in childhood. In J. Cassidy & P. R.
Shaver (Eds.), *Handbook of attachment: Theory, research, and clinical applications* (pp.
469–496). New York: Guilford.

Hackmann, A., Surawy, C., & Clark, D. M. (1998). Seeing yourself through others' eyes: A
study of spontaneously occurring images in social phobia. *Behavioural and Cognitive Psychotherapy, 26,* 3–12.

Hayward, C., Killen, J. D., Kraemer, H. C., & Taylor, C. B. (1998). Linking self-reported childhood behavioral inhibition to adolescent social phobia. *Journal of the American Academy of
Child and Adolescent Psychiatry, 37,* 1308–1316.

Heimberg, R. G., Klosko, J. S., Dodge, C. S., Shadick, R., Becker, R. E., & Barlow, D. H. (1989).
Anxiety disorders, depression, and attributional style: A further test of the specificity of
depressive attributions. *Cognitive Therapy and Research, 13,* 21–36.

Holt, C. S., Heimberg, R. G., Hope, D. A., & Liebowitz, M. R. (1992). Situational domains of
social phobia. *Journal of Anxiety Disorders, 6,* 63–77.

Hope, D. A., Heimberg, R. G., & Klein, J. F. (1990). Social anxiety and the recall of interpersonal information. *Journal of Cognitive Psychotherapy, 4,* 185–195.

Hope, D. A., Rapee, R. M., Heimberg, R. G., & Dombeck, M. J. (1990). Representations of the
self in social phobia: Vulnerability to social threat. *Cognitive Therapy and Research, 14,*
177–189.

Hope, D. A., Sigler, K. D., Penn, D. L., & Meier, V. (1998). Social anxiety, recall of interpersonal information, and social impact on others. *Journal of Cognitive Psychotherapy, 12,*
303–322.

Jacoby, L. L., Allan, L. G., Collins, J. C., & Larwill, L. K. (1988). Memory influences subjective
experience: Noise judgment. *Journal of Experimental Psychology: Learning, Memory, and
Cognition, 14,* 240–247.

Kagan, J., Reznick, J. S., & Snidman, N. (1988). Biological bases of childhood shyness. *Science,
240,* 167–171.

Kessler, R. C., McGonagle, K. A., Zhao, S., Nelson, C. B., Hughes, M., Eshleman, S., Wittchen,
H.-U., & Kendler, K. S. (1994). Lifetime and 12-month prevalence of *DSM–III–R* psychiatric disorders in the United States: Results from the National Comorbidity Survey. *Archives of General Psychiatry, 51,* 8–19.

Kimble, C. E., & Zehr, H. D. (1982). Self-consciousness, information load, self-presentation,
and memory in a social situation. *Journal of Social Psychology, 118,* 39–46.

La Greca, A. M., Dandes, S. K., Wick, P., Shaw, K., & Stone, W. L. (1988). Development of the
social anxiety scale for children: Reliability and concurrent validity. *Journal of Clinical
Child Psychology, 17,* 84–91.

Leung, A. W., & Heimberg, R. G. (1996). Homework compliance, perceptions of control, and outcome of cognitive-behavioral treatment of social phobia. *Behaviour Research and Therapy, 34*, 423–432.

Lieb, R., Wittchen, H.-U., Höfler, M., Fuetsch, M., Stein, M. B., & Merikangas, K. R. (2000). Parental psychopathology, parenting styles and the risk of social phobia in offspring. *Archives of General Psychiatry, 57*, 859–866.

Lucock, M. P., & Salkovskis, P. M. (1988). Cognitive factors in social anxiety and its treatment. *Behaviour Research and Therapy, 26*, 297–302.

Lundh, L. G., & Öst, L. G. (1996a). Recognition bias for critical faces in social phobics. *Behaviour Research and Therapy, 34*, 787–794.

Lundh, L. G., & Öst, L. G. (1996b). Stroop interference, self-focus, and perfectionism in social phobics. *Personality and Individual Differences, 20*, 725–731.

Lundh, L. G., & Öst, L. G. (1997). Explicit and implicit memory bias in social phobia: The role of subdiagnostic type. *Behaviour Research and Therapy, 35*, 305–317.

Lundh, L. G., & Öst, L. G. (2001). Attentional bias, self-consciousness and perfectionism in social phobia before and after cognitive-behavior therapy. *Scandanavian Journal of Behavior Therapy, 30*, 4–16.

Lundh, L., Thulin, U., Czyzykow, S., & Öst, L. (1998). Recognition bias for safe faces in panic disorder with agoraphobia. *Behaviour Research and Therapy, 36*, 323–337.

MacLeod, C., Mathews, A., & Tata, P. (1986). Attentional bias in emotional disorders. *Journal of Abnormal Psychology, 95*, 15–20.

Magee, W. J. (1999). Effects of negative life experiences on phobia onset. *Social Psychiatry and Psychiatric Epidemiology, 34*, 343–351.

Maidenberg, E., Chen, E., Craske, M., Bohn, P., & Bystritsky, A. (1996). Specificity of attentional bias in panic disorder and social phobia. *Journal of Anxiety Disorders, 10*, 529–541.

Mansell, W., Clark, D. M., Ehlers, A., & Chen, Y.-P. (1999). Social anxiety and attention away from emotional faces. *Cognition and Emotion, 13*, 673–690.

Mathews, A., & MacLeod, C. (1985). Selective processing of threat cues in anxiety states. *Behaviour Research and Therapy, 23*, 563–569.

Mattia, J. I., Heimberg, R. G., & Hope, D. A. (1993). The revised Stroop color-naming task in social phobics. *Behaviour Research and Therapy, 31*, 305–313.

McCabe, R. E., Antony, M. M., Summerfeldt, L. J., Liss, A., & Swinson, R. P. (2003). Preliminary examination of the relationship between anxiety disorders in adults and self-reported history of teasing or bullying experiences. *Cognitive Behaviour Therapy, 32*, 187–193.

McManus, F., Clark, D. M., & Hackmann, A. (2000). Specificity of cognitive biases in social phobia and their role in recovery. *Behavioural and Cognitive Psychotherapy, 28*, 201–209.

Mick, M. A., & Telch, M. J. (1998). Social anxiety and history of behavioral inhibition in young adults. *Journal of Anxiety Disorders, 12*, 1–20.

Mickelson, K. D., Kessler, R. C., & Shaver, P. R. (1997). Adult attachment in a nationally representative sample. *Journal of Personality and Social Psychology, 73*, 1092–1106.

Mogg, K., Mathews, A., & Weinman, J. (1987). Memory bias in clinical anxiety. *Journal of Abnormal Psychology, 96*, 94–98.

Muris, P., Merckelbach, H., Wessel, I., & van de Ven, M. (1999). Psychopathological correlates of self-reported behavioural inhibition in normal children. *Behaviour Research and Therapy, 37*, 575–584.

Pérez-López, J. R., & Woody, S. R. (2001). Memory for facial expressions in social phobia. *Behaviour Research and Therapy, 39*, 967–975.

Peterson, C., Semmel, A., von Baeyer, C., Abramson, L. Y., Metalsky, G. I., & Seligman, M. E. P. (1982). The Attributional Style Questionnaire. *Cognitive Therapy and Research, 6*, 287–299.

Rapee, R. M., & Hayman, K. (1996). The effects of video feedback on the self-evaluation of performance in socially anxious subjects. *Behaviour Research and Therapy, 34,* 315–322.

Rapee, R. M., & Heimberg, R. G. (1997). A cognitive-behavioral model of anxiety in social phobia. *Behaviour Research and Therapy, 35,* 741–756.

Rapee, R. M., & Lim, L. (1992). Discrepancy between self- and observer ratings of performance in social phobics. *Journal of Abnormal Psychology, 101,* 728–731.

Rapee, R. M., McCallum, S. L., Melville, L. F., Ravenscroft, H., & Rodney, J. M. (1994). Memory bias in social phobia. *Behaviour Research and Therapy, 32,* 89–99.

Rapee, R. M., & Spence, S. H. (2004). The etiology of social phobia: Empirical evidence and an initial model. *Clinical Psychology Review, 24,* 737–767.

Roediger, H. L., & McDermott, K. B. (1993). Implicit memory in normal human subjects. In H. Spinnler & F. Boller (Eds.), *Handbook of neuropsychology* (pp. 63–131). Amsterdam: Elsevier.

Rosenbaum, J. F., Biederman, J., Hirshfeld, D. R., Bolduc, E. A., & Chaloff, J. (1991). Behavioral inhibition in childhood: A possible precursor to panic disorder or social phobia. *Journal of Clinical Psychiatry, 52*(Suppl.), 5–9.

Roth, D. A., Antony, M. M., & Swinson, R. P. (2001). Interpretations for anxiety symptoms in social phobia. *Behaviour Research and Therapy, 39,* 129–138.

Roth, D., Coles, M., & Heimberg, R. G. (2002). The relationship between memories for childhood teasing and anxiety and depression in adulthood. *Journal of Anxiety Disorders, 16,* 151–166.

Rubin, K. H., & Mills, R. S. L. (1988). The many faces of social isolation in childhood. *Journal of Consulting and Clinical Psychology, 56,* 916–924.

Schacter, D. L. (1998). Memory and awareness. *Science, 280,* 59–60.

Schneier, F. R., Heckelman, L. R., Garfinkel, R., Campeas, R., Fallon, B. A., Gitow, A., Street, L., Del Bene, D., & Liebowitz, M. R. (1994). Functional impairment in social phobia. *Journal of Clinical Psychiatry, 55,* 322–331.

Schwartz, C. E., Snidman, N., & Kagan, J. (1996). Early temperamental predictors of Stroop interference to threatening information in adolescence. *Journal of Anxiety Disorders, 10,* 89–96.

Spence, S. H., Donovan, C., & Brechman-Toussaint, M. (1999). Social skills, social outcomes, and cognitive features of childhood social phobia. *Journal of Abnormal Psychology, 108,* 211–221.

Stopa, L., & Clark, D. M. (1993). Cognitive processes in social phobia. *Behaviour Research and Therapy, 31,* 255–267.

Stopa, L., & Clark, D. M. (2000). Social phobia and interpretation of social events. *Behaviour Research and Therapy, 38,* 273–283.

Storch, E., Roth, D., Coles, M. E., Heimberg, R. G., Bravata, E. A., & Moser, J. (2004). The measurement and impact of childhood teasing in a sample of young adults. *Journal of Anxiety Disorders, 18,* 681–694.

Strauss, C. C., Lahey, B. B., Frick, P., Frame, C. L., & Hynd, G. W. (1988). Peer social status of children with social anxiety disorders. *Journal of Consulting and Clinical Psychology, 56,* 137–141.

Stroop, J. R. (1935). Studies of interference in serial verbal reactions. *Journal of Experimental Psychology, 18,* 643–662.

Veljaca, K., & Rapee, R. M. (1998). Detection of negative and positive audience behaviors by socially anxious subjects. *Behaviour Research and Therapy, 36,* 311–321.

Vernberg, E. M., Abwender, D. A., Ewell, K. K., & Beery, S. H. (1992). Social anxiety and peer relationships in early adolescence: A prospective analysis. *Journal of Clinical Child Psychology, 21,* 189–196.

Wallace, S. T., & Alden, L. E. (1997). Social phobia and positive social events: The price of success. *Journal of Abnormal Psychology, 106,* 416–424.

Watson, D., & Friend, R. (1969). Measurement of social-evaluative anxiety. *Journal of Consulting and Clinical Psychology, 33*, 448–457.

Wells, A., Clark, D. M., & Ahmad, S. (1998). How do I look with my mind's eye? Perspective taking in social phobic imagery. *Behaviour Research and Therapy, 36*, 631–634.

Wells, A., & Papageorgiou, C. (1999). The observer perspective: Biased imagery in social phobia, agoraphobia, and blood/injury phobia. *Behaviour Research and Therapy, 37*, 653–658.

Wenzel, A., & Holt, C. S. (2002). Memory bias against threat in social phobia. *British Journal of Clinical Psychology, 41*, 73–79.

Williams, J. M. G., Mathews, A., & MacLeod, C. (1996). The emotional Stroop task and psychopathology. *Psychological Bulletin, 120*, 3–24.

Wittchen, H.-U., Stein, M. B., & Kessler, R. C. (1999). Social fears and social phobia in a community sample of adolescents and young adults: Prevalence, risk factors and co-morbidity. *Psychological Medicine, 29*, 309–323.

Yuen, P. K. (1994). *Social anxiety and the allocation of attention: Evaluation using facial stimuli in a dot-probe paradigm.* Unpublished research project, Department of Experimental Psychology, University of Oxford, England.

Cognitive Vulnerability to PTSD

Norah C. Feeny
Case Western Reserve University

Edna B. Foa
University of Pennsylvania

Large epidemiological studies have established the extremely high rates of trauma exposure among adults (about 70%, for a review see Solomon & Davidson, 1997). According to the *DSM–IV* (APA, 1994), a trauma is defined as an event that involves perceived or actual threat and elicits an extreme emotional response (i.e., helplessness, horror, or terror). The constellation of psychological difficulties that is observed most often following a trauma is posttraumatic stress disorder (PTSD). Among trauma survivors, the lifetime prevalence of PTSD has been estimated at 24%, and in the general population, the lifetime prevalence is estimated at 9% (Breslau, Davis, Andreski, & Peterson, 1991). The prevalence of current PTSD in trauma survivors varies by trauma type and by study, but has been reported to occur in from 12% to 65% of female assault victims (Resnick, Kilpatrick, Dansky, Saunders, & Best, 1993; Rothbaum, Foa, Riggs, Murdock, & Walsh, 1992), 15% of Vietnam combat veterans (Kulka et al., 1990), and up to 40% of people surviving serious motor vehicle accidents (Taylor & Koch, 1995). Women appear to be twice as likely to develop PTSD than men (10.4% of women vs. 5% of men in the general population; Kessler, Sonnega, Bromet, Hughes, & Nelson, 1995).

PTSD symptoms are organized into three general clusters: reexperiencing the trauma (e.g., intrusive and distressing thoughts, flashbacks, and nightmares), avoidance of trauma-related material (e.g., avoidance of trauma-related thoughts, feelings, and reminders; emotional numbing; sense of foreshortened future), and hyperarousal symptoms (e.g., sleep disturbance, irritability, and hypervigilance). Although many people experience the symptoms of PTSD shortly after exposure to a traumatic event, most will experience a natural reduction in symptoms over the course of the following several months (e.g., Riggs, Rothbaum, & Foa, 1995; Rothbaum et al., 1992). However, a substantial minority of trauma survivors continues to experience significant PTSD symptoms for months (Riggs et al., 1995; Rothbaum et al., 1992) and even years after the trauma (Kessler et al., 1995).

THE NATURAL COURSE OF PTSD SYMPTOMS
AFTER ASSAULT

Two studies, a sample of female rape victims (Rothbaum et al., 1992) and a sample of male and female victims of nonsexual assault (Riggs et al., 1995), have examined the prevalence of PTSD symptoms following assault. In both studies, participants were interviewed shortly after being assaulted and then assessed weekly over the subsequent 12 weeks. The results of the two studies were very similar, showing high levels of PTSD initially, and a gradual decline in symptoms over time for many. In the first study, 94% of the women met symptom criteria for PTSD within 2 weeks following the assault (Rothbaum et al., 1992). Rates of PTSD had declined considerably 3 months after the sexual assault, but 47% of these women continued to meet PTSD criteria. Women who did not meet criteria for PTSD 3 months after the assault showed steady improvement over the 12 weeks of the study. However, those women whose PTSD persisted 3 months after the assault did not show much symptom improvement after the 1-month assessment. Follow-up assessments conducted 6 and 9 months after the assault revealed that 41.7% of women met criteria for PTSD at each time point. In the second study, Riggs et al. (1995) found that within 2 weeks of an assault, 90% of rape victims and 62% of nonsexual assault victims met symptom criteria for PTSD. At the 1-month assessment, the rate had dropped to 60% for rape and 44% for nonsexual assault survivors. Three months after the index assault, the rate of PTSD had dropped to 51% and 21% for rape and nonsexual assault survivors, respectively.

Taken together, these results suggest that not all people who experience trauma go on to develop PTSD, and of those who develop acute PTSD, not everyone goes on to develop chronic PTSD. The important question remaining is why only some individuals develop chronic posttrauma disturbances. Several factors have been implicated in the development of PTSD, including type of assault (e.g., Weaver, Kilpatrick, Resnick, Best, & Saunders, 1997), severity of initial PTSD symptoms (e.g., Rothbaum et al., 1992), degree of dissociation (e.g., Bremner & Brett, 1997), anger (e.g., Feeny, Zoellner, & Foa, 2000; Riggs, Dancu, Gershuny, Greenberg, & Foa, 1992), and numbing (Feeny, Zoellner, Fitzgibbons, & Foa, 2000). The issue of understanding vulnerability to PTSD—that is, which factors are most important in determining response to trauma—is crucial. Recently, cognitive factors have received attention in attempts to understand the development and maintenance of this disorder.

THEORETICAL CONCEPTUALIZATIONS OF PTSD

The current cognitive behavioral conceptualization of the development and maintenance of PTSD was influenced by two major theories: learning theory and cognitive theory. This chapter reviews both cognitive behavioral theories of PTSD and research related to these theories, and introduces the notion of cognitive vulnerabilities to this disorder.

Learning Theory: Two-Factor Theory of Fear

Early behavioral theories of PTSD conceptualized the disorder within the framework of two-factor conditioning theory (Mowrer, 1960) in which both classical (Factor 1) and instrumental or operant (Factor 2) conditioning are viewed as the mechanisms underlying the acquisition and maintenance of pathological anxiety. Accordingly, fear is acquired via classical conditioning, in which a previously neutral stimulus (CS) is paired with an aversive stimulus (UCS), so that the CS alone can elicit the conditioned fear response (CR). In relation to PTSD, it has been posited that previously nonfeared stimuli associated with the traumatic event become able to generate anxiety themselves (e.g., Foa, Steketee, & Rothbaum, 1989). For example, the smell of cologne worn by a rapist may elicit anxiety when later smelled by the victim in a safe situation.

The second factor, operant conditioning, accounts for the maintenance of avoidance behavior; individuals learn that they can decrease trauma-related fear and anxiety though avoidance of the CSs. Such avoidance is established by its ability to reduce or eliminate the anxiety state (i.e., negative reinforcement). However, because avoidance prevents the realization that the CS is not in itself aversive, the fear and avoidance are maintained.

Within this conceptualization then, treatment for PTSD needs to facilitate exposure to the conditioned stimulus in the absence of the aversive stimulus, until anxiety is sufficiently reduced. Indeed, learning theory was the force behind the development of exposure techniques, which have become the treatment of choice for phobias (cf. Barlow, 1985) and obsessive-compulsive disorder (see Franklin & Foa, 1998).

COGNITIVE THEORIES OF PTSD

In contrast to learning theories, cognitive theories assert that it is the person's interpretation of an event, rather than the event itself, which produces emotional and behavioral reactions. Consequently, a given event can be interpreted in different ways and thus can evoke different emotions. Cognitive theory further hypothesizes that each emotion is associated with a particular class of thoughts; in anxiety, thoughts typically relate to the perception of danger.

Although typically people do experience situations that lead to negative emotions, cognitive theory focuses on emotional reactions that are more extreme and/or more prolonged than would be expected. Such "pathological" emotions are thought to be the result of distorted interpretations; for example, the overestimation of danger produces unrealistic fear. This theory was first developed to explain depression (Beck, Rush, Shaw, & Emery, 1979) and was later extended to the account for the anxiety disorders (e.g., Beck, Emery, & Greenberg, 1985; Clark, 1986).

SCHEMA THEORIES

Many trauma theorists have suggested that traumatic events cause changes in thoughts and beliefs, and these changes are important in determining one's emotional response to trauma (e.g., Ehlers & Clark, 2000; Epstein, 1991; Foa & Rothbaum, 1998; Horowitz, 1986; Janoff-Bulman, 1992; Resick & Schnicke, 1992). All of these theories highlight the role that cognitions play in reactions to trauma, but each focuses on different sets of cognitions. Epstein (1985, 1991), for example, suggested that four core beliefs change after a traumatic experience: the world is benign, the world is meaningful, the self is worthy, and people are trustworthy. Janoff-Bulman (1992) similarly posited that there are three categories of basic assumptions held by people in general—benevolence of the world, meaningfulness of the world, and worthiness of the self—and traumatic experiences violate these assumptions. Accordingly, to recover from trauma the victim must go through a "cognitive crisis," a struggle to either assimilate the traumatic experience into the old set of assumptions, or more often, to change the assumptions such that they can accommodate the traumatic experience. In an attempt to measure this hypothesis, Janoff-Bulman (1989, 1992) developed the World Assumptions Scale (WAS) to assess perceived self-worth and benevolence of the world. Interestingly, she found that the WAS discriminated between trauma victims and nonvictims. Janoff-Bulman's theory suggests that victims who prior to the trauma perceived the world as very safe and themselves as invulnerable, would be more likely to show posttrauma difficulties than those who did not have such views. However, evidence that individuals with previous traumas are more likely to develop PTSD (e.g., Resnick et al., 1993) is inconsistent with this notion; individuals with such histories are not likely to perceive the world as extremely safe or themselves as highly competent. Instead, it is more probable that such individuals would view the world as dangerous and themselves as incompetent.

EMOTIONAL PROCESSING THEORY

Foa and her colleagues (Foa & Riggs, 1993; Foa et al., 1989; Foa & Rothbaum, 1998) proposed that impaired "emotional processing" of the traumatic event underlies PTSD. Further, they suggested that in those who develop PTSD, memories of the trauma have pathological elements as a result of this impaired processing. According to Foa and Kozak's (1986) emotional processing theory, pathological fear is differentiated from typical fear by disruptive intensity, associations that do not accurately represent reality, and incorrect interpretations such as "my anxiety means I'm incompetent." Building on this theory, they proposed that two conditions are necessary for corrective emotional processing to occur: activation of the fear structure and the incorporation of new information that is incompatible with the pathological elements of the structure (e.g., overgeneralization of fear). Thus, from the perspective of emotional processing theory, treatment for PTSD should facilitate emotional engagement with traumatic memories in order to promote trauma-related fear reduction, reduce avoidance, and modify the distorted interpretations that contribute to the maintenance of PTSD.

Emotional processing theory suggests that, typically, there is a gradual decrease over time in the frequency and intensity of emotional responses to traumatic events. A recent sexual assault victim, for example, will experience a high level of fear when reminded of the rape. However, the fear usually lessens with the passage of time. Research findings lend support to this clinical observation. As was discussed earlier, two prospective studies that examined the process of recovery in women who had been recently assaulted found that assault victims reported fewer psychological difficulties with the passage time (Foa & Riggs, 1995; Rothbaum et al., 1992). Thus, not all individuals who experience a given trauma develop chronic PTSD, and several factors (e.g., type of assault, emotional numbing) mentioned earlier have been implicated in the development of PTSD. Foa and colleagues (e.g., Foa, Ehlers, Clark, Tolin, & Orsillo, 1999; Foa & Riggs, 1993; Foa & Rothbaum, 1998) hypothesized that certain erroneous cognitions underlie the development of PTSD. In addition, together with other trauma experts, they suggested that specific cognitive vulnerabilities may play a role in the development of PTSD.

COGNITIVE VULNERABILITIES

Schemas and Attributions

Beliefs about the self and the world that exist prior to a traumatic experience may constitute one specific area of cognitive vulnerability to PTSD. As discussed earlier, schema theorists suggest that individuals with very positive views (e.g., the world is a completely safe place) are more vulnerable to posttrauma disturbances because these beliefs are shattered by trauma. In contrast to some trauma theorists (e.g., Janoff-Bulman, 1992), Foa and her colleagues (Foa & Jaycox, 1999; Foa & Riggs, 1993) proposed that it is not the holding of overly positive perceptions about oneself and the world, but the holding of very rigid assumptions that disrupts an individual's ability to successfully recover from a trauma. More specifically, when trauma challenges the victim's perception that the world is a very safe place or the self is very competent, or alternatively, when the trauma confirms existing schemas of the self as incompetent, it will be more difficult to successfully recover from the trauma. They further suggested that specific dysfunctional cognitions underlie PTSD: the perception that the world is extremely dangerous and the self is totally incompetent. The hypothesized relation between these distorted cognitions and PTSD is shown in Fig. 11.1.

Support for the notion that these particular cognitions are important in PTSD was obtained in a recent study (Foa, Ehlers, et al., 1999) indicating that elevated perceptions of world dangerousness and self-incompetence distinguished individuals with PTSD from both trauma victims without PTSD and from nontraumatized individuals. In addition, higher scores on these scales were associated with PTSD severity. An investigation with recent trauma victims provides further support for the role of erroneous cognitions in posttrauma disturbances; victims with acute stress disorder (ASD) exaggerated both the probability of negative events happening and the cost of such events, as compared to those without ASD (Warda & Bryant, 1998). It follows that if PTSD is mediated by erroneous cognitions, then successful treatment should correct these exaggerated views about the self and world. Indeed, there is data suggesting that with cognitive behavioral intervention for PTSD, beliefs about the self and the world shift in a more positive direction (Foa, 1997; Resick, Nishith, Weaver, Astin, & Feuer, 2002; Resick & Schnicke, 1992; Tolin & Foa, 1999). Future research

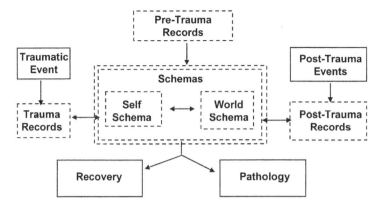

FIG. 11.1. Schematic model underlying posttraumatic stress disorder. From *Treating the Trauma of Rape* (p. 84), by E. B. Foa and B. O. Rothbaum, 1998, New York: Guilford Press. Copyright 1998 by Guilford Press. Reprinted with permission.

should investigate the specificity of these cognitions to PTSD, as opposed to other psychological disturbances (e.g., depression).

Coping

Adaptive coping strategies are thought to be important in successful recovery from traumatic events. On the other hand, maladaptive coping in response to trauma may reflect another area of cognitive vulnerability to PTSD. Indeed, coping style has been found to predict PTSD. In a study of coping among female assault victims, three coping scales were examined: Mobilizing Support, Wishful Thinking, and Positive Distancing (Valentiner, Foa, Riggs, & Gershuny, 1996). Three months after the assault, women who engaged in high levels of wishful thinking (e.g., self-blame and denial by fantasy) were more likely to have severe PTSD symptoms, which is consistent with the notion that dissociation following traumatic events impedes natural recovery.

Despite their apparent phenomenological differences, both dissociation and anger have been conceptualized to reflect coping via emotional disengagement from trauma memories, which has been thought to hinder recovery (Foa & Rothbaum, 1998; Horowitz, 1986; Putnam, 1989). Indeed, several studies suggest that both dissociation and anger hinder the processing of the traumatic event and subsequent natural recovery process. Trauma victims with PTSD exhibit more dissociative symptoms than those without PTSD (e.g., Bremner et al., 1992; Dancu, Riggs, Hearst-Ikeda, Shoyer, & Foa, 1996). Moreover, dissociation during or immediately after a trauma predicts later posttrauma psychopathology (Koopman, Classen, & Spiegel, 1994; Marmar et al., 1994; Tichenor, Marmar, Weiss, Metzler, & Ronfeldt, 1996). Similarly, acute stress disorder, which emphasizes dissociative symptoms, has been found to be predictive of later posttrauma symptoms (e.g., Bryant & Harvey, 1998; Classen, Koopman, Hales, & Spiegel, 1998; Harvey & Bryant, 1998).

Less attention has been given to the relation between anger and PTSD. Kilpatrick, Veronen, and Resick (1981) noted that a year after a rape, victims exhibited more hostility and anger than nonvictims. Studies have found a positive relation between anger and PTSD in combat veterans (Chemtob, Hamada, Roitblat, & Muraoka, 1994; Woolfolk & Grady, 1988) and women victims of various traumas (Koenen, Hearst-Ikeda, Caulfield, & Muldar, 1997). Riggs et al. (1992) reported results consistent with the hypothesis that elevated anger is positively related to the development of PTSD. In a prospective study of PTSD, they found that 1 week after an assault, victims were angrier than nonvictims; anger elevation at 1 week was predictive of PTSD severity 1 month later. In a similar study, early levels of anger were found to be predictive of PTSD severity 3 months after an assault (Feeny, Zoellner, & Foa, 2000).

Future research should explore the vulnerability that coping styles/ strategies that rely on disengagement from the trauma memory create following trauma; such work has potentially important clinical and theoretical implications.

Narrative Organization

The organization and elaboration of trauma narratives has also been implicated as an important cognitive feature related to the development of PTSD. Foa and Riggs (1993) suggested that the gradual organization and elaboration of the trauma memory is part of the natural recovery process. Consequently, individuals who do not successfully organize this memory will be more vulnerable to and thus evidence more trauma-related difficulties. To investigate this notion, Amir, Stafford, Freshman, and Foa (1998) examined the degree of complexity (i.e., articulation) of trauma narratives produced by recent sexual assault survivors (within 2 weeks). Results indicated that women who produced less articulate narratives were more likely to show high levels of anxiety shortly after the assault and were more likely to exhibit severe PTSD symptoms 12 weeks after the assault. Similarly, Halligan, Michael, Clark, and Ehlers (2003) found that assault survivors with current or past PTSD produced trauma narratives that were more disorganized than the narratives of assault survivors without PTSD, and disorganized trauma memories were associated with and predictive of PTSD symptoms. Further support for the role of narrative organization comes from a study of recent motor vehicle accident survivors with and without ASD (Harvey & Bryant, 1999). Again, memories for the trauma were more disorganized among those with ASD than among those without ASD.

It follows that, in order to be successful, treatment for PTSD should facilitate organization of the trauma narrative. In a study examining narrative changes over the course of exposure therapy, Foa, Molnar, and Cashman (1995) reported that trauma narratives obtained at the end of treatment were characterized by a greater percentage of organized thoughts, increased use of words denoting thoughts and feelings, and fewer references to specific actions or dialogue that occurred during the assault. Moreover, reduction of fragmentation (e.g., fillers, pauses) in the narratives was associated with decreases in anxiety and higher levels of organization were associated with a lower levels of depression. Thus, these studies suggest that the cognitive processes involved in the organization and articulation of the traumatic memories are important to understanding vulnerability for PTSD and successful treatment of this disorder.

Interpretation of Symptoms

Intrusions have long been considered a hallmark symptom of PTSD. Recently, attempts to cope with these symptoms, and the effects of such coping on the maintenance of PTSD, have been examined. Building on emotional processing theory, Ehlers and colleagues (Ehlers & Clark, 2000; Ehlers & Steil, 1995) suggested that dysfunctional meanings attributed to PTSD symptoms themselves (i.e., intrusive thoughts) play an important role in the maintenance of the disorder. This is hypothesized to happen in two ways: The negative meanings increase the level of distress associated with the intrusions, and they determine the extent of cognitive and behavioral avoidance. Support for this notion was obtained in a recent study in which dysfunctional meanings of intrusions predicted PTSD severity beyond intrusion frequency and the use of avoidance strategies (Steil & Ehlers, 2000). The authors hypothesized that this occurred in part because those who have negative interpretations of their symptoms are more likely to engage in cognitive avoidance (e.g., thought suppression) of the intrusions. As reviewed earlier, Foa and colleagues indicated that such cognitive strategies perpetuate, rather than reduce, intrusive symptoms. Indeed, there is evidence that active suppression of traumatic thoughts causes a delayed increase in such thoughts among those with acute stress disorder (Bryant & Harvey, 1998) and PTSD (Shipherd & Beck, 1999). Further, two correlational studies (Bryant & Harvey, 1995; Ehlers, Mayou, & Bryant, 1998) have found an association between self-reported thought suppression and the persistence of PTSD symptoms, supporting a role for thought suppression in producing and/or maintaining a cognitive vulnerability to PTSD.

CLINICAL IMPLICATIONS

Several types of psychosocial treatments have been used to treat posttrauma reactions, including psychodynamic psychotherapy, hypnotherapy, and cognitive behavioral therapy (CBT). Most outcome studies, however, have focused on the evaluation of CBT programs, the results of which have provided accumulating evidence for the efficacy of a number of such programs for chronic PTSD (see Foa & Meadows, 1997). CBT programs that have been developed to treat PTSD include: prolonged exposure (PE), stress inoculation training (SIT), cognitive restructuring (CR), eye movement desensitization and reprocessing (EMDR), and cognitive processing therapy (CPT). This section reviews selected outcome studies that evaluate the efficacy of these treatments. Keep in mind that the previous discussion of cognitive vulnerabilities to PTSD suggests that the success of a given treatment is dependent on facilitating several processes: the correction of erroneous cognitions associated with the disorder (i.e., that the world is extremely dangerous and the self is incompetent), the gradual elaboration and organization of the trauma narrative, and the reduction of trauma-related cognitive and behavioral avoidance.

Prolonged exposure (PE) is a set of procedures that involves confrontation, either imaginally (e.g., systematic desensitization), or in real life (in vivo), with feared stimuli. In the treatment of PTSD, exposure typically includes imaginally reliving the traumatic event repeatedly and in vivo confrontation with trauma-related situations that evoke fear, but are not objectively dangerous. In the first controlled study of exposure for rape-related PTSD, the efficacy of PE, SIT, supportive counseling (SC), and a wait-list control were compared for female victims of sexual assault (Foa, Rothbaum, Riggs, & Murdock, 1991). PTSD symptoms were assessed at pretreatment, posttreatment, and follow-up evaluations with psychometrically sound interviews and self-report measures administered by trained clinicians who were blind to treatment assignment. PE and SIT showed significant pre–post reductions on reexperiencing and avoidance clusters of PTSD, whereas SC and wait-list did not. Also, at the end of treatment, 50% of patients in SIT and 40% of PE no longer met criteria for PTSD; in contrast, only 10% of SC patients and none in the wait-list lost their diagnosis. At follow-up, there was a tendency for patients in the PE group to show further improvement in PTSD symptoms, whereas patients in SIT and SC did not show such further improvement.

In a second study, Foa, Dancu, et al. (1994) obtained further support for the efficacy of a modified PE in treating rape-related PTSD. This study compared the efficacy of PE to SIT, a combination of both treatments (PE/SIT), and a wait-list condition. All active treatments resulted in substantial symptom reduction, and were superior to the wait-list condition in ameliorating PTSD and related symptoms. On some indicators, however, PE seemed somewhat superior to the other treatments: It produced greater reductions of anxiety and depression and resulted in fewer dropouts than did SIT and PE/SIT. Also, the number of patients achieving good end-state functioning tended to be larger for PE than for SIT and PE/SIT.

In a third study, PE was compared with a program that included PE and cognitive restructuring (PE/CR) in female sexual and nonsexual assault survivors (Foa et al., 2004). Results provide additional support for the efficacy of PE across outcomes: PTSD severity and diagnosis, depression, general anxiety, and social functioning. Consistent with the PE/SIT results already described, combining PE with CR did not improve the efficacy or efficiency of PE.

In a fourth study, Marks, Lovell, Noshirvani, Livanou, and Thrasher (1998) compared PE to cognitive restructuring (CR), PE plus CR, and a relaxation control condition (R) in a sample of mixed trauma victims with chronic PTSD. Similar to the Foa et al. (1999) findings, PE, CR, and PE/CR were all quite effective and superior to the relaxation control. At posttreatment, good end-state functioning was found for 53% of clients in PE, 32% in CR and PE/CR, and 15% in relaxation. In another study, Tarrier et al. (1999) compared imaginal exposure to cognitive therapy among patients with PTSD resulting mostly from criminal victimization and automobile accidents. The two treatments were similarly effective in reducing PTSD symptoms.

Eye movement desensitization and reprocessing (EMDR; Shapiro, 1995) is a treatment for PTSD that has generated much interest, and controversy as well. In EMDR, the patient is asked to generate images, thoughts, and feelings about the trauma, to evaluate their negative qualities, and to generate alternative interpretations of the trauma. During this process, the therapist elicits rapid lateral eye movements by instructing the patient to visually track the therapist's finger as it is rapidly moved back and forth in front of the patient's face. Whereas multiple studies have evaluated the efficacy of EMDR, only some have utilized well-controlled designs and thus produced findings that are interpretable. One such study examined the efficacy of EMDR relative to a wait-list control condition for PTSD in female sexual assault survivors (Rothbaum, 1997). Three sessions of EMDR resulted in greater improvement for PTSD symptoms (57% reduction in independently evaluated PTSD at posttreatment and 71% in self-reported PTSD at follow-up), relative to the wait-list condition

(10% reduction at posttreatment). In a subsequent study, Devilly and Spence (1999) compared EMDR to a combined treatment of PE plus stress inoculation training (called trauma treatment protocol, TTP). Treatments reduced PTSD severity (TTP, 63%; EMDR, 46%), but those who received TTP maintained their gains at follow-up and those who received EMDR showed higher rates of relapse (symptom reduction at follow-up of 61% vs. 12%, respectively): At follow-up, the effect size of TTP was 1.13 and for EMDR it was 0.31.

Taylor et al. (2003) conducted the most recently published RCT examining the efficacy of EMDR. This study compared EMDR to exposure therapy and relaxation training. On average, the three treatments were efficacious in reducing PTSD, and did not differ in attrition rates or rates of symptom worsening. However, exposure was more effective than EMDR and relaxation in reducing avoidance and reexperiencing symptoms and tended to be faster in reducing avoidance. In addition, exposure therapy tended to yield a greater proportion of participants who no longer had symptoms meeting criteria for PTSD after treatment. EMDR did not differ from the control condition, relaxation. Similarly, a recent meta-analysis found EMDR no more effective than exposure therapy programs (Davidson & Parker, 2001). It is also important to note that the meta-analysis suggested that the eye movements integral to the treatment are not necessary (Davidson & Parker, 2001).

Cognitive processing therapy (CPT) is a program that was developed specifically for use with rape victims and includes cognitive restructuring and written exposure. In a quasi-experimental design, CPT was compared to a naturally occurring wait-list control group. Overall, women who received CPT improved significantly from pre to post treatment (about 50% reduction in PTSD symptoms), whereas the wait-list group did not evidence significant improvement (Resick & Schnicke, 1992). In a second study, Resick et al. (2002) compared the efficacy of a 12-session CPT, a 9-session PE, and a wait-list control in rape victims with chronic PTSD. Results of the RCT indicated that both treatments were highly effective in reducing PTSD: At posttreatment, 19.5% of completers in CPT and 17.5% in PE still met diagnostic criteria for PTSD. Among completers, 76% of the CPT and 58% of the PE clients met criteria for good end-state functioning (i.e., low PTSD and depression). Gains were maintained over time as well. At 9-month follow-up, 19.2% of CPT and 15.4% of PE clients met criteria for PTSD and 64% of the CPT and 68% of the PE participants experienced improvements meeting criteria for good end-state functioning.

In summary, at this point, evidence supports the efficacy of several treatments for PTSD (i.e., PE, SIT, CR, EMDR, and CPT). Prolonged exposure therapy is one of the best-validated treatments for PTSD. Notably, the importance of eye movements in EMDR has not been supported. This chapter has suggested that treatment for PTSD will be successful to the extent that it facilitates the correction of erroneous cognitions associated with the disorder, the elaboration and organization of the trauma narrative, and the reduction of trauma-related cognitive and behavioral avoidance.

———————

The majority of people in the United States are exposed to at least one traumatic experience in their lifetime, but only a large minority develops long-lasting psychological disturbances, including chronic PTSD. As we have suggested, understanding why some individuals recover successfully from a traumatic event and others develop chronic psychological difficulties is of the utmost importance. Cognitive behavioral theories, including emotional processing theory, have furthered our understanding of the development and maintenance of PTSD, and have suggested specific ways in which natural recovery from traumatic experiences may be impeded. Building on these theories and recent empirical work, this chapter has outlined several areas of hypothesized cognitive vulnerability to PTSD: overly rigid schemas that relate to perceiving the world as extremely dangerous and the self as incredibly incompetent, a maladaptive coping style that relies on emotional distancing, low levels of organization and articulation of the trauma narrative, and negative interpretations of PTSD symptoms (i.e., intrusions) and resultant trauma-related cognitive and behavioral avoidance. Future investigations need to build on existing cognitive theories and research to more clearly elaborate the role of specific cognitive vulnerabilities in the development, maintenance, and recovery from PTSD.

REFERENCES

American Psychiatric Association. (1994). *Diagnostic and statistical manual of mental disorders* (4th ed.). Washington, DC: Author.

Amir, N., Stafford, J., Freshman, M. S., & Foa, E. B. (1998). Relationship between trauma narratives and trauma pathology. *Journal of Traumatic Stress, 11*, 385–392.

Barlow, D. H. (1985). *Anxiety and its disorders*. New York: Guilford.

Beck, A. T., Emery, G., & Greenberg, R. L. (1985). *Anxiety disorders and phobias*. New York: Basic Books.

Beck, A. T., Rush, A. J., Shaw, B. F., & Emery, G. (1979). *Cognitive therapy of depression*. New York: Guilford.

Bremner, J. D., & Brett, E. (1997). Trauma-related dissociative states and long-term psychopathology in posttraumatic stress disorder. *Journal of Traumatic Stress, 10*(1), 37–49.

Bremner, J. D., Southwick, S., Brett, E., Fontana, A., Rosenheck, R., & Charney, D. S. (1992). Dissociation and posttraumatic stress disorder in Vietnam combat veterans. *American Journal of Psychiatry, 149*(3), 328–332.

Breslau, N., Davis, G. C., Andreski, P., & Peterson, E. (1991). Traumatic events and post-traumatic stress disorder in an urban population of young adults. *Archives General Psychiatry, 48,* 218–228.

Bryant, R. A., & Harvey, A. G. (1995). Avoidant coping style and posttraumatic stress following motor vehicle accidents. *Behaviour Research and Therapy, 33,* 631–635.

Bryant, R. A., & Harvey, A. G. (1998). Relationship between acute stress disorder and posttraumatic stress disorder following mild traumatic brain injury. *American Journal of Psychiatry, 155*(5), 625–629.

Chemtob, C. M., Hamada, R. S., Roitblat, H. L., & Muraoka, M. Y. (1994). Anger, impulsivity, and anger control in combat-related posttraumatic stress disorder. *Journal of Consulting and Clinical Psychology, 62*(4), 827–832.

Clark, D. M. (1986). A cognitive approach to panic. *Behaviour Research and Therapy, 24,* 461–470.

Classen, C., Koopman, C., Hales, R., & Spiegel, D. (1998). Acute stress disorder as a predictor of posttraumatic stress symptoms. *American Journal of Psychiatry, 155*(5), 620–624.

Dancu, C. V., Riggs, D. S., Hearst-Ikeda, D., Shoyer, B. G., & Foa, E. B. (1996). Dissociative experiences and posttraumatic stress disorder among female victims of criminal assault and rape. *Journal of Traumatic Stress, 9*(2), 253–267.

Davidson, P. R., & Parker, K. C. H. (2001). Eye movement desensitization and reprocessing (EMDR): A meta-analysis. *Journal of Consulting and Clinical Psychology, 69,* 305–319.

Devilly, G. J., & Spence, S. H. (1999). The relative efficacy and treatment distress of EMDR and a cognitive-behavior trauma treatment protocol in the amelioration of posttraumatic stress disorder. *Journal of Anxiety Disorders, 13,* 131–157.

Ehlers, A., & Clark, D. M. (2000). A cognitive model of persistent posttraumatic stress disorder. *Behaviour Research and Therapy, 38,* 319–345.

Ehlers, A., Mayou, R. A., & Bryant, B. (1998). Psychological predictors of chronic posttraumatic stress disorder after motor vehicle accidents. *Journal of Abnormal Psychology, 107,* 508–519.

Ehlers, A., & Steil, R. (1995). Maintenance of intrusive memories in posttraumatic stress disorder: A cognitive approach. *Behavioural and Cognitive Psychotherapy, 23,* 217–249.

Epstein, S. (1985). The implications of cognitive-experiential self-theory for research in social psychology and personality. *Journal of the Theory of Social Behavior, 15,* 283–310.

Epstein, S. (1991). The self-concept, traumatic neurosis, and the structure of personality. In D. Ozer, J. M. Healy, Jr., & A. J. Stewart (Eds.), *Perspectives on personality* (Vol. 3, pp. 63–98). London: Jessica Kingsley.

Feeny, N. C., Zoellner, L. A., Fitzgibbons, L. A., & Foa, E. B. (2000). Exploring the roles of emotional numbing, depression, and dissociation in PTSD. *Journal of Traumatic Stress, 13*(3), 489–498.

Feeny, N. C., Zoellner, L. A., & Foa, E. B. (2000). Anger, dissociation, and posttraumatic stress disorder among female assault victims. *Journal of Traumatic Stress, 13*(1), 89–100.

Feeny, N. C., Zoellner, L. A., & Foa, E. B. (2000, November). *Patterns of recovery women with chronic PTSD.* Symposium paper presented at annual AABT conference, New Orleans, LA.

Foa, E. B. (1997). Psychological processes related to recovery from a trauma and an effective treatment for PTSD. In R. Yehuda & A. McFarlane (Eds.), Psychobiology of PTSD. *Annals of the New York Academy of Sciences,* 410–424.

Foa, E. B., Dancu, C. V., Hembree, E. A., Jaycox, L. H., Meadows, E. A., & Street, G. P. (1999). A comparison of exposure therapy, stress inoculation training, and their combination for reducing posttraumatic stress disorder in female assault victims. *Journal of Consulting and Clinical Psychology, 67,* 194–200.

Foa, E. B., Ehlers, A., Clark, D., Tolin, D. F., & Orsillo, S. (1999). Posttraumatic cognitions inventory (PTCI): Development and comparison with other measures. *Psychological Assessment, 11,* 303–314.

Foa, E. B., Hembree, E. A., Cahill, S. P., Rauch, S. A., Riggs, D. S., & Feeny, N. C. (2004). *Prolonged exposure for PTSD with and without cognitive restructuring*. Manuscript submitted for publication.

Foa, E. B., & Jaycox, L. H. (1999). Cognitive-behavioral treatment of post-traumatic stress disorder. In D. Spiegel (Ed.), *Efficacy and cost-effectiveness of psychotherapy* (pp. 23–61). Washington, DC: American Psychiatric Press.

Foa, E. B., & Kozak, M. J. (1986). Emotional processing of fear: Exposure to corrective information. *Psychological Bulletin, 99*, 20–35.

Foa, E. B., & Meadows, E. A. (1997). Psychosocial treatments for post-traumatic stress disorder: A critical review. In J. Spence, J. M. Darley, & D. J. Foss (Eds.), *Annual review of psychology* (Vol. 48, pp. 449–480). Palo Alto, CA: Annual Reviews Inc.

Foa, E. B., Molnar, C., & Cashman, L. (1995). Change in rape narratives during exposure therapy for PTSD. *Journal of Traumatic Stress, 8*(4), 675–690.

Foa, E. B., & Riggs, D. S. (1993). Post-traumatic stress disorder in rape victims. In J. Oldham, M. B. Riba, & A. Tasman (Eds.), *American Psychiatric Press review of psychiatry* (Vol. 12, pp. 273–303). Washington, DC: American Psychiatric Press.

Foa, E. B., & Riggs, D. S. (1995). Posttraumatic stress disorder following assault: Theoretical considerations and empirical findings. *Current Directions in Psychological Science, 4*(2), 61–65.

Foa, E. B., & Rothbaum, B. O. (1998). *Treating the trauma of rape*. New York: Guilford.

Foa, E. B., Rothbaum, B. O., Riggs, D. S., & Murdock, T. (1991). Treatment of post-traumatic stress disorder in rape victims: A comparison between cognitive-behavioral procedures and counseling. *Journal of Consulting and Clinical Psychology, 59*, 715–723.

Foa, E. B., Steketee, G., & Rothbaum, B. (1989). Behavioral/cognitive conceptualizations of post-traumatic stress disorder. *Behavior Therapy, 20*, 155–176.

Franklin, M. E., & Foa, E. B. (2002). Cognitive behavioral treatments for obsessive compulsive disorder. In P. E. Nathan & J. M. Gorman (Eds.), *A guide to treatments that work* (pp. 367–386). New York: Oxford University Press.

Halligan, S. L., Michael., T., Clark, D. M., & Ehlers, E. (2003). Posttraumatic stress disorder following assault: The role of cognitive processing, trauma memory, and appraisals. *Journal of Consulting and Clinical Psychology, 71*, 419–431.

Harvey, A. G., & Bryant, R. A. (1998). The relationship between acute stress disorder and posttraumatic stress disorder: A prospective evaluation of motor vehicle accident survivors. *Journal of Consulting and Clinical Psychology, 66*(3), 507–512.

Harvey, A. G., & Bryant, R. A. (1999). A qualitative investigation of the organization of traumatic memories. *British Journal of Clinical Psychology, 38*, 401–405.

Horowitz, M. J. (1986). *Stress response syndromes* (2nd ed.). Northvale, NJ: Aronson.

Janoff-Bulman, R. (1989). Assumptive worlds and the stress of traumatic events: Applications of the schema construct. *Social Cognition, 7*, 113–136.

Janoff-Bulman, R. (1992). *Shattered assumptions: Towards a new psychology of trauma*. New York: The Free Press.

Kessler, R. C., Sonnega, A., Bromet, E., Hughes, M., & Nelson, C. B. (1995). Posttraumatic stress disorder in the National Comorbidity Survey. *Archives of General Psychiatry, 52*, 1048–1060.

Kilpatrick, D. G., Veronen, L. J., & Resick, P. A. (1981). Psychological sequelae to rape: Assessment and treatment strategies. In D. M. Dolays & R. L. Meredith (Eds.), *Behavioral medicine: Assessment and treatment strategies* (pp. 473–497). New York: Plenum.

Koenen, K., Hearst-Ikeda, D., Caulfield, M. B., & Muldar, R. (1997, November). *The relationship of anger and coping to PTSD symptoms in traumatized women*. Poster presented at the 31st annual meeting of the Association for the Advancement of Behavior Therapy (AABT), Miami, FL.

Koopman, C., Classen, C., & Spiegel, D. (1994). Predictors of posttraumatic stress symptoms among Oakland/Berkeley firestorm survivors. *American Journal of Psychiatry, 151,* 888–894.

Kulka, R. A., Schlenger, W. E., Fairbank, J. A., Hough, R. L., Jordan, B. K., Marmar, C. R., & Weiss, D. S. (1990). *Trauma and the Vietnam war generation.* New York: Brunner/Mazel.

Marks, I., Lovell, K., Noshirvani, H., Livanou, M., & Thrasher, S. (1998). Treatment of posttraumatic stress disorder by exposure and/or cognitive restructuring. *Archives of General Psychiatry, 55,* 317–325.

Marmar, C. R., Weiss, D. S., Schlenger, D. S., Fairbank, J. A., Jordan, B. K., Kulka, R. A., & Hough, R. L. (1994). Peritraumatic dissociation and posttraumatic stress in male Vietnam theater veterans. *American Journal of Psychiatry, 151,* 902–907.

Mowrer, O. A. (1960). *Learning theory and behavior.* New York: Wiley.

Putnam, F. W. (1989). Pierre Janet and modern views of dissociation. *Journal of Traumatic Stress, 2,* 413–429.

Resick, P. A., Nishith, P., Weaver, T., Astin, M. C., & Feuer, C. A. (2002). A comparison of cognitive processing therapy, prolonged exposure, and a waiting condition for the treatment of posttraumatic stress disorder in female rape victims. *Journal of Consulting and Clinical Psychology, 70,* 867–879.

Resick, P. A., & Schnicke, M. K. (1992). Cognitive processing therapy for sexual assault victims. *Journal of Consulting and Clinical Psychology, 60,* 748–756.

Resnick, H. S., Kilpatrick, D. G., Dansky, B. S., Saunders, B. E., & Best, C. L. (1993). Prevalence of civilian trauma and posttraumatic stress disorder in a representative national sample of women. *Journal of Consulting and Clinical Psychology, 61*(6), 984–991.

Riggs, D. S., Dancu, C. V., Gershuny, B. S., Greenberg, D., & Foa, E. B. (1992). Anger and posttraumatic stress disorder in female crime victims. *Journal of Traumatic Stress, 5*(4), 613–625.

Riggs, D. S., Rothbaum, B. O., & Foa, E. B. (1995). A prospective examination of symptoms of posttraumatic stress disorder in victims of non-assault. *Journal of Interpersonal Violence, 2,* 201–214.

Rothbaum, B. O. (1997). A controlled study of eye movement desensitization and reprocessing in the treatment of posttraumatic stress disordered sexual assault victims. *Bulletin of the Menninger Clinic, 61,* 317–334.

Rothbaum, B. O., Foa, E. B., Riggs, D. S., Murdock, T., & Walsh, W. (1992). A prospective examination of post-traumatic stress disorder in rape victims. *Journal of Traumatic Stress, 5,* 455–475.

Shapiro, F. (1995). *Eye movement desensitization and reprocessing: Basic principles, protocols, and procedures.* New York: Guilford.

Shipherd, J. C., & Beck, J. G. (1999). The effects of suppressing trauma-related thoughts on women with rape-related posttraumatic stress disorder. *Behavior Research and Therapy, 37,* 99–112.

Solomon, S. D., & Davidson, R. T. (1997). Trauma: Prevalence, impairment, service use, and cost. *Journal of Clinical Psychiatry, 58*(Suppl. 9), 5–11.

Steil, R., & Ehlers, A. (2000). Dysfunctional meaning of posttraumatic intrusions in chronic PTSD. *Behaviour Research and Therapy, 38,* 537–558.

Tarrier, N., Pilgrim, H., Sommerfield, C., Faragher, B., Reynolds, M., Graham, E., & Barrowclough, C. (1999). A randomized trial of cognitive therapy and imaginal exposure in the treatment of chronic posttraumatic stress disorder. *Journal of Consulting and Clinical Psychology, 67,* 13–18.

Taylor, S., & Koch, W. J. (1995). Anxiety disorders due to motor vehicle accidents: Nature and treatment. *Clinical Psychology Review, 15*(8), 721–738.

Taylor, S., Thordarson, D. S., Maxfield, L., Fedoroff, I. C., Lovell, K., & Ogrodniczuk, J. (2003). Comparative efficacy, speed, and adverse effects of three PTSD treatments: Exposure therapy, EMDR, and relaxation training. *Journal of Consulting and Clinical Psychology, 71,* 330–338.

Tolin, D. F., & Foa, E. B. (1999). Treatment of a police officer with PTSD using prolonged exposure. *Behavior Therapy, 30,* 527–538.

Tichenor, V., Marmar, C. R., Weiss, D. S., Metzler, T. J., & Ronfeldt, H. M. (1996). The relationship of peritraumatic dissociation and posttraumatic stress: Findings in female Vietnam theater veterans. *Journal of Consulting and Clinical Psychology, 64*(5), 1054–1059.

Valentiner, D. P., Foa, E. B., Riggs, D. S., & Gershuny, B. S. (1996). Coping strategies following traumatic assault: A predictive model of post-traumatic stress disorder symptomatology. *Journal of Abnormal Psychology, 105,* 455–458.

Warda, G., & Bryant, R. (1998). Cognitive bias in acute stress disorder. *Behaviour Research and Therapy, 36,* 1177–1183.

Weaver, T., Kilpatrick, D. G., Resnick, H. S., Best, C. L., & Saunders, B. E. (1997). An examination of physical assault and childhood victimization histories within a national probability sample of women. In G. K. Kantor & J. L. Jasinski (Eds.), *Out of darkness: Contemporary perspectives on family violence* (pp. 35–46). Thousand Oaks, CA: Sage.

Woolfolk, R. L., & Grady, D. A. (1988). Combat-related posttraumatic stress disorder: Patterns of symptomatology in help-seeking Vietnam veterans. *Journal of Nervous and Mental Disorders, 176,* 107–111.

12

Cognitive Vulnerability to Anxiety Disorders: An Integration

Adrian Wells
University of Manchester

Gerald Matthews
University of Cincinnati

Research on vulnerability to anxiety is difficult because of the multiplicity of possible vulnerability factors, such as early social learning, specific stressful events, and maladaptive cognition. As Schmidt and Woolaway-Bickel (chap. 8, this vol.) point out, a focus on only one or two factors is likely to be inadequate. This review features three central issues in conceptualizing vulnerability. The first is the discrimination of universal and specific distortions in cognition, within a conceptual scheme that integrates the roles of different vulnerability factors. For example, elevated levels of negative cognitions may be common to both anxiety and mood disorders, whereas specific content may discriminate different disorders (D. A. Clark & Beck, 1999). In panic, the content of thought is such that somatic symptoms are experienced as alarming; in obsessive-compulsive disorder, intrusive thoughts are interpreted as overly significant; in social phobia, anxiety responses are appraised as leading to possible rejection and loss of self-worth; and in PTSD, dysfunctional meanings are attributed to intruding thoughts.

A second theme is the role of dynamic factors. Anxiety disorders may reflect not just direct effects of discrete maladaptive cognitions, but patterns of interaction between person and environment, and between components of cognition and internal self-regulation that initiate and maintain pathology. For example, avoidance of threatening situations may block development of coping skills and prevent encoding of feedback that would disconfirm false beliefs (see Wells, 1997).

A third theme is the level of the cognitive architecture that supports distortions and bias in cognition. Attentional bias, for example, is common in anxiety disorders. However, it is unclear if bias emerges from unconscious and automatic cognitive processes or from volitional strategies for monitoring for threat (Matthews & Harley, 1996; Wells & Matthews, 1994a). The level of architectural representation for different vulnerabilities has implications for treatment and reducing risk of occurrence or reoccurrence of disorder. If vulnerability is located at the unconscious and reflexive level of processing it may be resistant to extinction, but its impact on self-regulation and adaptation to the outside world may be moderated. If, however, vulnerability is located primarily at a higher level of volitional processing, then it may be treated more permanently.

This chapter first outlines a general conceptual scheme for classifying vulnerability factors. This scheme offers a synopsis of some of the vulnerability concepts identified in the previous chapters. It discusses how cognitive behavioral vulnerability may be represented in both generic and disorder specific forms and identifies some general sources of vulnerability. Finally, it presents the Self-Regulatory Executive Function (S-REF) model as a useful architecture for representing cognitive vulnerability to emotional disorders, with reference to anxiety in particular. It is argued that vulnerability factors should be located predominantly at the level of volitional processing and represented in the propensity with which individuals activate negative self-perpetuating processing configurations and responses that fail to modify dysfunctional self-knowledge. A central feature of such configurations is perseverative thinking in the form of worry or rumination, and attentional strategies of threat monitoring driven by metacognitions.

Figure 12.1 presents a general outline scheme for vulnerability factors, compatible with previous cognitive psychological accounts (e.g., D. A. Clark & Beck, 1999; Ingram, Miranda, & Segal, 1998). Cognitive researchers have focused on stable *dysfunctional self-knowledge* as a key vulnerability factor. Self-knowledge may be explicit and declarative, in the form of negative self-beliefs, or it may be implicit and procedural, in the form of generic routines for coping (Wells & Matthews, 1994a). A third type of self-knowledge, metacognitive beliefs, in anxiety patients may specify an exaggerated importance for attending to internal thoughts, appraising such thoughts negatively, and engaging in unhelpful thought control strategies (Wells, 1994a, 1999). Typically, self-knowledge is seen as a distal factor that influences outcomes through more proximal factors such as processing of the immediate situation (e.g., Riskind & Williams, chap. 7, this vol.). However, what is seen as "distal" and what is "proximal" depends on the time span of interest, so the terms should be used with caution (Ingram et al., 1998).

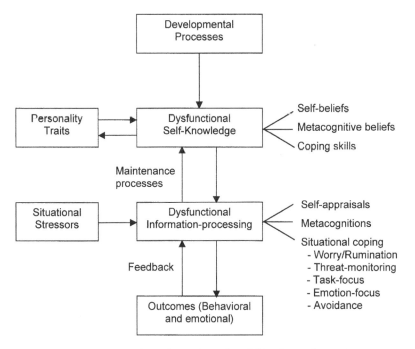

FIG. 12.1. An outline scheme for vulnerability factors for anxiety.

Within a dynamic conception of psychopathology, dysfunctional self-knowledge may be seen as both effect and cause. Over longer time spans, developmental processes such as childhood experiences of threatening situations may generate damaging self-referent cognitions. Stable personality traits such as neuroticism may also shape self-referent learning. Over shorter time spans, dysfunctional self-knowledge influences information processing elicited by specific stressors and demands, biasing self-appraisal, metacognition, and choice, as well as regulation of coping strategy. Thus, the vulnerability factor is latent until activated by some stressful event (Ingram et al., 1998). Under these circumstances, dysfunctional self-knowledge is expressed as dysfunctional information processing, including situational appraisals, metacognitions, and coping strategies. Coping strategies are often categorized as being task focused, emotion focused, or avoidant (Endler & Parker, 1990). Although more narrowly defined strategies such as thought suppression may play important roles in some disorders, more generally special importance has been attributed to worry/rumination (Wells & Matthews, 1994a; Wells, 2000). Figure 12.1 also includes hypervigilant "threat-monitoring" as a coping strategy (Matthews & Wells, 1996, 1999), expressed as bias in selective attention. Coping in this way reflects the accessibility of procedural self-knowledge that specifies maintaining attentional focus on potential sources of threat.

Recent research emphasizes the dynamic factors that contribute to pathology, such as "dynamic danger content" of cognition as an antecedent to various anxiety disorders (Riskind & Williams, chap. 7, this vol.). At a process level, Wells and Matthews (1994a, 1996) argued that it is not so much the availability or activation of specific negative cognitions that is pathological, but the development of self-perpetuating configurations of processing. Figure 12.1 identifies two types of dynamic processes. First, pathology may be perpetuated by dysfunctional information processing alone, which maintains dysfunctional self-knowledge. For example, attentional strategies such as threat monitoring, coping strategies such as sustained worrying, thought control strategies such as suppression and *cognitive* avoidance may actually increase the accessibility of dysfunctional self-knowledge that initiates threatening thoughts (Wells, 2000; Wells & Matthews, 1994a). Second, the processing of feedback derived from the person's interaction with the external environment may also contribute to pathology. For instance, *behavioral* avoidance may prevent exposure to experiences that disconfirm erroneous beliefs. Moreover, anxiety management behaviors may be problematic if the nonoccurrence of catastrophe is attributed to use of specific coping strategies and not to the fact that beliefs/appraisals concerning catastrophe are erroneous. By contrast, realistic appraisals of feared encounters, to which the patient may be guided by behavioral experiments in therapy, promote more positive information processing and adaptive modification of self-knowledge. The roles of self-knowledge, dynamic factors, and coping are considered further after reviewing some highlights of the preceding chapters.

COGNITIVE BEHAVIORAL ACCOUNTS OF ANXIETY DISORDERS: A SUMMARY

Obsessive-Compulsive Disorder

Rachman, Shafran, and Riskind (chap. 9, this vol.) identify several forms of dysfunctional self-knowledge typical of OCD, including self-beliefs related to personal responsibility and distortions that are essentially metacognitive. Other work (e.g., Lopatka & Rachman, 1995) implicates compulsive checking as a characteristic coping strategy. Rachman (1997, 1998) suggested that obsessions are caused by catastrophic misinterpretations of the significance of one's intrusive thoughts. Hence, the cognitive model of obsessions is anchored to a metacognitive context, an approach that concurs with our own view of OCD (Wells, 1997; Wells & Matthews,

1994a), in which we have argued that the distorted meanings that OCD patients assign to their own intrusions result from the influence of meta-cognitive beliefs concerning the importance of, or power of, such thoughts in representing or influencing events. Rachman's model encompasses the earlier concept of inflated responsibility that has been equated with OCD (Salkovskis, 1985), but, in our view, adds theoretical clarity by avoiding some of the problems that exist with the responsibility concept. In his framework, inflated responsibility is closely associated with a cognitive distortion labeled thought–action fusion (TAF). Two forms of TAF have been identified: *probability TAF*, in which experiencing intrusive thoughts is believed to increase the probability of an event, and *morality TAF*, in which experiencing intrusions is interpreted as morally equivalent to carrying out a prohibited action. Once an intrusive thought is misinterpreted as having negative personal significance, it will give rise to active resistance to the thought and neutralizing of potentially threatening outcomes. These acts preserve the negative misinterpretation.

Much of the work in this area is cross-sectional in nature: It identifies core cognitive attributes of the OCD patient, but vulnerability factors are not clearly distinguished from symptoms or concomitants. As Rachman, Shafran, and Riskind (chap. 9, this vol.) point out, exaggerated personal responsibility is not necessarily associated with clinical pathology, and multiple cognitive vulnerability factors may be implicated. However, these authors identify some of the possible longer term origins of elevated responsibility and TAF, such as exposure to rigid codes of conduct and anxious parents who convey a sense of imminent danger. A limitation is that the cognitive architecture for vulnerability is not conceptualized in detail. Does thought–action fusion represent an automatic bias in interpretations of intrusive thoughts or is it tapping a metacognitive strategy of assigning meaning to one's own thinking?

Panic Disorder

Cognitive behavioral models of panic disorder have placed a differential emphasis on behavioral and cognitive mechanisms such as interoceptive conditioning, misinterpretations of bodily sensations, and anxiety sensitivity. The basic premise in these approaches is that bodily sensations trigger anxiety responses through a conditioning or appraisal based mechanism. Beliefs that somatic arousal is harmful define a trait of anxiety sensitivity, which may influence whether or not someone will panic in response to bodily sensations (Reiss & McNally, 1985). In integrating the models of panic proposed by Barlow (1988), D. M. Clark (1986), and Reiss and McNally (1985), Schmidt and Woolaway-Bickel (chap. 8, this vol.) highlight three distal cognitive vulnerability factors for panic disorder:

anxiety sensitivity beliefs, predictability and control beliefs, and information-processing biases. In the context of our current conceptual framework, these factors relate to different aspects of dysfunctional self-knowledge: metacognitive knowledge of bodily symptoms (anxiety sensitivity), self-beliefs (related to predictability and control), and coping maladaptively through vigilant attention to somatic sensations.

Schmidt and Woolaway-Bickel suggest that catastrophic cognition operates as a specific proximal vulnerability for panic disorder. Catastrophic misinterpretations of bodily sensations are viewed as state variables required for the creation of panic attacks. Other cognitive risk factors, as already outlined, operate as more distal vulnerability factors. By comparison, Clark's cognitive model emphasizes proximal factors in the form of catastrophic misinterpretations of bodily responses, whereas the models of Barlow (1988) and of Reiss and McNally (1985) emphasize distal factors (i.e., anxiety sensitivity, predictability, and control). One of the strengths of the approach presented by Schmidt and Woolaway-Bickel is the examination of constellations of factors, both distal and proximal, and subcomponents of cognition (i.e., beliefs and cognitive processes) in explaining vulnerability to panic. It also recognizes dynamic factors appropriately (cf. D. M. Clark, 1986), and offers some plausible suggestions for longer term developmental processes such as biological factors, exposure to anxiety-related stressors, and childhood encounters with threatening situations. A limitation is that cognitive processes are not clearly integrated with concepts such as beliefs and anxiety sensitivity. For instance, is anxiety sensitivity a factor that emerges from unconscious and automatic cognitive processes or is it a product of strategies for self-evaluation and attentional monitoring? Is the activation of catastrophic cognitions a cause or effect of attentional bias, or are these factors linked within some dynamic processing configuration?

Social Phobia

Social phobics believe that others are likely to criticize them and evaluate them negatively (Rapee & Heimberg, 1997). These individuals tend to engage in cognitive processes and subtle safety behaviors that contribute to insecurity in presenting a favorable impression (D. M. Clark & Wells, 1995; Rapee & Heimberg, 1997). According to the D. M. Clark and Wells (1995) model, on entering feared social situations people with social phobia focus attention on the self and process the self as a social object. This self-processing often occurs as an image (or sometimes a felt-sense) from an observer perspective in which anxiety symptoms and failed performance is highly conspicuous. Rapee and Heimberg (1997) similarly asserted that social phobics tend to assume an audience perspective on themselves.

The focus of attention in social phobia appears to be biased in other ways as well. Roth, Fresco, and Heimberg (chap. 10, this vol.) review evidence of attentional biases in social anxiety that have used modified Stroop and dot-probe paradigms. The data reviewed are somewhat complex, but it seems that, under conditions of social threat, there is initial attention to threat-congruent stimuli, followed by avoidance. These bias effects in attention may support the maintenance of negative beliefs and appraisals in social anxiety. As in other anxiety disorders (Matthews & Wells, 2000), bias in social phobia may be at least partially strategic in nature. Holle, Neely, and Heimberg (1997) showed that a significant emotional Stroop effect for social threat words was found only when trials were blocked by word type, rather than randomized. The effect of blocking may be attributed to the role of expectancy (Richards, French, Johnson, Naparstek, & Williams, 1992); an automatic bias should operate on an individual trial basis. Roth et al. also review the informative literature on developmental factors that may influence the acquisition of dysfunctional cognition, although, as they point out, the bridge between studies focusing on longer term and shorter term processes remains to be constructed. The question remains as to whether socially anxious individuals show a general propensity to engage in biased attentional strategies that precedes the development of social anxiety. Moreover, research focusing predominantly on attentional biases for external stimuli neglects the wider constellation of attentional factors that may contribute to social anxiety. Further studies of the roles of heightened self-focused processing and attentional avoidance would be useful: For example, "avoidance" might actually represent shifting of attention to self-referent processing of social cues, such as the self-image, or self-monitoring necessary for the execution of self-control behaviors, rather than avoidance of external cues. The interplay between attentional processes and the memory and judgment biases described by Roth et al. also awaits elucidation.

PTSD

Feeny and Foa (chap. 11, this vol.) divide cognitive theories of PTSD into two subtypes, schema theories and emotional processing theories. Schema theories are based on the principle that changes in a victim's thoughts and beliefs induced by trauma determine subsequent emotional responses. Various theories (e.g., Epstein, 1985; Janoff-Bulman, 1992) identify core beliefs that may change, such as benevolence and meaningfulness of the world, and self-worthiness. Traumatic experiences violate these assumptions and victims must go through a cognitive crisis to assimilate these experiences into old assumptions or to change their assumptions.

Foa and Kozak (1986) developed an emotional processing framework for understanding maintenance of PTSD. According to this model, anxiety and fear represent activation of *fear networks*, or cognitive structures that serve as a program for escaping danger. Emotional processing is characterized by a decay of activity in fear networks established by the traumatic event. Fear networks have to be activated and incongruent information must be incorporated into them in order for emotional processing to take place. Several factors can interfere with these processes, including coping through avoidance and negative beliefs about anxiety symptoms.

Feeny and Foa's model integrates various aspects of vulnerability, beginning with the developmental processes that predispose the person to acquire a dysfunctional fear network in response to a traumatic stressor. Their model also specifies the nature of dysfunctional self-knowledge in PTSD, focusing especially on rigidly negative schematized beliefs and avoidant coping. Our view is that negative interpretations of PTSD symptoms, such as intrusions, are influenced by metacognitive styles and beliefs that focus attention on negative thoughts and images excessively. Moreover, we view the tendency to cope through the use of worry/rumination as an important factor interfering with emotional processing (Holeva, Tarrier, & Wells, 2001; Wells & Papageorgiou, 1995; Wells & Sembi, 2004a). The Feeny and Foa model is unique among those reviewed in its account of how situational information processing may modify self-knowledge maladaptively, through coping by attempting to suppress thoughts, or adaptively by elaborating and reorganizing the fear network to facilitate effective coping. As with other disorders, there remains a disconnection between studies of long- and short-term vulnerability.

Anxiety and the Looming Maladaptive Style

Riskind and Williams (chap. 7, this vol.) focus on maladaptive cognitions that may provide a common vulnerability factor for the various anxiety disorders. They identify a looming maladaptive style (LMS), which is essentially a type of danger schema that represents dynamically intensifying danger and rapidly escalating risk. Developmental factors that contribute to this vulnerability include modeling of parental anxieties, life events associated with "looming entrapment," and insecure attachment relationships. LMS is conceptualized as a distal vulnerability factor that interacts with additional factors in contributing to the etiology of the various anxiety disorders and their cognitive concomitants. The cognitive biasing initiated by the LMS includes danger-related cognitive content, hypervigilance for threat, imperative needs to avoid perceived threat, and self-protective behaviors. Maladaptive avoidance behaviors may serve to perpetuate the LMS dynamically, by creating a confirmatory bias that maintains exaggerated beliefs in intensifying danger. Riskind's (e.g., 1997) CVA project provides various lines of evidence in support of the LMS model, using experimental manipulations of looming and a questionnaire measure of vulnerability. Two features of this work are especially noteworthy. First, Riskind and colleagues showed that LMS predicts processing bias independently of anxiety. Second, looming vulnerability discriminates anxiety from depression. This finding is important in that levels of threat and danger cognitions often fail to discriminate anxious and depressed persons clearly (D. A. Clark & Beck, 1999).

Most models reviewed implicate some mixture of self-referent cognitions, metacognitions, and coping in vulnerability, although differing in the emphasis given to different components. The LMS model is different in giving primacy to schematized beliefs, which leads to subsequent changes in metacognition and coping. For example, Riskind and Williams state that the sense of escalating danger "should naturally lead" the person to search for danger stimuli. Our view (Matthews & Wells, 1999; Wells & Matthews, 1994a) is different, in that search for danger is seen as a form of coping represented independently from danger schemata, consistent with the modest magnitude of associations between pathological anxiety and attentional bias. Indeed, a propensity to search for threat guided by metacognitive knowledge might influence the development of the LMS, through raising awareness of potentially catastrophic threats. A further issue is the extent to which the sense of looming danger is "cognitive" or "metacognitive." Riskind and Williams appear to conceptualize looming cognitions as tied directly to external threat stimuli. However, anxiety patients often appraise their own uncontrollable thoughts as the source of threat, and metacognitive awareness of escalating loss of control over thoughts may be especially pathological (cf. Wells, 1999, 2000). It is conceivable that heightened metacognitions that lead to attentional monitoring for threat, and to the appraisal of uncontrollability of cognition and emotion, are antecedent to the sense of looming danger.

GENERIC AND DISORDER-SPECIFIC VULNERABILITY FACTORS

Some cognitive factors may confer generalized vulnerability to anxiety disorders, or even to both anxiety and depression. This section looks at early developmental processes that may generate dysfunctional self-beliefs, attentional bias, styles of coping, and personality traits (specifically, neuroticism, which is a dispositional vulnerability factor that has a strong basis in dysfunctional self-knowledge). Discussion of metacognitive vulnerability factors is postponed to the next section, on the S-REF model (Wells & Matthews, 1994a), which features metacognition as a central element of anxiogenic cognition.

Developmental Processes

Several chapters in Part II of this book describe childhood psychosocial factors that lead to an increased proneness to anxiety disorders. The major themes are faulty social learning from anxious parents, exposure to threatening events, and self-referent beliefs that create a vulnerability toward acquiring more generalized, schemalike dysfunctional self-knowledge. Rachman, Shafran, and Riskind (chap. 9, this vol.) suggest that exposure to rigid codes of conduct and anxious parents who convey a sense of imminent danger may contribute to elevated levels of responsibility in individuals and this may be the source of vulnerability to obsessive-compulsive problems. Riskind and Williams (chap. 7, this vol.) claim that the looming maladaptive style of processing, associated with dynamic threat awareness, may develop from learning histories such as faulty modeling, unresolved childhood fears, and insecure attachment experiences. Similarly, Schmidt and Woolaway-Bickel (chap. 8, this vol.) identify learning histories that may contribute to anxiety sensitivity, that is, beliefs about the harmfulness of symptoms, which is a vulnerability factor for panic (Reiss & McNally, 1985). High anxiety sensitivity may emerge from receiving misinformation about the harmfulness of sensations, or witnessing a catastrophic event. Feeny and Foa (chap. 11, this vol.) implicate rigidity of beliefs as a factor that promotes formation of a dysfunctional fear network in response to trauma, but the developmental antecedents of rigidity remain to be investigated. Turning to social anxiety, early experience with parents and peers may contribute to the origins of dysfunctional beliefs concerning the inflated likelihood of negative social feedback (Roth, Fresco, & Heimberg, chap. 10, this vol.). These authors review evidence that socially anxious children are more likely to experience negative peer relationships and that individuals high in social anxiety report more frequent teasing in childhood. They also indicate that people who develop social anxiety grow up in families where great importance is placed on making a good impression and children learn by watching parent relationships. Moreover, parents with social anxiety themselves may isolate their children from social experiences, and hence the opportunity to acquire social skills.

Overall, it appears that both learning experiences early in life and subsequent experiences surrounding stress occurrences are recurring themes in several of the contributions offered here. The evidence cited in support of this proposition tends to be cross-sectional or retrospective in nature. In each of these cases, learning experiences have been translated into vulnerability for specific subtypes of anxiety disorder. So, in obsessive-compulsive disorder, learning experiences are translated into inflated responsibility, and cognitive bias typified by thought–action fusion. In social phobia, learning experiences are translated into the belief that other people are likely to be critical and that negative evaluation is probable in social situations. In panic disorder, learning experiences are translated into beliefs that underlie anxiety sensitivity.

Developmental processes are clearly important, but there are also some limitations in the picture offered by existing research. First, content and process are not well-distinguished. Most authors focus on children's beliefs rather than the styles of processing that influence the self-knowledge they acquire. For example, anxiety-related attentional bias is evident in children as young as 4 to 5 years (Martin & Jones, 1995), and it might influence self-knowledge acquisition. Second, the role of metacognitive development has been largely ignored. To what extent does vulnerability reflect the child's beliefs about its own thought processes? Third, the child tends to be viewed as a passive receptacle for knowledge, leading to a rather unfortunate trend toward blaming the parents for faulty learning. More complex patterns of person–environment interaction may be involved (see Caspi & Bem, 1990). Children of differing temperament may differ in their style of exploring and interacting with the external environment. Temperament may also influence the ways in which parents and peers act toward children. The role of the child as an active participant in its own development may explain why "within-family" environmental influences on traits related to anxiety and neuroticism are often minor (Loehlin, 1992).

Attentional Biases

Cognitive biases such as selective attention to threat, biases of memory, and judgments may also be vulnerability factors for anxiety disorders. Selective attention to threat, as indexed by the emotional Stroop and other tasks, appears to be a general feature of both anxiety and mood disorders, with the content of the stimuli that attract attention varying from disorder to disorder (Matthews & Wells, 1999). The role of attentional biases are most clearly evident in the chapters reviewed, through studies of looming maladaptive style (Riskind & Williams, chap. 7, this vol.), the Integrated Anxiety Sensitivity Model of Panic (Schmidt & Woolaway-Bickel, chap. 8, this vol.), and the discussion of cognitive factors associated with social phobia (Roth, Fresco, & Heimberg, chap. 10, this vol.). A few studies suggest that attentional bias may operate as a vulnerability factor. For example, when emotionally primed, recovered depressives show attentional bias in dichotic listening (Ingram, Bernet, & McLaughlin, 1994) and visual attention (McCabe, Gotlib, & Martin, 2000). Studies of nonclinical samples suggest that the emotional Stroop may predict anxiety responses to threatening events (Van den Hout, Tenney, Huygens, Merckelbach, & Kindt, 1995). Although recovered patients typically do not show attentional abnormality, Ingram et al. (1998) correctly pointed to the need to assess attention in primed conditions that may activate latent dysfunctional self-knowledge. However, more evidence is required in order to establish that attentional biases contribute to vulnerability or, alternatively, that they emerge primarily as a consequence of the development of anxiety disorders and serve to maintain disorder.

Coping

Anxious and depressed individuals show a typical pattern of coping: heightened use of emotion-focused strategies such as self-blame and avoidance, and lower levels of problem- or task-focused coping (Matthews & Wells, 1996). This coping style tends to be linked to symptoms of pathology and other negative outcomes, in both nonclinical samples (Zeidner & Saklofske, 1996) and in patient groups (Vollrath, Alnæs, & Torgersen, 1996). Moreover, as discussed later in this chapter, anxiety and depression can be linked to perseverative styles of coping through worry or rumination driven by metacognitive beliefs (Wells, 2000; Wells & Matthews, 1994a). Chapters in this book highlight both commonalities and differences in coping across anxiety disorders. Riskind and Williams (chap. 7, this vol.) link the looming maladaptive style to "coping rigidity," in that the imperative need for action and time urgency leads to selection of fast acting but potentially maladaptive default coping strategies. Other chapters identify more disorder specific coping styles. Posttrauma pathology appears to relate to cognitive-emotional avoidance, wishful thinking, and dissociation during and immediately after trauma (Feeny & Foa, chap. 11, this vol.). However, metacognitions and thinking style also appear important. Holeva, Tarrier, and Wells (2001), in a longitudinal study, found that thought control strategies of worry predicted PTSD following road accidents. Morgan, Matthews, and Winton (1995), in a study of flood victims, found that emotion-focus and thought suppression were more predictive of anxiety and depression than a generalized avoidance measure. Coping is not much emphasized in the chapters on panic and on social phobia, other than the threat monitoring and avoidance strategies common to various anxiety disorders. OCD is associated with the rather more specific coping strategy of checking.

It is plausible that styles of coping constitute vulnerability factors, but it is often difficult to draw strong conclusions from coping studies. Most studies are cross-sectional, and the efficacy of coping strategies varies with the type of encounter to which the strategy is applied (Zeidner & Saklofske, 1996). However, there is increasing evidence from longitudinal studies for the validity of coping measures as predictors of future outcomes (Lazarus, 2000). For example, a recent longitudinal study of 154 former psychiatric outpatients in Norway (Vollrath et al., 1996; Vollrath, Alnæs, & Torgersen, 1998) found that coping style measures predicted clinical syndromes assessed 6 or 7 years later. Several conditions, including anxiety, dysthymia, depression, and somatoform disorder, were associated with greater use of disengagement and venting of emotions, and reduced use of active goal-oriented coping and seeking social support. Modeling of data suggested that anxiety was especially related to low active goal-oriented coping, and depression to low social support seeking (Vollrath et al., 1996). One difficulty is the overlap between coping and other cognitive constructs, because choice of coping strategy may reflect metacognitions and appraisals of control (Wells, 2000; Wells & Matthews, 1994a). For example, Matthews, Hillyard, and Campbell (1999) found that use of maladaptive coping strategies correlated with various aspects of metacognition, but coping and metacognition predicted test anxiety independently of one another. More multivariate research discriminating coping from other aspects of cognitive vulnerability is required.

Personality Traits

Dispositional factors are perhaps rather neglected by the contributors to this volume as vulnerability factors, except as confounds to be controlled (e.g., Riskind & Williams, chap. 7). Neuroticism, especially, is reliably elevated in anxiety and mood disorders and, although bidirectional causal links between neuroticism and psychopathology are likely, this trait appears to operate as a fairly general risk factor (Matthews, Schwean, Campbell, Saklofske, & Mohamed, 2000; Vollrath et al., 1998). Neglect of neuroticism may reflect the view that basic dispositions are essentially biological in nature. In fact, there is considerable evidence that bias in self-knowledge is central to neuroticism and related traits such as optimism-pessimism, although bias may be a product of both biological and social-cognitive influences on cognitive development (Matthews, Derryberry, & Siegle, 2000; Matthews, Schwean, et al., 2000). Neuroticism is substantially correlated with negative self-appraisals—presumably reflecting stable negative self-beliefs, metacognitive beliefs, and use of emotion-focused and avoidant coping strategies—and with dispositional worry (Matthews, Schwean, et al., 2000; Wells, 1994b; Wells & Davies, 1994). Several authors have explored how coping factors might mediate neuroticism effects on pathology (e.g., Matthews, Derryberry, et al., 2000; Vollrath et al., 1998), although much work remains to be done. On the one hand, it is important to discriminate individual vulnerability factors that may be central to pathology in general, or to specific disorders. On the other hand, some cognitive vulnerability factors seem to co-occur as a complex of maladaptive cognitions, and may sometimes be treated as a syndrome closely related to personality.

AN INTEGRATED ACCOUNT OF VULNERABILITY: THE S-REF MODEL

The question of cognitive vulnerability concerns how multiple, cognitive, and behavioral factors interact dynamically in rendering individuals susceptible to anxiety disorders. As discussed, cognitive factors include stable schemas or beliefs, metacognitions, individual differences in coping, and biases in attention, memory, and judgment. What is often lacking in theoretical accounts of emotional disorder is a model of the dynamic interplay between multiple cognitive factors, and between these factors and behavior, that contributes to vulnerability and disorder maintenance. Important issues remain unresolved, including the relation between beliefs and cognitive biases, the roles of attention and metacognition in maintaining vulnerability, and the relative importance of strategic and automatic processes. Our own theoretical work on cognitive-attentional vulnerability to emotional disorders addresses these questions. The Self-Regulatory Executive Function (S-REF) theory (Wells, 2000; Wells & Matthews, 1994a) links emotional disorder to a cognitive-attentional syndrome consisting of activation of negative self-beliefs, heightened self-focused processing, the diversion of attention to worry and ruminative appraisal, and maladaptive coping strategies (e.g., threat monitoring) that fail to restructure negative beliefs. Vulnerability can be viewed in part in terms of the distally acquired metacognitive knowledge that when activated by critical incidents gives rise to the cyclical worry, threat monitoring, and coping that maintain disturbance.

Two components of the S-REF syndrome that maintain emotional pathology are perseverative worry/rumination, and the use of threat monitoring (maintenance of attention on threat-related stimuli). Worry/rumination-based strategies and attentional bias are a function of the anxious or depressed individual's choice of coping strategies for dealing with threat, which in turn derives from proceduralized self-knowledge (Matthews & Wells, 1996, 1999; Wells & Matthews, 1994a). This theory has a number of distinctive features. First, processing is conceptualized within a cognitive architecture of three interacting levels. These levels consist of an upper level of beliefs or stored knowledge, online executive processing that is dependent on activation of stored knowledge for its operation, and lower level processing that is largely automatic and stimulus driven. Dysfunction at any one of these levels or dynamic disturbances in the interaction between levels can increase vulnerability and maintain psychological disorder. For instance, high levels of self-consciousness may increase vulnerability to overload of attention in demanding situations, such that performance or coping is impaired or biased (Matthews, Mohamed, & Lochrie, 1998; Wells & Matthews, 1994b).

A further distinctive feature is that beliefs are conceptualized as containing a metacognitive component that guides processing. Beliefs are not only represented as propositional information as in schema theory (e.g., "I'm bad; if I show signs of weakness everyone will reject me"), but as knowledge that guides processing. For example, patients believe that it is imperative to worry, ruminate, attend to threat, or use particular mental strategies in order to cope. In the case of an obsessive-compulsive disorder patient troubled by intrusive thoughts of the Devil, metacognitions guiding coping were as follows: "If intrusion of devil occurs, then stop current behavior. If behavior is stopped, then activate memory of Jesus. If memory activated, then construct perfect image of Jesus. If image constructed, then exclude all thoughts of the devil." The S-REF model gives particular prominence to metacognitions for appraisal and coping in determining emotional disorder vulnerability and maintenance.

Metacognitions and Anxiety

Metacognition is defined as any knowledge or cognitive process supporting the appraisal, monitoring, or control of thinking (Flavell, 1979). It has two basic aspects. *Metacognitive knowledge* is the information that individuals have about their own cognition and about the factors that affect it. *Metacognitive regulation* refers to a range of executive functions, such as the allocation of attention, monitoring, checking, and planning (Brown, Bransford, Campione, & Ferrara, 1983). Until the advent of the S-REF model (Wells, 2000; Wells & Matthews, 1994a), metacognition was largely ignored in cognitive behavioral theory of psychological disturbance. The S-REF model sees beliefs as having a metacognitive component consisting of knowledge about cognitions, such as beliefs about the meaning of particular types of thoughts (e.g., "worrying is harmful"), and knowledge about the use of styles of thinking for coping (e.g., "worrying will make me more prepared to deal with threat").

In anxiety disorders, many of the negative appraisals and coping strategies used by individuals are metacognitive in nature and/or origin. Generalized anxiety disorder (GAD) is generated proximally by "metaworry," or worry about worry that feeds into a vicious circle in which anxiety symptoms generate further metaworry and further anxiety (Wells, 1994, 1995). Individuals with GAD are distinguishable from other anxiety reactions by heightened negative metacognitions (Wells, 2005; Wells & Carter, 2001). In obsessive-compulsive disorder, metacognitive beliefs concerning the meaning and power of thoughts lead to negative interpretations of obsessional thoughts and coping strategies that perpetuate intrusions (Wells, 1997). Metacognitive beliefs about intrusions still contribute to obsessive-compulsive symptoms when belief domains capturing responsibility are statistically controlled (Gwilliam, Wells, & Cartwright-Hatton, 2004; Myers & Wells, in press). In PTSD, metacognitive beliefs are hypothesized to underlie the activation of mental regulation strategies such as worry/rumination, threat monitoring, and negative appraisal of symptoms that are problematic for emotional processing (Wells & Sembi, 2004a, 2004b).

An important issue is whether maladaptive metacognitions, either at the knowledge or regulation level, precede the onset of psychopathology. Positive associations have been found between measures of metacognition and trait anxiety, proneness to pathological worry and obsessive-compulsive symptoms in cross-sectional studies (Cartwright-Hatton & Wells, 1997; Wells & Carter, 1999; Wells & Papageorgiou, 1998). Rassin, Merchelback, Muris, and Spaan (1999) used an experimental induction of thought–action fusion. Individuals who were led to believe that their thoughts would lead to negative outcomes report significantly more obsessive intrusions, greater discomfort, and greater efforts to avoid thinking than subjects receiving a neutral manipulation. Negative metacognitive beliefs about the uncontrollability and dangers of worrying have also been found to predict the development of GAD in prospective analyses of nonpatients (Nassif, 1999). Thus, there is some emerging evidence that maladaptive metacognitive beliefs may precede emotional dysfunction.

Further evidence supports the damaging role of metacognitive coping strategies that seek to control the content of thought. Attempts to suppress target thoughts are ineffective and may in some instances be counterproductive (Wenzlaff, Wegner, & Roper, 1988). However, paradoxical effects of suppression have not been consistently detected (see Purdon, 1999, for a review). A limitation of suppression research is that it has tended to rely on general instructions not to think about target thoughts, but different thought control strategies may be more ineffective or problematic under some circumstances than others. The Thought Control Questionnaire (TCQ; Wells & Davies, 1994) assesses the use of five thought control strategies: distraction, social control, worry, punishment, and reappraisal. Studies suggest that punishment and worry strategies are elevated in various anxiety disorders and are positively correlated with vulnerability. Strategies of distraction, social control, and reappraisal show nonsignificant but negative associations with anxiety and worry (see Wells, 2000). Reynolds and Wells (1999) explored relations between thought control strategies and psychiatric symptoms in patients with major depression and patients with PTSD, with or without major depression. TCQ predictors of recovery from PTSD and depression were investigated. Recovered and unrecovered patients differed in both baseline TCQ scores, and change over time. At baseline, recovered patients were higher in distraction and reappraisal. At follow-up, recovered patients showed improvements in the ability to use distraction and reappraisal, and showed reduced use of punishment. Unrecovered patients failed to show these beneficial changes, and obtained higher worry scores at both baseline and follow-up. In a recent prospective study of PTSD following motor vehicle accidents, Holeva et al. (2001) administered self-report measures of stress symptoms, the TCQ and Social Support measures, within 4 weeks of an accident and individuals were reassessed within 6 months. PTSD at Time 2 was predicted not just by acute stress disorder at Time 1, but also by the use of TCQ worry at Time 1, a change in perceived social support from Time 1 to Time 2 and an interaction between social support and the use of TCQ social control. Taken together, the results of these studies suggest that individual differences in the choice of strategies for controlling thoughts are associated with trait measures of anxiety and appear to be causally linked to emotional disturbance.

Worry and Rumination

The S-REF model links a generic cognitive-attentional syndrome consisting in part of active worry or rumination to stress vulnerability and disorder maintenance. Consistent with this idea, a growing body of research supports the view that worry or ruminative styles of thinking are indeed problematic for emotional self-regulation (see Papageorgiou & Wells, 2004). In early work on worry, Borkovec, Robinson, Pruzinsky, and De-Pree (1983) showed that brief periods of worrying in contrast to longer periods lead to more anxiety and more negative thoughts during a basic breathing task. Perseverative rumination also predicts future depression in longitudinal studies, for example, in recently bereaved adults (Nolen-Hoeksema, Parker, & Larson, 1994). As already pointed out, worry is associated longitudinally with PTSD-type symptoms (Holeva et al., 2001). In a direct study of the effects of worrying on intrusive images following stress, Butler, Wells, and Dewick (1995) asked three groups of subjects to watch a gruesome film about a workshop accident. Subjects were then asked to do one of the following for a 4-minute period: settle down, image the events in the film, and worry in verbal form about the events in the film. Participants who were asked to worry about the film reported significantly more intrusive images related to the film over the next 3 days as compared to subjects who had imaged or settled down. In a larger study, Wells and Papageorgiou (1995) extended these findings, again showing that worry led to the most number of intrusions compared with other mentation conditions.

COGNITIVE ARCHITECTURE: INTERACTION BETWEEN LEVELS

In general, the S-REF model sees emotional disorder as being initiated and maintained through dynamic interaction between levels of cognition: self-knowledge, online strategic processing (i.e., appraisal & coping), and lower level processing. However, in contrast to some other theoretical formulations, the model places special emphasis on strategy use, and lower level processing is important primarily through its interactions with strategic processing. As previously indicated, the issue of whether vulnerabilities are located at "automatic" or "controlled" levels of representation is potentially clinically significant.

The S-REF model equates vulnerability with strategic processes driven by the individuals' self-knowledge, of which metacognitive knowledge or plans for guiding cognition and action are of particular importance. However, this position is not intended to rule out the involvement of lower level automatic or reflexive processes in vulnerability. In particular, lower level networks may become dysfunctional as a result of repeated consistent stimulus–response mapping leading to strong interconnections among low-level processing units. Such negative associations could be learned through repeated exposure to aversive events early in life, prior to the development of more complex upper level knowledge. These low level networks would shape the development of upper level knowledge, and could still operate even if the upper level were modified. The lower level may be most sensitive to innate fear stimuli rather than to the complex and ambiguous stimuli (often of a social nature), which are open to misinterpretation during the elicitation of anxiety. The S-REF model sees cognitive biases that constitute vulnerability as predominantly strategy driven, representing an outcome of the individual's volitional plan for coping and appraising threat. Strategies such as worrying, or rumination (as in the case of depression), are problematic for self-regulation because they drain the resources necessary for cognitive restructuring and the more attentionally demanding forms of problem-focused coping. Worry and rumination may disrupt lower level processes, such as exposure to imagery, which is necessary for habituation effects. Worry may also prime lower level processing so that worry congruent information is more likely to intrude into consciousness.

Coping strategies that lead to avoidance of danger also maintain erroneous self-beliefs and metacognitions. For instance, individuals with anxiety disorders may engage in subtle forms of coping behavior that are designed to prevent feared catastrophes. The social phobic who fears shaking uncontrollably and spilling a drink may avoid drinking in public or engage in behaviors such as gripping a cup tightly, moving slowly, or trying to relax. Some of these behaviors will enhance self-consciousness and its attendant problems of overload of attention, thereby compromising performance or compromising belief change. Some coping responses may inadvertently exacerbate unwanted symptoms. For instance, trying to relax by taking deep breaths may lead to hyperventilation and increase sensations of unsteadiness and dizziness. Finally, the nonoccurrence of catastrophes can be attributed to use of the coping behavior, so that individuals may inadvertently reinforce or maintain their negative predictions and negative beliefs. Each exposure becomes a "near miss" rather than a disconfirmatory experience. Thus, the results of online processing in the form of execution of coping can feed back to changes in or failures to change the person's self-knowledge.

Even if behavior leads to disconfirmatory experiences, successful transformation of the schema or knowledge base may not follow. Individuals may lack the knowledge or control of processes that undertake such metacognitive change. Such biases present a latent vulnerability to emotional disturbance, and give rise to ineffective or inflexible means of cognitive self-regulation. These factors are discussed in detail elsewhere (Wells, 2000).

The preceding chapters provide many insights into the causes of clinical anxiety, and the multiple sources of vulnerability involved. In attempting a synthesis of work on cognitive vulnerability, the focus was put on different categories of stable self-knowledge (nonmetacognitive and metacognitive) that bias situational information processing; the role of dynamic factors in promoting pathological cognitive-attentional processing configurations; and the underlying cognitive architecture. Our S-REF model places vulnerability factors within an explicit multilevel architecture. The sources of vulnerability reside in dysfunctional self-knowledge, including self-beliefs, metacognitions, and coping processes. Self-knowledge underpins personality traits such as neuroticism. Proximally, vulnerability to anxiety and other emotional disturbances depend on the likelihood that self-relevant threat stimuli activate executive processing associated with the maladaptive cognitive-attentional syndrome (i.e., worry/rumination, threat monitoring, avoidance). Distally, vulnerability emerges from the developmental processes that give rise to dysfunctional self-knowledge in the generic and metacognitive domains. Self-knowledge biases the appraisal of external events, emotional and somatic symptoms, and intrusive thoughts, and influences the selection and regulation of coping strategies. Multiple processes may contribute directly to anxiety. They include exaggerated negative appraisals of external threats and of the self, and anxiogenic coping strategies. Such strategies include fixating attention on potential threat sources (i.e., attentional bias), worry, excessive self-criticism, attempts at thought control, and avoidant strategies that fail to restructure maladaptive self-knowledge or prevent exposure to disconfirmatory experiences. Additionally, the dynamic configuration of processing that maintains worry may generate pathological anxiety beyond the influence of its component processes. More specifically, metacognitive appraisals and beliefs about negative emotions and thoughts contribute to reciprocal links between emotional experience and cognition that perpetuate worry and anxiety. Reciprocal links between cognition and feedback from the external environment also serve to maintain worry and anxiety dynamically. This analysis adds to existing cognitive behavioral accounts in identifying attentional focus, metacognition, perseverative thinking, and behaviors that lead to failure of disconfirmation of dysfunctional beliefs as suitable targets for therapy. Modification of cognitive styles and the maladaptive metacognitions underlying them provide a new focus for treatment that supplements or offers an alternative to approaches focused on the content of general social cognitions. This chapter has outlined an integrative perspective on anxiety, but the metacognitive and perseverative factors highlighted are likely to be important in most forms of psychological disorder.

REFERENCES

Barlow, D. H. (1988). *Anxiety and its disorders: The nature and treatment of anxiety and panic.* New York: Guilford.

Borkovec, T. D., Robinson, E., Pruzinsky, T., & DePree, J. A. (1983). Preliminary exploration of worry: Some characteristics and processes. *Behaviour Research and Therapy, 21,* 9–16.

Brown, A. L., Bransford, J. D., Campione, J. C., & Ferrara, R. A. (1983). Learning, remembering and understanding. In J. Flavell & E. Markman (Eds.), *Handbook of child psychology: Vol. 3. Cognitive development.* New York: Wiley.

Butler, G., Wells, A., & Dewick, H. (1995). Differential effects of worry and imagery after exposure to a stressful stimulus: A pilot study. *Behavioural and Cognitive Psychotherapy, 23,* 45–56.

Cartwright-Hatton, S., & Wells, A. (1997). Beliefs about worry and intrusions: The Metacognitions Questionnaire and its correlates. *Journal of Anxiety Disorders, 11,* 279–296.

Caspi, A., & Bem, D. J. (1990). Personality continuity and change across the life course. In L. A. Pervin (Ed.), *Handbook of personality: Theory and research* (pp. 549–575). New York: Guilford.

Clark, D. A., & Beck, A. T. (1999). *Scientific foundations of cognitive theory and therapy of depression.* New York: Wiley.

Clark, D. M. (1986). A cognitive model of panic. *Behaviour Research and Therapy, 24,* 461–470.

Clark, D. M., & Wells, A. (1995). A cognitive model of social phobia. In R. Heimberg, M. Liebowitz, D. A. Hope, & F. R. Schneier (Eds.), *Social phobia: Diagnosis, assessment and treatment* (pp. 69–93). New York: Guilford.

Endler, N., & Parker, J. (1990). Multi dimensional assessment of coping: A critical review. *Journal of Personality and Social Psychology, 58,* 844–854.

Epstein, S. (1985). The implications of cognitive-experiential self-theory for research in social psychology and personality. *Journal of the Theory of Social Behavior, 15,* 283–310.

Flavell, J. H. (1979). Metacognition and metacognitive monitoring: A new area of cognitive-developmental inquiry. *American Psychologist, 34,* 906–911.

Foa, E. B., & Kozak, M. J. (1986). Emotional processing and fear: Exposure to corrective information. *Psychological Bulletin, 99,* 20–35.

Gwilliam, P., Wells, A., & Cartwright-Hatton, S. (2004). Does meta-cognition or responsibility predict obsessive-compulsive symptoms: A test of the metacognitive model. *Clinical Psychology and Psychotherapy, 11,* 137–144.

Holeva, V., Tarrier, N., & Wells, A. (2001). Prevalence and predictors of acute PTSD following road traffic accidents: Thought control strategies and social support. *Behavior Therapy, 32,* 65–84.

Holle, C., Neely, J. H., & Heimberg, R. G. (1997). The effects of blocked versus random presentation and semantic relatedness of stimulus words on response to a modified Stroop task among social phobics. *Cognitive Therapy and Research, 21,* 681–697.

Ingram, R. E., Bernet, C. Z., & McLaughlin, S. C. (1994). Attentional allocation processes in individuals at risk for depression. *Cognitive Therapy and Research, 18,* 317–332.

Ingram, R. E., Miranda, J., & Segal, Z. V. (1998). *Cognitive vulnerability to depression.* New York: Guilford.

Janoff-Bulman, R. (1992). *Shattered assumptions: Towards a new psychology of trauma.* New York: The Free Press.

Lazarus, R. S. (2000). Toward better research on stress and coping. *American Psychologist, 55,* 665–673.

Loehlin, J. C. (1992). *Genes and environment in personality development.* Newbury Park, CA: Sage.

Lopatka, C., & Rachman, S. (1995). Perceived responsibility and compulsive checking: An experimental analysis. *Behaviour Research and Therapy, 33,* 673–684.

Martin, M., & Jones, G. V. (1995). Integral bias in the cognitive processing of emotionally linked pictures. *British Journal of Psychology, 86,* 419–435.

Matthews, G., Derryberry, D., & Siegle, G. J. (2000). Personality and emotion: Cognitive science perspectives. In S. E. Hampson (Ed.), *Advances in personality psychology* (Vol. 1, pp. 199–237). London: Routledge.

Matthews, G., & Harley, T. A. (1996). Connectionist models of emotional distress and attentional bias. *Cognition and Emotion, 10,* 561–600.

Matthews, G., Hillyard, E. J., & Campbell, S. E. (1999). Metacognition and maladaptive coping as components of test anxiety. *Clinical Psychology and Psychotherapy, 6,* 111–125.

Matthews, G., Mohamed, A., & Lochrie, B. (1998). Dispositional self-focus of attention and individual differences in appraisal and coping. In J. Bermudez, A. M. Perez, A. Sanchez-Elvira, & G. L. van Heck (Eds.), *Personality psychology in Europe* (Vol. 6, pp. 278–285). Tilburg: Tilburg University Press.

Matthews, G., Schwean, V. L., Campbell, S. E., Saklofske, D. H., & Mohamed, A. A. R. (2000). Personality, self-regulation and adaptation: A cognitive-social framework. In M. Boekarts, P. R. Pintrich, & M. Zeidner (Eds.), *Handbook of self-regulation* (pp. 171–207). New York: Academic Press.

Matthews, G., & Wells, A. (1996). Attentional processes, coping strategies and clinical intervention. In M. Zeidner & N. S. Endler (Eds.), *Handbook of coping: Theory, research, applications* (pp. 573–601). New York: Wiley.

Matthews, G., & Wells, A. (1999). The cognitive science of attention and emotion. In T. Dalgleish & M. Power (Eds.), *Handbook of cognition and emotion* (pp. 171–192). New York: Wiley.

Matthews, G., & Wells, A. (2000). Attention, automaticity and affective disorder. *Behavior Modification, 24,* 69–93.

McCabe, S. B., Gotlib, I. H., & Martin, R. A. (2000). Cognitive vulnerability for depression: Deployment of attention as a function of history of depression and current mood state. *Cognitive Therapy and Research, 24,* 427–444.

Morgan, I. A., Matthews, G., & Winton, M. (1995). Coping and personality as predictors of post-traumatic intrusions, numbing, avoidance and general distress: A study of victims of the Perth flood. *Behavioural and Cognitive Psychotherapy, 23,* 251–264.

Myers, S., & Wells, A. (in press). Obsessive-compulsive symptoms: The contribution of metacognitions and responsibility. *Journal of Anxiety Disorders.*

Nassif, Y. (1999). *Predictors of pathological worry.* Unpublished master's thesis, University of Manchester, England.

Nolen-Hoeksema, S., Parker, L. E., & Larson, J. (1994). Ruminative coping with depressed mood following loss. *Journal of Personality and Social Psychology, 67,* 92–104.

Papageorgiou, C., & Wells, A. (2004). *Depressive rumination: Nature, theory, and treatment.* Chichester, England: Wiley.

Purdon, C. (1999). Thought suppression and psychopathology. *Behaviour Research and Therapy, 37,* 1029–1054.

Rachman, S. (1997). A cognitive theory of obsessions. *Behaviour Research and Therapy, 35,* 793–802.

Rachman, S. (1998). *Anxiety.* East Sussex, England: Psychology Press.

Rapee, R. M., & Heimberg, R. G. (1997). A cognitive-behavioral model of anxiety in social phobia. *Behaviour Research and Therapy, 35,* 741–756.

Rassin, E., Merckelbach, H., Muris, P., & Spaan, V. (1999). Thought–action fusion as arousal factor in the development of intrusions. *Behaviour Research and Therapy, 37,* 231–237.

Reiss, S., & McNally, R. J. (1985). Expectancy model of fear. In S. Reiss & R. R. Bootzin (Eds.), *Theoretical issues in behavior therapy* (pp. 107–121). San Diego, CA: Academic Press.

Reynolds, M., & Wells, A. (1999). The Thought Control Questionnaire—psychometric properties in a clinical sample, and relationships with PTSD and depression. *Psychological Medicine, 29,* 1089–1099.

Richards, A., French, C. C., Johnson, W., Naparstek, J., & Williams, J. (1992). Effects of mood manipulation and anxiety on performance of an emotional Stroop task. *British Journal of British Psychology, 83,* 479–491.

Riskind, J. H. (1997). Looming vulnerability to threat: A cognitive paradigm for anxiety. *Behaviour Research and Therapy, 35*(5), 386–404.

Salkovskis, P. M. (1985). Obsessional-compulsive problems: A cognitive-behavioural analysis. *Behaviour Research and Therapy, 23,* 571–583.

Van Den Hout, M., Tenney, N., Huygens, K., Merckelbach, H., & Kindt, M. (1995). Responding to subliminal threat cues is related to trait anxiety and emotional vulnerability: A successful replication of Macleod and Hagan (1992). *Behaviour Research and Therapy, 33,* 451–454.

Vollrath, M., Alnæs, R., & Torgersen, S. (1996). Differential effects of coping in mental disorders: A prospective study in psychiatric outpatients. *Journal of Clinical Psychology, 52,* 125–135.

Vollrath, M., Alnæs, R., & Torgersen, S. (1998). Neuroticism, coping and change in MCMI–II clinical syndromes: Test of a mediator model. *Scandinavian Journal of Psychology, 39,* 15–24.

Wells, A. (1994a). Attention and the control of worry. In G. C. L. Davey & F. Tallis (Eds.), *Worrying: Perspectives on theory, assessment and treatment* (pp. 90–114). Chichester, UK: Wiley.

Wells, A. (1994b). A multi-dimensional measure of worry: Development and preliminary validation of the Anxious Thought Inventory. *Anxiety, Stress and Coping, 6,* 280–299.

Wells, A. (1995). Meta-cognition and worry: A cognitive model of generalised anxiety disorder. *Behavioural and Cognitive Psychotherapy, 23,* 301–320.

Wells, A. (1997). *Cognitive therapy of anxiety disorders: A practice manual and conceptual guide.* Chichester, England: Wiley.

Wells, A. (1999). A metacognitive model and therapy for generalized anxiety disorder. *Clinical Psychology and Psychotherapy, 6,* 86–95.

Wells, A. (2000). *Emotional disorders and metacognition: Innovative cognitive therapy.* Chichester, England: Wiley.

Wells, A. (2005). The metacognitive model of GAD: Assessment of meta-worry and relationship with DSM IV generalized anxiety disorder. *Cognitive Therapy and Research, 29,* 108–121.

Wells, A., & Carter, K. (1999). Preliminary tests of a cognitive model of GAD. *Behaviour Research and Therapy, 37,* 585–594.

Wells, A., & Carter, K. (2001). Further tests of a cognitive model of generalized anxiety disorder: Metacognitions and worry in GAD, panic disorder, social phobia, depression, and non-patients. *Behavior Therapy, 32,* 85–102.

Wells, A., & Davies, M. (1994). The Thought Control Questionnaire: A measure of individual differences in the control of unwanted thoughts. *Behaviour Research and Therapy, 32,* 871–878.

Wells, A., & Matthews, G. (1994a). *Attention and emotion: A clinical perspective.* Hove, England: Lawrence Erlbaum Associates.

Wells, A., & Matthews, G. (1994b). Self-consciousness and cognitive failures as predictors of coping is stressful episodes. *Cognition and Emotion, 8,* 279–295.

Wells, A., & Matthews, G. (1996). Modelling cognition in emotional disorders: The S-REF model. *Behaviour Research and Therapy, 34,* 881–888.

Wells, A., & Papageorgiou, C. (1995). Worry and the incubation of intrusive images following stress. *Behaviour Research and Therapy, 33,* 579–583.

Wells, A., & Papageorgiou, C. (1998). Relationships between worry, obsessive-compulsive symptoms, and meta-cognitive beliefs. *Behaviour Research and Therapy, 36,* 899–913.

Wells, A., & Sembi, S. (2004a). Metacognitive therapy for PTSD: A core treatment manual. *Cognitive and Behavioral Practice, 11,* 365–377.

Wells, A., & Sembi, S. (2004b). Metacognitive therapy for PTSD: A preliminary investigation of a new brief treatment. *Journal of Behavior Therapy and Experimental Psychiatry, 35,* 307–318.

Wenzlaff, R. M., Wegner, D. M., & Roper, D. W. (1988). Depression and mental control: The resurgence of unwanted negative thoughts. *Journal of Personality and Social Psychology, 55,* 882–892.

Zeidner, M., & Saklofske, D. S. (1996). Adaptive and maladaptive coping. In M. Zeidner & N. S. Endler (Eds.), *Handbook of coping* (pp. 505–531). New York: Wiley.

III

EATING DISORDERS

13

Cognitive Vulnerability to Bulimia

Lyn Y. Abramson
University of Wisconsin–Madison

Anna M. Bardone-Cone
University of Missouri–Columbia

Kathleen D. Vohs
University of British Columbia

Thomas E. Joiner, Jr.
Florida State University

Todd F. Heatherton
Dartmouth College

Clinicians (e.g., Pacht, 1984) and researchers (e.g., Flett & Hewitt, 2002) alike have linked perfectionism and psychological maladjustment. The role of perfectionism has been especially underscored in the development and maintenance of eating disorders (see Shafran & Mansell, 2001). For example, Goldner, Cockell, and Srikameswaran (2002) described the quest for the "perfect diet, perfect exercise regime, perfect body shape, or perfect weight" (p. 319) of individuals suffering from eating disorders. Indeed, the very nature of eating disorders—relentlessly striving toward an impossible standard of thinness—is perfectionistic. On the one hand, then, the link between perfectionism and eating disorders makes sense, especially for individuals with anorexia nervosa who are successful, albeit maladaptively, in their relentless pursuit of thinness. But what about individuals suffering from bulimia nervosa, an eating disorder characterized not only by strict dieting and extreme compensatory behaviors (e.g., self-induced vomiting) to prevent weight gain, but also by recurrent episodes of binge eating? There is a paradox here because the binge eating component of bulimia severely contradicts and undermines bulimic individuals' goals for bodily perfection. Why would a bulimic individual with highly perfectionist goals for thinness engage in the very behavior—binge eating—that most profoundly sabotages these goals?

This chapter integrates work on bulimia with theories and research on self-regulation (e.g., Bandura, 1977; Carver & Scheier, 1998; Heatherton & Baumeister, 1991; Pyszczynski & Greenberg, 1987; Tice, Bratslavsky, & Baumeister, 2001) to resolve the intriguing paradox of perfectionism and binge eating among bulimic individuals. Ironically, for reasons outlined later in this chapter, individuals who are vulnerable to bulimia may be especially likely to resort to binge eating in a desperate attempt to decrease overwhelming negative emotion, aversive self-awareness, and self-loathing when they feel helpless to meet their perfectionistic standards. According to this view, binge eating among bulimic individuals represents a short-term strategy for attempting to regulate negative emotion and an aversive sense of self that is self-defeating over the long run (see Baumeister & Scher, 1988).

DESCRIPTIVE ASPECTS OF BULIMIA

Bulimia nervosa, a self-defeating eating disorder, consists of three key components: binge eating, during which large quantities of food are consumed uncontrollably in a short period of time (e.g., 2 hours); recurrent inappropriate compensatory behavior to prevent weight gain from calories consumed during a binge, such as self-induced vomiting, misuse of laxatives, diuretics, enemas, fasting, or excessive exercise; and excessive concern about body shape and weight (American Psychiatric Association, 2000).

Because the paradox of perfectionism and bulimia relates to the binge eating component of bulimia, it is useful to describe the characteristics of a typical binge (American Psychiatric Association, 2000). Binge eating usually occurs in secrecy or as inconspicuously as possible. The food consumed during a binge varies, often depending on what is available. Typically, binges contain sweet, high-calorie foods like ice cream and cookies, but the binge appears to be characterized more by the excessive amount of food eaten rather than by a craving for a specific type of food. Binges may be planned or spontaneous, but a common factor is the feeling of a lack of control. Many binge eaters describe being in a frenzied state while bingeing and feeling unable to stop. Another common feeling reported during a binge is dissociation. Often a binge eating episode ends only when the individual is painfully full or when there is an interruption (e.g., a family member comes home unexpectedly). Binge eating is a self-defeating behavior because, in addition to whatever good it serves, there are also distressing short- and long-term consequences (e.g., bloated feeling, movement away from dietary goals, and the negative consequences of compensatory behaviors such as vomiting to expel the calories consumed during a binge).

The following composite of illustrative quotations from different individuals (Fairburn, 1995) vividly illustrates the characteristics and contexts of typical binges:

> It all starts with the way I feel when I wake up. If I am unhappy or someone has said something to upset me, I feel a strong urge to eat . . . and I automatically move toward food. . . . First of all it is a relief and a comfort to eat, and I feel quite high. But then I can't stop, and I binge. I eat and eat frantically until I am absolutely full. . . . The food I eat usually consists of all my "forbidden" foods: chocolate, cake, cookies . . . and improvised sweet food like raw cake mixture. . . . (Sometimes) I randomly grab whatever food I can and push it into my mouth, sometimes not even chewing it. . . . I eat really quickly, as if I'm afraid that by eating slowly I will have too much time to think about what I am doing. . . . And binge eating does numb the upset feelings. It blots out whatever it was that was upsetting me. The trouble is that it is replaced with feeling stuffed and guilty and drained. (pp. 3–17)

DEMOGRAPHIC CONTEXT OF BULIMIA

Bulimia typically begins in late adolescence or early adult life (American Psychiatric Association, 2000). Based on retrospective reports with clinical samples, the typical age of onset for clinically diagnosable bulimia appears to be 18–19 years (e.g., Fairburn & Cooper, 1984). However, the age of onset for the emergence of the subclinical components of bulimia (bingeing and purging) may be even younger. In this regard, Stice, Killen, Hayward, and Taylor (1998) conducted a prospective study of the age of onset of bingeing and purging among an initially asymptomatic sample of adolescents over a follow-up period from age 14 to 19 and found that the peak risk for onset of binge eating occurred at age 16 and peak risk for onset of purging occurred at age 18. Insofar as individuals exhibiting eating disorder symptoms at the outset of the study were excluded, it is possible that the modal age of onset of the components of bulimia is even lower than found in this study. Consistent with findings that disordered eating patterns are largely in place by late adolescence, Vohs, Heatherton, and Herrin (2001) reported that disordered eating symptoms and attitudes are established before college.

Although individuals meeting diagnostic criteria for bulimia are overwhelmingly female (about 90% female; American Psychiatric Association,

2000), the gender difference for binge eating is less disproportionate (about 60% female; American Psychiatric Association, 1994). The lifetime prevalence of bulimia nervosa among women is about 1%–3% (American Psychiatric Association, 2000). However, the prevalence of subclinical but significant bulimic symptoms is higher (e.g., 14% in a female college sample; Kurth, Krahn, Nairn, & Drewnowski, 1995).

AN INCONSISTENT EMPIRICAL LINK BETWEEN PERFECTIONISM AND BULIMIA

As described earlier, there has been much interest in linking perfectionism to eating disorders. That a relation would exist between perfectionism and bulimia is intuitively compelling given the undue emphasis placed on body weight and shape by bulimic individuals. The bulimic individual's relentless striving toward an impossible standard of thinness is inherently perfectionistic. Moreover, clinical researchers have linked perfectionism to bulimia and its components. As Fairburn (1995) put it, "Another common longstanding characteristic is perfectionism; many who binge tend to set unduly demanding standards for themselves" (p. 60). Finally, theoretical accounts of the development of eating disorders have featured perfectionism (e.g., Beebe, 1994; Goldner et al., 2002; Heatherton & Baumeister, 1991). For example, Levine and Smolak (1992) emphasized the importance of the "superwoman ideal" in the etiology of eating disorders.

Despite the plausibility of a link between perfectionism and bulimia, empirical work has revealed an inconsistent relation between the two. On the one hand, some work has indicated that bulimic individuals do exhibit high levels of perfectionism. For example, Joiner, Heatherton, and Keel (1997) reported that scores on the Perfectionism subscale of the Eating Disorders Inventory (EDI; Garner, Olmstead, & Polivy, 1983), a measure of global perfectionism, predicted *DSM*-based bulimic symptoms 10 years later (see also Rosch, Crowther, & Graham, 1991; Steiger, Leung, Puentes-Neuman, & Gottheil, 1992, for positive findings). However, other studies have questioned the relation between perfectionism and bulimia (e.g., Blouin, Bushnik, Braaten, & Blouin, 1989; Fryer, Waller, & Kroese, 1997; Hurley, Palmer, & Stretch, 1990). Work in our own laboratory has highlighted the inconsistent relation between perfectionism and bulimic symptoms. Whereas Vohs, Bardone, Joiner, Abramson, and Heatherton (1999) found a positive relation between EDI-perfectionism scores and EDI-bulimia scores, Vohs, Voelz, et al. (2001) did not.

A TWO-FACTOR MODEL TO UNDERSTAND
THE INCONSISTENT EMPIRICAL LINK
BETWEEN PERFECTIONISM AND BULIMIA

Why is perfectionism only inconsistently related to bulimia? When a variable of interest (e.g., perfectionism) sometimes relates to another variable (e.g., bulimia) but other times does not, psychologists often look for "moderator" variables (Baron & Kenny, 1986; Kraemer, Stice, Kazdin, Offord, & Kupfer, 2001). That is, perhaps perfectionism predicts bulimia only in some contexts or only for a subgroup of people. Consistent with this approach, Joiner, Heatherton, Rudd, and Schmidt (1997) proposed a two-factor vulnerability–stress model in which perfectionism (the vulnerability) predicts bulimia only if individuals feel that they are overweight (the stressor).

According to Joiner et al.'s two-factor model, perfectionism only leads to negative mental health outcomes when the perfectionist's high standards go unmet. As Joiner et al. (1997) stated, "Perfection, if both desired and obtained, is a positive state of affairs" (p. 146). On this view, then, perfectionism is not necessarily a bad thing and it does not necessarily lead to psychological maladjustment. Supporting this general perspective, work on perfectionism as a vulnerability factor for depression has shown that perfectionistic people became depressed only when their standards were unmet (i.e., when negative life events occurred; Hewitt & Flett, 1993; Joiner & Schmidt, 1995).

Drawing on the well-documented link between body dissatisfaction/ weight concern and bulimia (e.g., Killen et al., 1994; Killen et al., 1996; Ruderman, 1986; also see Jacobi, Hayward, de Zwaan, Kraemer, & Agras, 2004, for a review), Joiner et al. (1997) reasoned that the perception of being overweight would be a particularly potent stressor in their vulnerability (perfectionism)–stress model of bulimia. In two separate studies, Joiner et al. (1997) obtained support for this hypothesis. Perfectionism appeared to serve as a vulnerability factor for bulimic symptoms for women who perceived themselves to be overweight, but not for those who did not see themselves in that way. Specifically, women who were both perfectionistic and perceived themselves as overweight exhibited greater levels of bulimic symptoms than perfectionistic women who did not perceive themselves as overweight and nonperfectionistic women who either did or did not perceive themselves to be overweight. It is interesting to note that, among women who did not perceive themselves to be overweight, those who were perfectionistic exhibited similar levels of bulimic symptoms to those who did not exhibit this trait. In the study, only perceived weight, but not actual weight, interacted with perfectionism to predict bulimic symptoms. Thus, it is perfectionistic individuals' *perceptions* of not meeting their weight standards, rather than an objective discrepancy in this domain, that best predicts when they will exhibit bulimic symptoms. Because Joiner et al.'s (1997) study was cross-sectional, a replication with a longitudinal design is needed to confirm the most plausible temporal interpretation of the findings; namely, perfectionism paired with the perception of being overweight provides risk for development of or increase in bulimic symptoms.

The vulnerability–stress model proposed by Joiner et al. (1997) and the results supporting it help explain why perfectionism has been linked to bulimia in some studies but not others. Presumably, the perfectionists in the studies obtaining positive results were more likely to have perceived themselves as overweight than the perfectionists in the studies failing to obtain a relation between perfectionism and bulimia.

PERFECTIONISM AND BULIMIA: A PARADOX

Although Joiner et al.'s two-factor vulnerability–stress model helps explain the empirical inconsistencies in the link between perfectionism and bulimia, it also highlights the paradox with which this chapter began: The binge eating component of bulimia severely contradicts and undermines bulimic individuals' goals for bodily perfection. Specifically, Joiner et al.'s model and supporting results suggest that perfectionists are especially likely to engage in bulimic behaviors, including bingeing when they perceive themselves to be overweight. This is maladaptive and self-defeating! For an individual with perfectionistic weight and body shape goals, the very worst time to binge would be when feeling overweight. Yet, Joiner et al.'s (1997) model and results suggest that this is precisely when perfectionists engage in bulimic bingeing. Clearly, there is a paradox to be explained here.

TOWARD EXPLAINING THE PARADOX OF BULIMIC BINGEING: A THREE-FACTOR MODEL

To help resolve the paradox of bulimic bingeing among individuals with perfectionistic bodily standards, it is useful to consider the possible response options of individuals with perfectionistic weight and body shape goals who perceive that they are overweight. Surely, there must be some perfectionists who would respond to this self–body standard discrepancy with instrumental behaviors to remedy the situation rather than with self-defeating bulimic bingeing. The two-factor model fails to account for the reasonable possibility of perfectionists who, upon perceiving themselves to be overweight, redouble their efforts to lose weight and approach perfection rather than engage in binge eating behavior, which is self-defeating for attaining "perfection" in appearance. More generally, some perfectionists likely do respond to perceived bodily flaws in an adaptive way. As an example, the combination of having perfectionistic bodily goals and responding adaptively to remedy perceived bodily flaws would seem to be critical for athletes to win the highest titles in bodybuilding such as Mr. and Ms. Olympia (see also Parker, 2002).

A case study of a highly visible celebrity, Arnold Schwarzenegger (the world-renowned bodybuilder and now governor of California), demonstrates that the combination of perfectionism and the perception that one falls short of an important bodily standard does not inevitably lead to a maladaptive behavior. Schwarzenegger's autobiography (Schwarzenegger & Hall, 1977) reveals that he exhibited the "vulnerability" of perfectionism, "One word was constantly on my mind: *perfection*. . . . I wanted to be the best-built man in the world" (pp. 68–69). Moreover, Arnold perceived that he had some serious bodily flaws, "I had weak points—glaring weak points— . . . in the beginning everybody said, 'Arnold has no calves . . . his calves aren't developed at all.' One look in the mirror told me they were right" (p. 68). Yet, unlike the perfectionists in Joiner et al.'s (1997) study who succumbed to maladaptive behaviors when confronted with a bodily discrepancy, Arnold responded adaptively to his "skinny calves" by developing an exercise program to build them up. Indeed, Arnold confronted many significant bodily discrepancies in his quest to be the "best-built man in the world." But, in each case, he developed new exercises, workout programs, and dietary changes to slowly overcome his "glaring weak points." It is likely that Arnold Schwarzenegger would have been a "bad data point" for Joiner et al.'s (1997) vulnerability (perfectionism)–stress (perceived overweight) hypothesis if he had been in their study. If the perfectionist Arnold had perceived himself to be overweight, then he likely would have focused on developing and following a program to lose weight rather than engaging in self-defeating behavior such as bulimic bingeing.

In fact, Arnold (Schwarzenegger & Hall, 1977) stated, "Before competition I would always walk into the gym to train with no shirt on. Why? Because the instant I sat down I'd see my stomach and say, 'Wait a minute, Arnold, you can't go into a contest with a stomach like that, with so much fat on it you get wrinkles.' So I would train my waist harder and stay on my diet" (pp. 161–162). There must be a third factor, an additional moderator, that identifies perfectionists, like Arnold Schwarzenegger as an extreme, who do not succumb to maladaptive behaviors (e.g., bulimic bingeing) when they are dissatisfied with their bodies.

The Third Factor: Low Self-Efficacy

What additional vulnerability factor distinguishes the perfectionist who responds to an unmet body standard with bulimic symptoms from the perfectionist who, when faced with the same unmet standard, persists in attempts to achieve the standard or positively accepts the situation? Building on Joiner et al.'s (1997) two-factor model, we (Bardone-Cone, Abramson, Vohs, Heatherton, & Joiner, 2004a, 2004b) hypothesized that low self-efficacy would function as such a vulnerability factor in a three-factor (i.e., high perfectionism, low self-efficacy, perceived overweight or body dissatisfaction) model of bulimia. Specifically, perfectionists who have low self-efficacy may be especially likely to succumb to self-defeating behaviors such as bulimic binge eating rather than respond adaptively when they perceive themselves to be overweight. In contrast, perfectionists who are not meeting their standards of body weight but who have high self-efficacy will respond to the discrepancy from their standards with goal-directed weight reduction strategies or perhaps self-acceptance (e.g., I can show people that a large woman can be the most beautiful of all).

Inclusion of low self-efficacy as the third factor in the model is consistent with a number of studies showing an association between low self-efficacy and bulimic behaviors (Etringer, Altmaier, & Bowers, 1989; Gordon, Denoma, Bardone, Abramson, & Joiner, in press; Gormally, Black, Daston, & Rardin, 1982; Striegel-Moore, Silberstein, Frensch, & Rodin, 1989). Similarly, in the treatment outcome literature, a number of treatments for bulimia target low self-efficacy directly or appear to contribute to symptom reduction via improved self-efficacy (Garner & Garfinkel, 1997; Schneider, O'Leary, & Agras, 1987; Wilson, Fairburn, Agras, Walsh, & Kraemer, 2002).

Because self-efficacy involves a cognitive appraisal of one's abilities, it is particularly well suited to the scenario of being perfectionistic and failing to meet one's standards (e.g., perceiving that one is overweight). According to Bandura and Cervone (1986), "Whether perceived discrepancies between personal standards and attainments are motivating or discouraging is likely to be determined by the strength of people's perceived capabilities to attain the standards they have been pursuing. Those who distrust their capabilities are easily discouraged by failure, whereas those who are highly assured of their efficacy for goal attainment will intensify their efforts when their performances fall short and persevere until they succeed" (p. 93). Thus, Bandura and Cervone postulated that self-efficacy plays an important role in determining cognitive, affective, and behavioral responses to a discrepancy between standards and attainments.

Similarly, drawing on objective self-awareness theory (S. Duval & Wicklund, 1972), T. S. Duval, V. H. Duval, and Mulilis (1992) suggested that when people perceive a discrepancy between their goals and actual attainments, they are motivated to reduce either the discrepancy or the level of increased self-focus engendered by the perceived discrepancy. Attempts to reduce self-focus can include physical (e.g., moving away from a mirror) or mental (e.g., distraction) avoidance of the self-focusing situation. Self-regulation theorists (e.g., Carver & Scheier, 1981; Pyszczynski & Greenberg, 1987) have elaborated this line of thought by arguing that when people have high expectations that they can reduce the discrepancy, they will engage in behavior aimed at eliminating it. In contrast, when people believe that they will not be able to reduce the discrepancy, they quit trying to do so and instead attempt to minimize or escape self-focus because it has become an aversive reminder that they are not meeting their standards.

Also underscoring the importance of people's beliefs about their abilities to reduce discrepancies, Higgins, Vookles, and Tykocinski (1992) reported that the extent of people's distress when they perceive discrepancies between their current self and their standards for themselves depends on whether they believe that they will be able to attain the standard in the future (i.e., future self). Finally, an extensive body of work on learned helplessness (Seligman, 1975) echoes the importance of belief in one's capabilities in influencing response to discrepancies. Both animal and human studies have found that organisms who expect to control outcomes persist in their endeavors, whereas those who do not expect to have control give up (Abramson, Seligman, & Teasdale, 1978).

According to the three-factor model, then, for perfectionists with high self-efficacy, perceptions of being overweight will be resolved by effectively engaging in activities aimed at achieving their weight goal or perhaps finding a way to positively accept the weight discrepancy. High self-efficacy perfectionists who feel overweight would not resort to a maladaptive response like bulimic binge eating because they are likely to view an unmet goal as a temporary, changeable situation rather than as an uncontrollable failure. In contrast, for low self-efficacy perfectionists, perceptions of being overweight will be resolved in less productive and less goal-directed ways because they are likely to view the situation as an uncontrollable devastating reality. Low self-efficacy perfectionists will doubt that they can rectify the situation and perhaps succumb to bulimic binge eating.

To go back to our case study, Arnold Schwarzenegger's autobiography (Schwarzenegger & Hall, 1977) underscores his extraordinarily high sense of self-efficacy, "Never was there even the slightest doubt in my mind that I would make it. . . . I knew I had what it took" (pp. 67–68). Thus, according to our three-factor model, Arnold's high sense of self-efficacy led him to develop and implement effective strategies to overcome his "glaring weak points" in his quest for bodily perfection. In contrast, the logic of the three-factor model would suggest that a bodybuilder with equally high perfectionism but low self-efficacy would succumb to self-defeating behaviors when confronted with body standard discrepancies.

In sum, the three-factor model specifies two cognitive/personality vulnerability factors (high perfectionism and low self-efficacy) that, when paired, identify *who* will exhibit bulimic symptoms, given a requisite "occasion setter." The additional factor of perceiving that one is overweight or being dissatisfied with one's body is the occasion setter that marks *when* such vulnerable individuals actually will engage in bulimic behaviors.

Empirical Tests of the Three-Factor Model

The core prediction of the three-factor model is straightforward: The three factors of high perfectionism, low self-efficacy, and perceived overweight/body dissatisfaction should interact (high perfectionism × low self-efficacy × perceived overweight/body dissatisfaction) to predict bulimic symptoms. Specifically, individuals with the profile of high perfectionism, low self-efficacy, and perceived overweight or body dissatisfaction should exhibit the highest level of bulimic symptoms.

In early tests of the three-factor model, self-esteem was used in place of self-efficacy because self-esteem and self-efficacy are strongly related conceptually and empirically (Judge, Erez, Bono, & Thoresen, 2002). In addition, investigators have emphasized that self-esteem is a multifaceted construct that includes self-efficacy as an integral component (Bardone, Perez, Abramson, & Joiner, 2003; Tafarodi & Swann, 1995; Vohs & Heatherton, 2001). The initial study (Vohs et al., 1999) used a longitudinal design to test whether late adolescent females who were high in perfectionism and low in self-esteem would be especially likely to show an increase in bulimic symptoms during the transition from high school to college if they also perceived themselves to be overweight. Consistent with the three-factor model, we found a three-way interaction among perfectionism, self-esteem, and perceived weight status in predicting increases in bulimic symptoms over the prospective follow-up period (average length of follow-up = 9 months). Young women high in perfectionism who perceived a self–standard weight discrepancy exhibited bulimic symptoms only if they also had low self-esteem. Women who had high self-esteem were buffered from bulimic symptoms even if they were high in perfectionism and felt overweight.

To examine the robustness of the three-factor model and the replicability of Vohs et al.'s (1999) findings, an additional longitudinal study

(Vohs, Voelz, et al., 2001) was conducted with a different sample, time frame, and measures. First, whereas Vohs et al. (1999) conducted their study with a sample of young women attending a selective northeastern college, Vohs, Voelz, et al. (2001) employed a sample of young women from a southern state university. Testing the three-factor model on a different sample of participants provides information about the model's generalizability. Second, Vohs et al. (1999) examined change in bulimic symptoms from participants' senior year of high school to first year of college. In contrast, Vohs, Voelz, et al. (2001) assessed change in bulimic symptoms over 5 weeks during a college semester. Testing the model's ability to predict change over only 5 weeks is a strong test of the model's sensitivity. Third, Vohs, Voelz, et al. (2001) utilized different measures of the predictor variables in the three-factor model. For example, the original Vohs et al. (1999) study operationalized the stressor variable as perceived overweight, whereas Vohs, Voelz, et al. (2001) looked at body dissatisfaction as the stressor. Finally, Vohs, Voelz, et al. (2001) tested the specificity of the three-factor model to bulimia. Given the comorbidity of bulimia with both depression (e.g., Lee, Rush, & Mitchell, 1985) and anxiety (e.g., Brewerton, Lydiard, Ballenger, & Herzog, 1993), as well as the role of perfectionism in depression and anxiety (Hewitt & Flett, 1991), Vohs, Voelz, et al. (2001) tested whether the interaction of perfectionism, low self-efficacy, and body dissatisfaction predicted increases not only in bulimic symptoms but also in depression and/or anxiety symptoms.

Consistent with the three-factor model and the results of Vohs et al. (1999), Vohs, Voelz, et al. (2001) found that the three-way interaction of perfectionism, low self-esteem, and body dissatisfaction predicted increases in bulimic symptoms. Of great interest, this interaction also predicted increases in depression, but not anxiety, symptoms. Thus, perfectionistic individuals with low self-esteem who were dissatisfied with their bodies showed increases in both depressive and bulimic symptoms. These results suggest that the well-documented comorbidity between bulimia and depression may, in part, be due to overlapping causal factors.

Denoma et al. (in press) further tested the generalizability of the three-factor model to a sample of women of diverse ages (mean age approximately 45 years). Replicating Vohs et al. (1999) and Vohs, Voelz, et al. (2001), Denoma et al. (in press) used a longitudinal design and found that the three-way interaction of perfectionism, low self-esteem, and perceived overweight predicted increases in bulimic symptoms in this sample over 2½ years. The form of the interaction was as expected (perfectionistic women with low self-esteem who perceived themselves to be overweight were the most likely to show increases in bulimic symptoms over the follow-up period). These results are important because they show that the three-factor model holds over different parts of the life span among women. Moreover, the results support the conclusions of Cosford and Arnold (1992) that bulimic symptom presentation of women over age 50 is similar to that of adolescents and young women.

Similarly to Vohs, Voelz, et al. (2001), Denoma et al. (in press) examined the specificity of the three-factor model for predicting bulimic symptoms versus symptoms of depression and/or anxiety. In contrast to Vohs, Voelz, et al. (2001), Denoma et al. (in press) found specificity with respect to depression, but not anxiety, symptoms. Specifically, in Denoma et al.'s older sample, perfectionistic women with low self-esteem who perceived themselves to be overweight were especially likely to show increases in bulimic and anxiety, but not depression, symptoms over the 2½-year follow-up. Taken together, the findings of Vohs, Voelz, et al. (2001) and Denoma et al. (in press) show that the three-factor model consistently predicts bulimic symptoms and negative affect, but the form of the negative affect, depression versus anxiety, varies from one study to the next. Future work is needed to illuminate when the three-factor model predicts depression versus anxiety.

In the studies testing our three-factor model presented so far, we used low self-esteem in place of low self-efficacy because the two constructs are highly related (Bardone et al., 2003; Judge et al., 2002; Tafarodi & Swann, 1995; Vohs & Heatherton, 2001) and the data sets available included measures of self-esteem. However, given that low self-efficacy is featured as the "third factor" in the model, it is important to see if it indeed "works" as hypothesized. Do perfectionists with low self-efficacy respond to an unmet body standard with self-defeating bulimic symptoms, whereas perfectionists with high self-efficacy do not? A second question not answered by the studies presented so far concerns whether or not the three-factor model predicts both components of bulimia: bingeing and inappropriate compensatory behaviors such as vomiting. This is an especially important question because it is the bingeing component of bulimia that is so paradoxical in the context of the bulimic's perfectionism. Although inappropriate compensatory behaviors like vomiting following a binge are highly maladaptive in many ways, it does not seem paradoxical for individuals with perfectionist goals for weight and body shape to engage in drastic measures to rid their body of the excess calories consumed in a binge.

Bardone-Cone, Abramson, Vohs, Heatherton, and Joiner (in press) conducted a study to address these two questions. A methodological advantage of this longitudinal study is that symptoms of bulimia were assessed weekly over an 11-week interval, thereby reducing recall difficulties and providing more accurate responses; prior work has been limited to two time points of data collection. This study found that the three-factor model predicted the binge eating component of bulimia. Young college women who exhibited the profile of high perfectionism, low self-efficacy, and perceived overweight scored highest on binge eating measures over the 11-week prospective follow-up. Women with the opposite profile (low perfectionism, high self-efficacy, no perception of overweight) exhibited some of the lowest levels of binge eating in the sample.

A strikingly different pattern of results emerged for the inappropriate compensatory behaviors component of bulimia. Bardone-Cone et al. (in press) assessed three inappropriate compensatory behaviors—two purging behaviors (vomiting and laxative use) and one nonpurging behavior (fasting). The three-factor model did not predict inappropriate compensatory behaviors, whether assessed separately (e.g., vomiting alone) or as a group. Although no main effect was significant across all analyses to predict inappropriate compensatory behaviors, the perception of being overweight was most consistently related to vomiting, and perfectionism was most consistently related to fasting. However, nonsignificant findings for predicting inappropriate compensatory behaviors with the three-factor model could be due to predicting behaviors with low base rates (base rates of vomiting, laxative use, and fasting were 6%, 1%, and 4%, respectively). Future studies should use a larger sample size of individuals engaging in inappropriate compensatory behaviors (to avoid low base rates) and an even more comprehensive assessment of various kinds of inappropriate compensatory behaviors (e.g., excessive exercise) to investigate the predictive value of the three-factor model for the inappropriate compensatory behavior component of bulimia.

Perhaps most importantly, the binge eating and inappropriate compensatory behavior components of bulimia were examined independently. It is likely that some women exhibited inappropriate "compensatory" behaviors in the absence of binge eating. For example, some women with an anorexic profile likely exhibited vomiting, laxative use, or fasting while never engaging in binge eating (American Psychiatric Association, 2000). The predictors of inappropriate "compensatory" behaviors not accompanied by binge eating (as in some cases of anorexia) may differ from the predictors of such behaviors accompanied by binge eating (as in bulimia). Indeed, for a bulimic who always exhibits inappropriate compensatory behaviors following a binge and never in the absence of a binge, there is a perfect correlation between bingeing and engaging in inappropriate compensatory behaviors. In such cases, the predictors of binge eating should be identical to those of inappropriate compensatory behaviors. Thus, in future studies, it will be important to look separately at the predictors of inappropriate compensatory behaviors "comorbid" with binge eating (the bulimic pattern) versus such behaviors not comorbid with binge eating (an anorexic pattern). In this regard, it is useful to note that only 3% of Bardone-Cone et al.'s (in press) sample (young adult female Introductory

Psychology students) reported both binge eating and inappropriate compensatory behaviors (vomiting, laxative use, or fasting) during the 11-week follow-up period.

Summary of Empirical Tests of the Three-Factor Model

Previously, four longitudinal studies were presented providing consistent and strong support for the three-factor model of bulimia. Perfectionistic women with low self-efficacy or low self-esteem were especially likely to exhibit bulimic symptoms when they perceived themselves to be overweight or were dissatisfied with their bodies. Across diverse samples and follow-up intervals, the three-factor model proved to be robust and generalizable. All four studies obtained the critical three-way interaction (perfectionism × low self-efficacy/low self-esteem × body dissatisfaction/perceived overweight), which is impressive given that detecting moderator effects is very difficult, especially in prospective field research (McClelland & Judd, 1993). We are aware of only one prospective study (Shaw, Stice, & Springer, 2004) that failed to obtain this three-way interaction in predicting bulimic symptoms. Moreover, levels of bulimic symptoms were quite stable across the various prospective follow-up periods used in the studies obtaining the three-way interaction (e.g., the correlation of Time 1 and Time 2 bulimic symptoms in Vohs, Voelz, et al., 2001, was $r = .63$), making prediction of increases in such symptoms potentially difficult. Insofar as we controlled for initial levels of bulimic symptoms in predicting subsequent bulimic symptoms, tests of the three-factor model were conservative (see Alloy, Abramson, Raniere, & Dyller, 1999). Although the effect sizes for the predicted three-way interaction across the studies were not large, inspection of the figures from the studies shows that the effect was nonetheless dramatic.

A limitation of these studies is that we measured perceived weight status/body dissatisfaction as if it were "traitlike." That is, we measured this factor, along with the hypothesized cognitive/personality vulnerability factors of perfectionism and low self-efficacy, at the outset of the follow-up interval in each study. However, greater fidelity to the three-factor model would be obtained if perceived weight status/body dissatisfaction were measured frequently during the follow-up interval. Obviously, bulimic individuals do not engage in a chronic binge lasting the whole follow-up interval. Instead, such individuals go for a period without bingeing and then something triggers a binge. According to the three-factor model, it is the perception of being overweight or body dissatisfaction that triggers a binge among vulnerable women. Thus, better temporal sequencing would be obtained if both perceived weight status/body dissatisfaction and bulimic behaviors were assessed frequently over the follow-up interval. Such an assessment strategy would enable a test of whether the perception of being overweight or being dissatisfied with her body is a proximal trigger of an episode of binge eating among highly perfectionistic women with low self-efficacy. Of course, the possibility exists that some women do exhibit chronic perceptions of being overweight or feeling dissatisfied with their bodies. We suspect that, among such women, a binge is triggered by an event that brings these body dissatisfactions to mind (e.g., getting on the scale, seeing a beautiful model on TV, etc.).

We are intrigued by Bardone-Cone et al.'s (in press) result that the three-factor model predicted the binge eating, but not the inappropriate compensatory behaviors (e.g., vomiting), component of bulimia. Although the finding is preliminary and may have been influenced by the low base rates of inappropriate compensatory behaviors in the sample, we suspect that the main reason for the failure to find support for the three-factor model in predicting compensatory behaviors was that we looked at compensatory behaviors separately from binge eating. The three-factor model always may predict binge eating, regardless of whether or not it is accompanied by compensatory behaviors. In contrast, the predictors of "compensatory" behaviors not accompanied by binge eating (an anorexic profile) may be different from the predictors of true compensatory behaviors accompanying binge eating that are in the service of undoing the damage of a binge. In the latter case, the compensatory behaviors are linked to the binge in a one-to-one fashion and should be predicted by the same factors. Over time, as the binge and inappropriate compensatory behaviors become inextricably linked in the bulimic cycle, prediction of the two components should become more and more similar. It will be important for future research to look at the predictors of compensatory behaviors comorbid with binge eating separately from "compensatory" behaviors not occurring in the wake of binge eating.

Two studies (Denoma et al., in press; Vohs, Voelz, et al., 2001) examined whether the three-factor model predicted negative affect (depression and anxiety) and bulimic symptoms. Although the form of negative affect (depression vs. anxiety) predicted differed across the studies, it is noteworthy that in each case negative affect was predicted by the same model predicting bulimic symptoms. As argued later, this is important because the negative affect engendered by the confluence of perfectionism, low self-efficacy, and body dissatisfaction may set the stage for the self-defeating binge eating of women exhibiting these three factors.

In sum, the three-factor model goes a long way in resolving the paradox of perfectionism and binge eating. In fact, perfectionism per se does not reliably predict binge eating. Women with high perfectionistic goals for themselves do not necessarily engage in binge eating. Moreover, even when perfectionistic women perceive themselves to be overweight or are dissatisfied with their bodies, they do not necessarily binge (Denoma et al., in press; Vohs, Voelz, et al., 2001). Instead, perfectionistic women binge when they perceive they are overweight or are dissatisfied with their bodies and feel that they cannot resolve the discrepancy between their high standards and their current state. Consistent with work on self-efficacy (Bandura & Cervone, 1986), self-regulation (e.g., Carver & Scheier, 1981; Pyszczynski & Greenberg, 1987), self-discrepancies (Higgins et al., 1992), and learned helplessness (Seligman, 1975; Abramson et al., 1978), it becomes less paradoxical that a perfectionistic woman would binge precisely when she perceives herself to be overweight if she also has low self-efficacy. The low self-efficacy of the woman prevents her from engaging in what would seem to be a more adaptive response to the discrepancy, such as redoubling her efforts or changing her strategy to lose weight or positively accepting the situation as might a woman with higher self-efficacy.

But the three-factor model, as presented so far, provides only a partial resolution to the paradox. Why doesn't a perfectionistic woman who perceives that she is overweight but feels helpless to reduce this discrepancy between her high standards and current self simply become depressed, anxious, or passive as might be predicted by learned helplessness theory (Abramson et al., 1978; Abramson, Metalsky, & Alloy, 1989; Seligman, 1975)? Depression or passivity in the situation, albeit distressing, does not seem paradoxical given the low self-efficacy of the woman. Indeed, Vohs, Voelz, et al. (2001) and Denoma et al. (in press) showed that perfectionistic women who have low self-efficacy do become depressed or anxious when they are dissatisfied with their bodies or perceive that they are overweight. But why do these woman go the next step of engaging in the very behavior, binge eating, that so effectively sabotages their perfectionistic goals for body weight and shape? We now turn to this final issue in resolving the paradox.

BINGE EATING AS A SELF-DEFEATING ATTEMPT TO REGULATE NEGATIVE EMOTION AND AVERSIVE SELF-AWARENESS

Giving Priority to Short-Term Emotion Regulation

Tice et al. (2001) presented theory and evidence suggesting that when people are distressed, they may indulge immediate impulses (e.g., eating) to make themselves feel better. That is, when people are not distressed, they direct their behavior to attaining their long-term goals. For example, when not distressed, individuals with perfectionistic goals for weight and body shape will engage in behaviors to achieve their ideal body (e.g., not eating fattening foods). However, Tice et al. suggested that when people are overwhelmed with negative emotion, they strategically may divert their behavior away from achievement of their long-term goals to the more immediate goal of reducing negative emotion. In essence, in such situations, people are giving short-term emotion regulation priority over other self-regulatory goals. It is important to emphasize that Tice et al. were not suggesting that emotional distress impairs the ability or the motivation to regulate oneself. Instead, the idea is that when people are distressed, the immediate self-regulatory goal of decreasing negative emotion may conflict with and win out over more long-term goals (e.g., eating "comfort foods" such as cheesey macaroni to feel better conflicts with adhering to a healthy diet to achieve more long-term weight and body shape goals; Baumeister & Heatherton, 1996). People are still self-regulating when they indulge immediate impulses to make themselves feel better. In this situation, however, the goal of self-regulation has changed from long-term attainment of ideals to short-term improvement of mood. Thus, people may engage in behaviors such as overeating that are self-defeating in the long run but possibly functional in reducing negative emotion in the short run.

Particularly pertinent to the paradox of binge eating among bulimics, Tice et al. (2001) presented an experiment demonstrating that people will eat fattening, unhealthy foods that taste good as a strategy to regulate negative emotion even though ordinarily they would refrain from eating such foods. In the study, college students had either a negative or positive mood induced in the laboratory. Further, half of the participants were told that eating would not improve their moods, whereas the other participants were given no information about the supposed effects of eating on mood. Insofar as our culture promotes the belief that eating can reduce emotional distress (e.g., drowning one's sorrows in a chocolate bar), participants not given any information about the supposed effects of eating on mood should be more likely to eat unhealthy foods (e.g., chocolate chip cookies) when distressed than participants given information debunking the popular idea that eating can make a bad mood go away. Results supported Tice et al.'s hypothesis. In the experimental condition similar to everyday life in which participants were not disabused of the belief that eating can make you feel better, emotional distress led participants to increase their consumption of snack food. In contrast, those participants who were instructed that eating does not make people feel better did not show increased consumption of unhealthy food when distressed. These results show that negative emotion does not necessarily impair regulation of behavior to achieve long-term goals (even though distressed, participants instructed that, contrary to popular lore, eating doesn't improve moods did not overeat). Overeating occurred when participants were distressed and believed that eating could make them feel better. Thus, giving in to immediate impulses (e.g., overeating) when distressed appeared to reflect a strategic shift from pursuit of long-term goals to the immediate goal of emotion regulation rather than a breakdown of regulation per se.

Escape Theory

Tice et al.'s (2001) hypothesis that people may engage in behaviors that are self-defeating in the long run in order to control negative emotions in the short run is consistent with the "escape" theory proposed by Baumeister (1991; Baumeister & Scher, 1988). In brief, Baumeister (1991) suggested that many apparently self-defeating behaviors such as alcoholism, drug abuse, binge eating, self-mutilation, and even masochism may represent attempts to escape from aversive self-awareness and negative emotion. Although such behaviors may sabotage an individual's long-term goals, they may serve the short-term purpose of providing an escape from distressing thoughts and images of the self. According to Baumeister, the common denominator across these apparently self-defeating behaviors is that they enable a state of "cognitive deconstruction." In a state of cognitive deconstruction, a person's focus is on the immediate present rather than the past or the future, on movements and sensations rather than broad thoughts and emotions, and on immediate goals rather than more long-term goals. Heatherton and Baumeister (1991) suggested that the essence of this deconstructed state is the abandonment of the kind of higher level thought necessary to compare oneself negatively to one's standards or to others and to consider the negative implications of failure. In short, a state of cognitive deconstruction provides an escape from aversive self-awareness. For example, a woman motivated to escape bad thoughts and feelings about herself after a perceived failure to meet a body standard (i.e., seeing cellulite on her thighs in the mirror) may focus on some concrete, physical activity that will prevent her mind from drifting to meaningful thought about her flawed appearance, self-loathing, and associated negative emotion.

Heatherton and Baumeister (1991) suggested that binge eating may provide a particularly potent form of escape because it affords reduction of awareness to the immediate, concrete motions and sensations of tasting, chewing, and swallowing. A deconstructed cognitive state of low self-awareness in which meaningful (negative) thoughts about the self are banished can arise from the absorbing activity of eating. Thus, at least for some individuals, eating may indeed provide, or at least promise, emotional comfort. Integration of Baumeister's (1991) original escape theory with his more recent work on the diversion of regulatory behaviors from the achievement of long-term goals to the reduction of immediate overwhelming negative emotion (Tice et al., 2001) suggests that individuals for whom food is particularly "reinforcing" or who believe that eating can make you feel better may be particularly prone to overeat when emotionally distressed.

Integration

Recall that Duval et al. (1992) drew on objective self-awareness theory (S. Duval & Wicklund, 1972) to suggest that when people perceive a discrepancy between their goals and actual attainments, they are motivated to reduce either the discrepancy or the level of self-focus engendered by the perceived discrepancy. Self-regulation theorists (e.g., Carver & Scheier, 1981; Pyszczynski & Greenberg, 1987) further indicated that people who believe they can reduce the discrepancy (high self-efficacy) will engage in behaviors aimed at eliminating it. In contrast, people who feel inadequate to reduce the discrepancy (low self-efficacy) will give up and instead attempt to escape self-focus because it has become aversive.

Consistent with this view, Steenbarger and Aderman (1979) reported that individuals who were led to perceive large self-discrepancies on the dimension of "self-expression" and told that such discrepancies were not remediable (low self-efficacy) exhibited negative emotion and sought to avoid a self-focusing cue (an audio recording of themselves giving a speech). In contrast, individuals who were led to perceive an equally large discrepancy in self-expression but told that they could effectively remedy the discrepancy (high self-efficacy) did not show any more negative emotion or avoidance of the self-focusing cue than individuals who were not led to perceive self-discrepancies. Carver, Blaney, and Scheier (1979) presented similar results from an experiment in which the self-focusing cue was a mirror. Moreover, Carver et al.'s (1979) results further suggested that self-focus actually increases attempts to reduce discrepancies when people believe they can reduce the discrepancy (high self-efficacy). Taken together, these two studies demonstrate that people find self-awareness (e.g., listening to a tape of oneself giving a speech, seeing one's reflection in a mirror) especially aversive and seek to escape from it when they are confronted with a discrepancy that they feel inadequate to reduce. However, self-awareness in the face of a discrepancy that is perceived as reducible is not so aversive and may facilitate attempts to reduce the discrepancy.

According to this line of reasoning, a highly perfectionistic woman with high self-efficacy who perceives herself to be overweight is likely to redouble her efforts to lose weight or find a way to positively accept the situation. For such a woman, self-focus or self-awareness should not be highly aversive because she believes that she will meet her goals in one way or another. In contrast, a highly perfectionistic woman with low self-efficacy who similarly perceives herself to be overweight is more likely to be focused on escaping from negative emotion and aversive self-awareness than her high self-efficacy counterpart because she believes that she will not be able to remedy her current overweight problem. Thus, women exhibiting the maladaptive profile featured in our three-factor model (high perfectionism, low self-efficacy, perceived overweight or body dissatisfaction) may be particularly prone to divert behavior away from achievement of the long-term goal of weight regulation to try to reduce the immediate negative emotions and aversive self-awareness engendered by their failure to meet perfectionistic body standards. If food were particularly reinforcing for such a woman or if she believed that eating can reduce distress, then it would not be surprising if she overate or even engaged in an eating binge. Indeed, Heatherton and Baumeister (1991) argued that binge eating is motivated by a desire to escape aversive self-awareness.

Consistent with this line of reasoning, our case study of Arnold Schwarzenegger reveals that a perfectionistic individual with high self-efficacy does not engage in dramatic attempts to escape aversive self-awareness when confronted with a discrepancy between perfectionistic bodily standards and a body that falls short of such standards. To the contrary, Arnold sought out situations that would promote self-focus in order to facilitate reducing his body discrepancies. For example, in his autobiography (Schwarzenegger & Hall, 1977), Arnold said, "Personally, I prefer to train in as few clothes as possible so I can see my faults. I try to see the specific areas that have fallen behind or that I've neglected. I like to expose them so I have to look at them all the time. For instance, in the beginning my calves were underdeveloped. When I understood how really weak they were, I cut the bottoms off my pants so everybody would see. And that made me eager to train hard and build them up. . . . It's very important that you expose your weaknesses, that you constantly point them up to yourself. Let the mirror be your reminder" (pp. 161–162). Given Arnold's extraordinarily high sense of self-efficacy, his advice to seek out self-focusing cues, such as a mirror, to be a reminder of your weaknesses is wholly consistent with Carver et al.'s (1979) results that self-awareness in the face of a discrepancy that is perceived as reducible is not so aversive and may facilitate attempts to reduce the discrepancy.

This anecdote vividly illustrates that far from avoiding self-focus, an individual with high self-efficacy actually may seek it out when perceiving bodily flaws, even "glaring weaknesses," in order to remedy the flaws and thereby attain perfectionistic bodily goals. In contrast, a perfectionistic individual with low self-efficacy who is dissatisfied with her body may try to avoid self-awareness or self-focus at all costs because it is so aversive. The last thing such an individual would want is to seek out a mirror to be a reminder of bodily flaws. Such an individual may divert behavior to trying to reduce the overwhelming negative emotion and aversive self-awareness engendered by falling short of her high bodily standard that she believes she never can attain. Ironically, such an attempt to escape from aversive self-awareness and negative emotion may take the form of an eating binge for a bulimic individual. Is there evidence that negative emotions and aversive self-awareness do precipitate eating binges among bulimic individuals?

Aversive Emotional States and Binge Eating

Considerable empirical and clinical evidence suggests that negative emotional states do precipitate eating binges (e.g., Abraham & Beumont, 1982; Beebe, 1994; Herman & Polivy, 1975; Johnson, Stuckey, Lewis, & Schwartz, 1982; Schotte, Cools, & McNally, 1990). For example, Johnson et al. (1982) surveyed by mail women who met binge eating criteria for bulimia and who had contacted a medical center because of disturbed eating. They found that 40% of the 316 women in their sample attributed the onset of bulimia to problems coping with negative emotions such as depression, loneliness, boredom, and anger. Abraham and Beumont (1982) interviewed 32 binge eating patients and found that all of them reported typically feeling anxious and tense before a binge. Internal feelings of tension, boredom, and loneliness were endorsed as precipitants to binge eating episodes by at least 59% of the patients. Finally, in a series of laboratory studies, Heatherton, Striepe, and Wittenberg (1998) found that negative mood states implicating the self promoted excessive eating among chronic dieters.

The emotion regulation (Tice et al., 2001) and escape (Heatherton & Baumeister, 1991) theories suggest that people engage in behavior that is self-defeating over the long run in order to decrease current aversive mood states, so it is important to additionally know whether or not binge eating reduces negative emotion and aversive self-awareness. Beebe's (1994) summary of studies of self-reported affective changes across the binge–purge cycle indicates that the high levels of anxiety and general emotional distress that appear to precipitate eating binges often are alleviated temporarily during the binge episode. Similarly, in their study of the temporal changes in affective states associated with bulimic behaviors, Tachi, Murakami, Murotsu, and Washizuka (2001) reported that irritation, frustration, and depression were alleviated during bingeing. Further, Abraham and Beumont (1982) found that the majority of their bulimic subjects reported feelings of depersonalization and derealization during eating binges. Finally, most of these bulimic individuals also reported experiencing a reduction in negative emotion during the binge. Thus, initial evidence based mainly on self-report suggests that binge eating may indeed provide relief, albeit temporary, from negative emotions and aversive self-awareness for bulimic individuals. However, future research employing other methods will be important to more fully characterize the mental state during a binge and to determine if binge eating truly leads to a state of cognitive deconstruction and, in turn, a reduction in aversive self-awareness as featured in Heatherton and Baumeister's (1991) escape theory of binge eating (see Curtin & Fairchild, 2003, for the ingenious use of event-related potential, ERP, measures to assess cognitive functions following alcohol intoxication, another hypothesized form of escape).

The Choice of Binge Eating as an Escape Route

But why would a bulimic individual select the very behavior, binge eating, that so conflicts with her long-term perfectionistic bodily goals to try to escape aversive self-awareness and emotion? Given that there are multiple ways to escape from aversive self-awareness and negative emotion, why wouldn't such an individual select a form of escape that does not undermine attainment of her long-term perfectionistic weight goals? Consider six factors that may increase the likelihood of choosing binge eating as an escape route and how these factors likely characterize bulimic individuals (see Bardone-Cone et al., 2004).

First, differences in the *reward value* of food and eating may partly explain the choice of binge eating. That is, individual differences in the degree to which eating "soothes" negative feelings and promotes a state of cognitive deconstruction are relevant to the choice of escape. For example, for individuals who are relatively indifferent to food (i.e., enjoy it in a natural way and don't "get into" food or eating), binge eating may not be an effective escape route because eating likely would not lead to cognitive deconstruction and reduction of distress. In contrast, individuals who greatly enjoy food and find food highly reinforcing in reducing negative feelings/thoughts may be especially likely to turn to food in response to these aversive states. Bulimic individuals often diet (Heatherton & Polivy, 1992), which suggests that they do find food reinforcing (which may be why they need to diet). In this regard, Stice (2001) speculated that the reinforcement value of food may be especially high for bulimic individuals (possibly mediated by dopaminergic or serotonergic systems). An interesting avenue for future research would be exploration of activity in regions of the brain implementing approach behavior (e.g., Davidson, Jackson, & Kalin, 2000) in bulimic and nonbulimic individuals when food is presented.

Second, individual differences in *expectancies* that eating will provide a temporary escape from thinking about the self and feeling badly ought to influence choice of escape route. Those who expect that eating can soothe emotional distress should be especially likely to overeat to regulate negative emotion. Accordingly, recall that Tice et al. (2001) manipulated people's beliefs about the potential comfort value of food and found that distressed people overate when they believed that eating would alleviate their distress but not when they had been disabused of this belief by the experimenter. Evidence suggests that bulimic individuals indeed hold expectancies that eating can reduce distress. For example, Smith, Hohlstein, and Atlas (1989) reported that individuals with eating disorders held food-related expectancies such as "Eating can help me bury my emotions" and "Eating helps me forget or block out negative feelings like depression." In addition, Bardone, Jaffee, Krahn, and Baker (1996) found that approximately 60% of their clinical sample of bulimics reported "very typically" using a binge to numb their feelings.

Third, *modeling* may affect the choice of escape method. Individuals from families in which children observed a parent turn to food for emotional relief may be likely to select eating as the escape route from negative emotions. In this regard, Pike and Rodin (1991) found that mothers of eating disordered daughters were more eating disordered themselves than mothers of noneating disordered daughters. However, there currently are no studies looking directly at parental modeling above and beyond or separate from genetic influences (e.g., adoption studies). Studies investigating peer modeling find some evidence that peers' disordered eating is associated with individuals' bulimic symptoms (Crandall, 1988; Stice, 1998).

Fourth, in contrast to alcohol and illicit drugs, food does not involve *legality* issues. Also, compared with excessive alcohol and drug use (which could increase risk for unwanted sexual experiences, accidents, etc.), binge eating is less likely to put one in harm's way. The subset of women who are high in harm avoidance and low in general impulsivity, but seeking escape from aversive self-states, would be more likely to choose binge eating than other forms of substance use as an escape behavior. Significant comorbidity exists between bulimia and substance abuse (Herzog, Nussbaum, & Marmor, 1996), and it may be that individuals who both binge eat and drink excessively are those who are less harm avoidant and more impulsive or who are especially desperate to escape.

Fifth, *dieting* may stack the deck in favor of choosing binge eating as an escape behavior. Supporting this hypothesis, Polivy and Herman (1985) argued that dieting increases the likelihood of binge eating based on evidence that dieting precedes binge eating in diverse study designs including studies of binge eaters (e.g., Pyle, Mitchell, & Eckert, 1981), human starvation (Keys, Brozek, Henschel, Mickelsen, & Taylor, 1950), and animals (Coscina & Dixon, 1983). Dieters place themselves in a constant state of deprivation, especially from attractive foods that they consider "bad" or "forbidden" (e.g., desserts). In a state of deprivation and self-imposed hunger, food can become even more appealing and salient. It also may be that for many dieters, food and eating have a high reward value to begin with (which is why they need to diet), making food that much more appealing. In addition to the other factors likely to promote selection of binge eating as a means to escape negative emotion and aversive self-awareness, bulimic individuals also exhibit dieting. For example, bulimic individuals typically engage in dieting between binges (American Psychiatric Association, 2000; Heatherton & Polivy, 1992). Moreover, studies have shown that dieting predicted onset of bulimic symptoms (e.g., Stice, Killen, Hayward, & Taylor, 1998).

Finally, because bulimia and binge eating are predominantly experienced by women, it is important to ask why *women* would choose binge eating over other escape routes such as alcohol abuse. Wilson, Brick, Adler, Cocco, and Breslin (1989) indicated that alcohol did not reduce self-awareness nor reliably reduce anxiety for female social drinkers. They suggested that alcohol may be a less effective means of escaping negative emotion and aversive self-awareness for women than men, thus making alcohol a less appealing escape route for women. However, some evidence suggests that women may turn from binge eating to alcohol for escape if they reduce the behavior of binge eating without developing more adaptive ways to cope with the aversive emotional states that motivate some sort of escape (i.e., "symptom substitution"; Yager, Landsverk, Edlestein, & Jarvik, 1988).

In sum, these six factors may increase an individual's likelihood of choosing binge eating as a preferred route to escape from negative emotions: high reward value of food, high expectancies that eating can assuage negative emotional states, exposure to models who eat to assuage negative emotional states, legality of obtaining and eating food, dieting, and being female. Many, if not all, of these factors characterize bulimic individuals. Thus, the deck seems to be stacked against bulimic individuals when they are overwhelmed with negative emotion and they want to escape. Such individuals exhibit the very characteristics likely to make eating, and even binge eating, the preferred escape route from negative emotion, even though it so profoundly sabotages their long-term perfectionistic body standards.

Three Patterns of Eating to Reduce Negative Emotion and Aversive Self-Awareness

Whereas some individuals seeking to escape from negative emotion and aversive self-awareness by eating may embark on a full-blown eating binge right off, others initially may begin to eat in a way that is qualitatively different from mealtime eating (i.e., eating to distract or zone out instead of to satisfy hunger) but not yet quantitatively equal to a binge. For this latter group of individuals, the initial "distractive"[1] eating to relieve negative emotion and aversive self-awareness may escalate into a full-blown binge. Specifically, through this distractive eating, awareness is reduced to the immediate, concrete motions and sensations of tasting, chewing, and swallowing. More importantly, meaningful thoughts about the self are banished. In short, the deconstructed cognitive state of low self-awareness will emerge from the absorbing activity of eating. Although low self-awareness will provide relief from negative emotion and cognitions, it also will further interfere with self-regulation of eating because an individual in a state of cognitive deconstruction no longer will be comparing current behaviors to standards. Individuals who normally inhibit eating (i.e., restrained eaters; Herman & Mack, 1975) may experience the removal of restraints and the disinhibition of eating in this state of cognitive deconstruction. Such disinhibited eating may escalate into a full-blown binge among restrained eaters. In contrast, binge eating should not be disinhibited among unrestrained eaters (i.e., individuals who are not inhibiting eating) who engage in distractive eating to escape from aversive self-awareness and negative emotion. Instead, for these individuals, distractive eating may provide an escape, although perhaps only temporary, from negative emotions that does not escalate into a full-blown binge.

Thus, three distinct patterns of eating to escape from negative emotions and aversive self-awareness may exist. In the first, individuals respond to negative emotion with a full-blown binge. In the second, individuals, particularly restrained eaters, respond to negative emotion with distractive eating that escalates into a full-blown binge. Finally, in the third, individuals respond to negative emotion with distractive eating that does not escalate into a binge. The first two patterns may be particularly troublesome.

RESOLUTION OF THE PARADOX OF PERFECTIONISM AND BULIMIA: A RECAPITULATION

Our integration of work on bulimia with theories and research on self-regulation provides a resolution of the intriguing paradox of perfectionism and binge eating among bulimic individuals. We first presented the three-factor theory and evidence supporting it suggesting that highly

---

[1]To our knowledge, "distractive" is not a proper word, but it captures our intended meaning of eating in order to distract.

perfectionistic individuals with low self-efficacy are especially likely to exhibit bulimic symptoms when they perceive themselves to be over-weight or are dissatisfied with their bodies. Then to explain *why* such indi-viduals engage in bulimic behaviors, we expanded on Heatherton and Baumeister's (1991) escape theory of binge eating and suggested that indi-viduals exhibiting the cognitive/personality profile associated with bulimia in the three-factor model (high perfectionism paired with low self-efficacy) may become overwhelmed by negative emotion, aversive self-awareness, and self-loathing when they believe they cannot meet their perfectionistic standards (e.g., when they perceive themselves to be overweight or are dissatisfied with their bodies). In these situations, such individuals are so distressed that they temporarily may abandon pursuit of their long-term goals (e.g., pursuit of the perfect body weight and shape) to divert behavior to the immediate goal of trying to decrease their negative emotion and aversive self-awareness (Tice et al., 2001). If such in-dividuals exhibit factors biasing them to select binge eating as a preferred escape route (e.g., high reward value of food, high expectancies that food will assuage negative emotions, etc.), then they will turn to eating, and even overeating, to relieve distress. According to this view, then, binge eating among bulimic individuals represents a short-term strategy for at-tempting to regulate negative emotion and an aversive sense of self that is self-defeating over the long run (see Baumeister & Scher, 1988).

When Does the Three-Factor Profile Not Lead to Bulimia?

The resolution of the paradox of perfectionism and bulimia implies that there will not be a perfect mapping between the three-factor profile (high perfectionism, low self-efficacy, perceptions of being overweight or body dissatisfaction) and display of bulimic symptoms. As described earlier, an individual with this profile might not exhibit the factors biasing toward selection of binge eating as a preferred route to escape negative emotion (e.g., high reward value of food). Instead, some individuals with the three-factor profile may be biased to select another type of escape from negative emotion. For example, an individual who finds the effects of alcohol pleasant and grew up in a home with alcoholic parents who drank when stressed may turn to alcohol to escape negative emotion. Of course, the possibility exists that some individuals exhibiting the three-factor profile may be biased toward more than one escape behavior (e.g., binge eating and drug abuse). This scenario is consistent with the significant comor-bidity of bulimia and other maladaptive behaviors, such as substance abuse and self-mutilation, that have been hypothesized to provide tempo-rary escape (e.g., Dansky, Brewerton, & Kilpatrick, 2000; Garfinkel & Gar-ner, 1982; Holderness, Brooks-Gunn, & Warren, 1994).

Also consider that not all individuals exhibiting the three-factor profile may be motivated or able to divert behavior to the short-term goal of affect regulation when distressed. In this regard, Abramson and Alloy (1981) speculated that depressed individuals may suffer from a breakdown or absence of the motivation to maintain self-esteem. Following this line of reasoning, there may be a subset of individuals exhibiting the three-factor profile who become depressed (or anxious) but who do not go the additional step of engaging in some behavior to escape their negative emotions. Such individuals would suffer from "pure" more persistent depression or anxiety. Perhaps these individuals are less impulsive than their counterparts who engage in dramatic attempts such as binge eating, substance abuse, or self-mutilation to escape their negative emotions.

Alternative Accounts of Bulimic Symptoms in Response to Negative Emotions

It is worth noting that two alternative accounts exist of why bulimic symptoms tend to occur in the presence of negative emotion. Although related, each is different in important ways from the expanded escape theory view presented here. One account, the *disinhibition* theory, suggests that negative emotion serves to disinhibit dietary restriction (e.g., Herman & Polivy, 1980; Stice, 2001). According to this theory, negative emotion interferes with the cognitive control of eating such that impulses to eat no longer are held in check. Although similar to the expanded escape theory in highlighting the role of negative emotion as a proximal cause of binge eating, the two theories differ because our expanded escape theory further posits that individuals prone to bulimia binge eat in order to reduce distress. In contrast, binge eating serves no strategic function in disinhibition theory. It has been argued elsewhere (Bardone-Cone et al., 2004) that Heatherton and Baumeister's (1991) original escape theory of binge eating actually is a hybrid escape–disinhibition theory. Note that the hypothesis that distractive eating may escalate into a full-blown binge among restrained eaters relies on disinhibition of eating due to cognitive deconstruction. However, the escalation of distractive eating to a full-blown binge is in the escape theory genre because the initial distractive eating is a strategic attempt to relieve negative emotion and aversive self-awareness.

Related to the disinhibition idea, Baumeister and Heatherton (1996) invoked the concept of self-regulatory strength as a limited resource to provide another explanation of why emotional distress may precipitate episodes of self-regulatory failure (e.g., binge eating by a person with highly perfectionistic weight and body shape goals). According to this idea, when people are emotionally distressed, they deplete their regulatory resources dealing with their distress, which in turn leaves them unable to effectively regulate behavior to achieve their long-term goals (e.g., a slim body). Thus, this theory suggests that emotional distress reduces the capacity for self-regulation in the service of long-term goals. As with the disinhibition theory, binge eating serves no strategic function in this *depleted capacity* account of self-regulation failure.

A challenge for future research will be to empirically distinguish among our expanded escape theory and the disinhibition and depleted capacity accounts of binge eating among individuals exhibiting the three-factor profile. The results presented supporting this model do not distinguish among the three theories. None of the studies tested whether binge eating, in fact, was a strategic attempt to reduce distress as opposed to being the result of disinhibition or depleted self-regulatory capacity due to the distress. Work disentangling these theories promises to be important.

CLINICAL IMPLICATIONS

Identification of the three-factor profile (high perfectionism, low self-efficacy, perceptions of being overweight or body dissatisfaction) predictive of bulimic symptoms has implications for the treatment and prevention of bulimia. The fact that these three factors interact (i.e., a three-way interaction) to predict bulimic symptoms suggests that altering any of them will alter the likelihood of bulimic symptoms. This provides flexibility in where to focus therapeutic and preventive efforts (Bardone, Vohs, Abramson, Heatherton, & Joiner, 2000).

However, we suggest that modification of some of the targets may be more defensible than modification of others. In particular, as the anecdotes from Arnold Schwarzenegger's autobiography vividly illustrated, the high standards inherent in perfectionism, in and of themselves, may not be bad, which is a harder stance to argue for low self-efficacy. Decreasing perfectionism may have the undesirable side effect of putting a ceiling on achievement and accomplishments. As emphasized in this chapter and argued elsewhere (Abramson et al., 2002), perfectionism may be a problem only when it is paired with low self-efficacy and/or low ability. When perfectionism is paired with high self-efficacy and/or high ability, it may be an asset. Thus, it may be more appropriate to focus therapeutic and preventive efforts on increasing self-efficacy and abilities rather than on decreasing perfectionism, unless the perfectionism is extremely rigid or completely unrealistic (but who is to say whether an individual's standards are unrealistic?). This approach to intervention is consistent with the general argument of Kraemer et al. (2001) that selection of appropriate targets of intervention must be based on knowledge of how risk factors work together (e.g., perfectionism is a problem only in the context of other risk factors such as low self-efficacy). From this perspective, it would be inappropriate, and prohibitively expensive, to target all perfectionistic adolescent females in a prevention program for bulimia because perfectionism only predicts bulimia when it is paired with low self-efficacy and perceptions of being overweight or body dissatisfaction.

The expanded escape theory that we have developed has additional therapeutic implications related to the escape component itself (Bardone-Cone et al., 2004). Specifically, the following interventions should reduce the likelihood that individuals will engage in binge eating to escape from negative emotion and aversive self-awareness: increase the repertoire of skills to cope with negative emotions and cognitions to include more effective problem-solving skills and/or healthy distractions/escape behaviors; increase ability to tolerate negative emotion so that a dramatic escape like binge eating is not required; decrease the tendency to give priority to short-term emotion regulation over other more long-term self-regulatory goals; educate about the association between chronic dieting and binge eating, encourage moderate eating, and discourage the mentality of good versus bad foods; and provide family therapy to address family modeling and dynamics that may be supporting binge eating. Interventions promoting increases in both perceived and actual self-efficacy will likely have the desirable consequence of promoting the goals described in the first three interventions. As individuals increase their perceived and actual self-efficacy, they will feel and be empowered to resolve discrepancies and, thus, will suffer less negative emotion, aversive self-awareness, and self-loathing when encountering discrepancies. In turn, they should be less motivated to give priority to short-term emotion regulation over other more long-term goals and less motivated to seek dramatic, maladaptive escapes from negative emotion and aversive self-awareness.

According to our theoretical perspective (see Bardone-Cone et al., 2004), interventions that seek only to decrease binge eating (e.g., strictly behavioral therapies) but fail to address the factors giving rise to binge eating (e.g., low self-efficacy, inability to tolerate negative emotion, etc.) might encourage "symptom substitution." If the same pre-conditions for a binge remain following therapy focused on binge eating per se, individuals theoretically still would be motivated to escape and may turn to other means of escape, benign or maladaptive (Yager et al., 1988). Such "at risk" individuals who do not choose substitute escapes like drug abuse because they are low in harm avoidance likely would remain in aversive states longer and may develop more severe, persistent symptoms of anxiety and depression. Thus, interventions that do not address the factors giving rise to binge eating will leave individuals likely to seek

alternative maladaptive escapes from negative emotion or more depressed and anxious.

This chapter has integrated work on bulimia with theories and research
on self-regulation to resolve the intriguing paradox of perfectionism and
binge eating among bulimic individuals. The resolution emphasized that
perfectionism is not always bad and does not inevitably lead to bulimia or
maladjustment. Instead, the three-factor model and empirical work testing it showed that it is the combination of high perfectionism and low self-
efficacy that provides risk for bulimic symptoms when perfectionistic
standards (e.g., for weight and body shape) are not met. Individuals with
high perfectionism and low self-efficacy may be especially likely to resort
to binge eating in a desperate attempt to decrease overwhelming negative
emotion, aversive self-awareness, and self-loathing when they feel helpless to meet their perfectionistic standards. According to this view, binge
eating among bulimic individuals represents a short-term strategy for attempting to regulate negative emotion and an aversive sense of self that is
self-defeating over the long run.

The view that perfectionism is not necessarily maladaptive, and indeed
can be very adaptive, is consistent with emerging work in clinical (e.g.,
Alden, Ryder, & Mellings, 2002) and social (e.g., Campbell & Di Paula,
2002) psychology, suggesting that the context in which perfectionism occurs determines whether it is deleterious. The profile of high perfectionism
and low self-efficacy/low abilities is psychologically toxic, whereas the
profile of high perfectionism and high self-efficacy/high abilities is not and
may well fuel superior achievement. Consistent with the perspective that
perfectionism sometimes is psychologically beneficial and other times deleterious, some writers have distinguished between "good" and "bad" perfectionism—for example, normal versus neurotic perfectionism (Hamachek, 1978); positive achievement strivings versus maladaptive evaluation
concerns (Frost, Heimberg, Holt, Mattia, & Neubauer, 1993); positive versus negative perfectionism (Terry-Short, Owens, Slade, & Dewey, 1995);
healthy versus unhealthy perfectionism (Terry-Short et al., 1995); and satisfied versus dissatisfied perfectionism (Slade & Dewey, 1996).

Early views emphasizing that perfectionism is inherently bad and almost inevitably linked to psychopathology (e.g., Pacht, 1984) were likely
grounded in clinical observation without benefit of research on "normal"
and "superior" individuals. Indeed, many patients with psychological
disorders, especially eating disorders, do exhibit high levels of perfectionism (see Shafran & Mansell, 2001), so it is not surprising that clinicians
would come to vilify perfectionism. What is understandably harder for
clinicians to see, given that they rarely do therapy with individuals who

do not have problems, is that it is the *context* in which perfectionism occurs that determines whether it is deleterious to psychological health. As the case history of Arnold Schwarzenegger so vividly illustrated, perfectionism paired with high self-efficacy and high abilities may promote high, and even extraordinary, achievement with no maladjustment. The clinician does not have the opportunity to observe high achieving, well-adjusted perfectionists because such individuals do not seek treatment (see Dykman & Abramson, 1990, and Dykman, Abramson, Alloy, & Hartlage, 1989, for a discussion of parallel "baseline" problems in early clinically based formulations of information-processing biases and depression that were not informed by relevant basic work in psychology on normal human cognition). This chapter has shown that the paradox of perfectionism and bulimia can be resolved by integrating work on bulimia with contemporary theory and research in social and personality psychology.

ACKNOWLEDGMENT

Preparation of this chapter was supported by National Institute of Mental Health Grant Nos. MH 43866 and MH 52662 to Lyn Y. Abramson.

REFERENCES

Abraham, S., & Beumont, P. J. V. (1982). How patients describe bulimia or binge eating. *Psychological Medicine, 12,* 625–635.

Abramson, L. Y., & Alloy, L. B. (1981). Depression, nondepression, and cognitive illusions: A reply to Schwartz. *Journal of Experimental Psychology: General, 110,* 436–447.

Abramson, L. Y., Alloy, L. B., Hankin, B. L., Haeffel, G. J., MacCoon, D. G., & Gibb, B. E. (2002). Cognitive vulnerability–stress models of depression in a self-regulatory and psychobiological context. In I. H. Gotlib & C. L. Hammen (Eds.), *Handbook of depression* (pp. 268–294). New York: Guilford.

Abramson, L. Y., Metalsky, G. I., & Alloy, L. B. (1989). Hopelessness depression: A theory-based subtype of depression. *Psychological Review, 96,* 358–372.

Abramson, L. Y., Seligman, M. E., & Teasdale, J. D. (1978). Learned helplessness in humans: Critique and reformulation. *Journal of Abnormal Psychology, 87,* 49–74.

Alden, L. E., Ryder, A. G., & Mellings, T. M. B. (2002). Perfectionism in the context of social fears: Toward a two-component model. In G. L. Flett & P. L. Hewitt (Eds.), *Perfectionism: Theory, research, and treatment* (pp. 373–391). Washington, DC: American Psychological Association.

Alloy, L. B., Abramson, L. Y., Raniere, D., & Dyller, I. (1999). Research methods in adult psychopathology. In P. C. Kendall, J. N. Butcher, & G. N. Holmbeck (Eds.), *Handbook of research methods in clinical psychology* (2nd ed., pp. 466–498). New York: Wiley.

American Psychiatric Association. (1994). *Diagnostic and statistical manual of mental disorders* (4th ed.). Washington, DC: Author.

American Psychiatric Association. (2000). *Diagnostic and statistical manual of mental disorders* (4th ed., text rev.). Washington, DC: Author.

Bandura, A. (1977). Self-efficacy: Toward a unifying theory of behavioral change. *Psychological Review, 84,* 191–215.

Bandura, A., & Cervone, D. (1986). Differential engagement of self-reactive influences in cognitive motivation. *Organizational Behavior and Human Decision Processes, 38,* 92–113.

Bardone, A. M., Jaffee, S., Krahn, D., & Baker, T. (1996, April). *A validation study of the Bulimia Expectancy Scale.* Paper presented at the International Conference on Eating Disorders, New York.

Bardone, A. M., Perez, M., Abramson, L. Y., & Joiner, T. E., Jr. (2003). Self-competence and self-liking in the prediction of change in bulimic symptoms. *International Journal of Eating Disorders, 34,* 361–369.

Bardone, A. M., Vohs, K. D., Abramson, L. Y., Heatherton, T. F., & Joiner, T. E., Jr. (2000). The confluence of perfectionism, body dissatisfaction, and low self-esteem predicts bulimic symptoms: Clinical implications. *Behavior Therapy, 31,* 265–280.

Bardone-Cone, A. M., Abramson, L. Y., Vohs, K. D., Heatherton, T. F., & Joiner, T. E., Jr. (2004). *The expanded escape theory of binge eating.* Manuscript submitted for publication.

Bardone-Cone, A. M., Abramson, L. Y., Vohs, K. D., Heatherton, T. F., & Joiner, T. E., Jr. (in press). Predicting bulimic symptoms: An interactive model of self-efficacy, perfectionism, and perceived weight status. *Behavior Research and Therapy.*

Baron, R. M., & Kenny, D. A. (1986). The moderator–mediator variable distinction in social psychological research: Conceptual, strategic, and statistical considerations. *Journal of Personality and Social Psychology, 51,* 1173–1182.

Baumeister, R. F. (1991). *Escaping the self: Alcoholism, spirituality, masochism, and other flights from the burden of selfhood.* New York: Basic Books.

Baumeister, R. F., & Heatherton, T. F. (1996). Self-regulation failure: An overview. *Psychological Inquiry, 7,* 1–15.

Baumeister, R. F., & Scher, S. J. (1988). Self-defeating behavior patterns among normal individuals: Review and analysis of common self-destructive tendencies. *Psychological Bulletin, 104,* 3–22.

Beebe, D. W. (1994). Bulimia nervosa and depression: A theoretical and clinical appraisal in light of the binge–purge cycle. *British Journal of Clinical Psychology, 33,* 259–276.

Blouin, A. G., Bushnik, T., Braaten, J., & Blouin, J. H. (1989). Bulimia and diabetes: Distinct psychosocial profiles. *International Journal of Eating Disorders, 8,* 93–100.

Brewerton, T. D., Lydiard, R. B., Ballenger, J. C., & Herzog, D. B. (1993). Eating disorders and social phobia. *Archives of General Psychiatry, 50,* 70.

Campbell, J. D., & Di Paula, A. (2002). Perfectionistic self-beliefs: Their relation to personality and goal pursuit. In G. L. Flett & P. L. Hewitt (Eds.), *Perfectionism: Theory, research, and treatment* (pp. 181–198). Washington, DC: American Psychological Association.

Carver, C. S., Blaney, P. H., & Scheier, M. F. (1979). Reassertion and giving up: The interactive role of self-directed attention and outcome expectancy. *Journal of Personality and Social Psychology, 37,* 1859–1870.

Carver, C. S., & Scheier, M. F. (1981). *Attention and self-regulation: A control-theory approach to human behavior.* New York: Springer-Verlag.

Carver, C. S., & Scheier, M. F. (1998). *On the self-regulation of behavior.* Cambridge, England: Cambridge University Press.

Cosford, P., & Arnold, E. (1992). Eating disorders in later life: A review. *International Journal of Geriatric Psychiatry, 7,* 491–498.

Coscina, D. V., & Dixon, L. M. (1983). Body weight regulation in anorexia nervosa: Insights from an animal model. In P. L. Darby, P. E. Garfinkel, D. M. Garner, & D. V. Coscina (Eds.), *Anorexia nervosa: Recent developments* (pp. 207–220). New York: Allan R. Liss.

Crandall, C. S. (1988). Social contagion of binge eating. *Journal of Personality and Social Psychology, 55,* 588–598.

Curtin, J. J., & Fairchild, B. A. (2003). Alcohol and cognitive control: Implications for regulation of behavior during response conflict. *Journal of Abnormal Psychology, 112,* 424–436.

Dansky, B. S., Brewerton, T. D., & Kilpatrick, D. G. (2000). Comorbidity of bulimia nervosa and alcohol use disorders: Results from the National Women's Study. *International Journal of Eating Disorders, 27,* 180–190.

Davidson, R. J., Jackson, D. C., & Kalin, N. H. (2000). Emotion, plasticity, context, and regulation: Perspectives from affective neuroscience. *Psychological Bulletin, 126,* 890–909.

Denoma, J. M., Gordon, K. H., Bardone, A. M., Vohs, K. D., Abramson, L. Y., Heatherton, T. F., & Joiner, T. E., Jr. (in press). A test of an interactive model of bulimic symptomatology in adult women. *Behavior Therapy.*

Duval, S., & Wicklund, R. A. (1972). *A theory of objective self-awareness.* San Diego, CA: Academic Press.

Duval, T. S., Duval, V. H., & Mulilis, J. P. (1992). Effects of self-focus, discrepancy between self and standard, and outcome expectancy favorability on the tendency to match self to standard or to withdraw. *Journal of Personality and Social Psychology, 62,* 340–348.

Dykman, B. M., & Abramson, L. Y. (1990). Contributions of basic research to the cognitive theories of depression. *Personality and Social Psychology Bulletin, 16,* 42–57.

Dykman, B. M., Abramson, L. Y., Alloy, L. B., & Hartlage, S. (1989). Processing of ambiguous feedback among depressed and nondepressed college students: Schematic biases and their implications for depressive realism. *Journal of Personality and Social Psychology, 56,* 431–445.

Etringer, B. D., Altmaier, E. M., & Bowers, W. (1989). An investigation into the cognitive functioning of bulimic women. *Journal of Counseling and Development, 68,* 216–219.

Fairburn, C. G. (1995). *Overcoming binge eating.* New York: Guilford.

Fairburn, C. G., & Cooper, P. J. (1984). Clinical features of bulimia nervosa. *British Journal of Psychiatry, 144,* 238–246.

Flett, G. L., & Hewitt, P. L. (2002). Perfectionism and maladjustment: An overview of theoretical, definitional, and treatment issues. In G. L. Flett & P. L. Hewitt (Eds.), *Perfectionism: Theory, research, and treatment* (pp. 5–31). Washington, DC: American Psychological Association.

Frost, R. O., Heimberg, R. G., Holt, C. S., Mattia, J. I., & Neubauer, A. L. (1993). A comparison of two measures of perfectionism. *Personality and Individual Differences, 14,* 119–126.

Fryer, S., Waller, G., & Kroese, B. S. (1997). Stress, coping, and disturbed eating attitudes in teenage girls. *International Journal of Eating Disorders, 22,* 427–436.

Garfinkel, P. E., & Garner, D. M. (1982). *Anorexia nervosa: A multidimensional perspective.* New York: Brunner/Mazel.

Garner, D. M., & Garfinkel, P. E. (Eds.). (1997). *Handbook of treatment for eating disorders.* New York: Guilford.

Garner, D. M., Olmstead, M. P., & Polivy, J. (1983). Development and validation of a multidimensional eating disorder inventory for anorexia nervosa and bulimia. *International Journal of Eating Disorders, 2,* 15–34.

Goldner, E. M., Cockell, S. J., & Srikameswaran, S. (2002). Perfectionism and eating disorders. In G. L. Flett & P. L. Hewitt (Eds.), *Perfectionism: Theory, research, and treatment* (pp. 319–340). Washington, DC: American Psychological Association.

Gordon, K. H., Denoma, J. M., Bardone, A. M., Abramson, L. Y., & Joiner, T. E., Jr. (in press). Self-competence and the prediction of bulimic symptoms in older women. *Behavior Therapy.*

Gormally, J., Black, S., Daston, S., & Rardin, D. (1982). The assessment of binge eating severity among obese persons. *Addictive Behaviors, 7,* 47–55.

Hamachek, D. E. (1978). Psychodynamics of normal and neurotic perfectionism. *Psychology: A Journal of Human Behavior, 15*, 27–33.

Heatherton, T. F., & Baumeister, R. F. (1991). Binge eating as escape from self-awareness. *Psychological Bulletin, 110*, 86–108.

Heatherton, T. F., & Polivy, J. (1992). Chronic dieting and eating disorders: A spiral model. In J. H. Crowther, S. E. Hobfall, & M. A. P. Tennenbaum (Eds.), *The etiology of bulimia nervosa: The individual and familial context* (pp. 133–155). Washington, DC: Hemisphere.

Heatherton, T. E., Striepe, M., & Wittenberg, L. (1998). Emotional distress and disinhibited eating: The role of self. *Personality and Social Psychology Bulletin, 24*, 301–313.

Herman, C. P., & Mack, D. (1975). Restrained and unrestrained eating. *Journal of Personality, 43*, 647–660.

Herman, C. P., & Polivy, J. (1975). Anxiety, restraint, and eating behavior. *Journal of Abnormal Psychology, 84*, 666–672.

Herman, C. P., & Polivy, J. (1980). Restrained eating. In A. J. Stunkard (Ed.), *Obesity* (pp. 208–225). Philadelphia: Saunders.

Herzog, D. B., Nussbaum, K. M., & Marmor, A. K. (1996). Comorbidity and outcome in eating disorders. *The Psychiatric Clinics of North America, 19*, 843–859.

Hewitt, P. L., & Flett, G. L. (1991). Perfectionism in the self and social contexts: Conceptualization, assessment, and association with psychopathology. *Journal of Personality and Social Psychology, 60*, 456–470.

Hewitt, P. L., & Flett, G. L. (1993). Dimensions of perfectionism, daily stress, and depression: A test of the specific vulnerability hypothesis. *Journal of Abnormal Psychology, 102*, 58–65.

Higgins, E. T., Vookles, J., & Tykocinski, O. (1992). Self and health: How "patterns" of self-beliefs predict types of emotional and physical problems. *Social Cognition, 10*, 125–150.

Holderness, C. G., Brooks-Gunn, J., & Warren, M. P. (1994). Co-morbidity of eating disorders and substance abuse review of the literature. *International Journal of Eating Disorders, 16*, 1–34.

Hurley, J. B., Palmer, R. L., & Stretch, D. (1990). The specificity of the Eating Disorder Inventory: A re-appraisal. *International Journal of Eating Disorders, 9*, 419–424.

Jacobi, C., Hayward, C., de Zwaan, M., Kraemer, H. C., & Agras, W. S. (2004). Coming to terms with risk factors for eating disorders: Application of risk terminology and suggestions for a general taxonomy. *Psychological Bulletin, 130*, 19–65.

Johnson, C., Stuckey, M., Lewis, L., & Schwartz, D. (1982). Bulimia: A descriptive survey of 316 cases. *International Journal of Eating Disorders, 2*, 3–16.

Joiner, T. E., Jr., Heatherton, T. F., & Keel, P. K. (1997). Ten-year stability and predictive validity of five bulimia-related indicators. *American Journal of Psychiatry, 154*, 1133–1138.

Joiner, T. E., Jr., Heatherton, T. F., Rudd, M. D., & Schmidt, N. B. (1997). Perfectionism, perceived weight status, and bulimic symptoms: Two studies testing a diathesis–stress model. *Journal of Abnormal Psychology, 106*, 145–153.

Joiner, T. E., Jr., & Schmidt, N. B. (1995). Dimensions of perfectionism, life stress, and depressed and anxious symptoms: Prospective support for diathesis–stress but not specific vulnerability among male undergraduates. *Journal of Social and Clinical Psychology, 14*, 165–183.

Judge, T. A., Erez, A., Bono, J. E., & Thoresen, C. J. (2002). Are measures of self-esteem, neuroticism, locus of control, and generalized self-efficacy indicators of a common core construct? *Journal of Personality and Social Psychology, 83*, 693–710.

Keys, A., Brozek, J., Henschel, A., Mickelsen, O., & Taylor, H. L. (1950). *The biology of human starvation.* Minneapolis, MN: University of Minnesota Press.

Killen, J. D., Taylor, C. B., Hayward, C., Haydel, K. F., Wilson, D. M., Hammer, L., et al. (1996). Weight concerns influence the development of eating disorders: A 4-year prospective study. *Journal of Consulting and Clinical Psychology, 64*, 936–940.

Killen, J. D., Taylor, C. B., Hayward, C., Wilson, D. M., Haydel, K. F., Robinson, T. N., et al. (1994). Pursuit of thinness and onset of eating disorder symptoms in a community sample of adolescent girls: A three year prospective analysis. *International Journal of Eating Disorders, 16,* 227–238.

Kraemer, H. C., Stice, E., Kazdin, A., Offord, D., & Kupfer, D. (2001). How do risk factors work together?: Mediators, moderators, and independent, overlapping, and proxy risk factors. *American Journal of Psychiatry, 158,* 848–856.

Kurth, C. L., Krahn, D. D., Nairn, K., & Drewnowski, A. (1995). The severity of dieting and bingeing behaviors in college women: Interview validation of survey data. *Journal of Psychiatric Research, 29,* 211–225.

Lee, N. F., Rush, A. J., & Mitchell, J. E. (1985). Bulimia and depression. *Journal of Affective Disorders, 9,* 231–238.

Levine, M. P., & Smolak, L. (1992). Toward a model of the developmental psychopathology of eating disorders: The example of early adolescence. In J. H. Crowther & D. L. Tennenbaum (Eds.), *The etiology of bulimia nervosa: The individual and familial context* (pp. 59–80). Washington, DC: Hemisphere.

McClelland, G. H., & Judd, C. M. (1993). Statistical difficulties of detecting interactions and moderator effects. *Psychological Bulletin, 114,* 376–390.

Pacht, A. R. (1984). Reflections on perfection. *American Psychologist, 39,* 386–390.

Parker, W. D. (2002). Perfectionism and adjustment in gifted children. In G. L. Flett & P. L. Hewitt (Eds.), *Perfectionism: Theory, research, and treatment* (pp. 133–148). Washington, DC: American Psychological Association.

Pike, K. M., & Rodin, J. (1991). Mothers, daughters, and disordered eating. *Journal of Abnormal Psychology, 100,* 198–204.

Polivy, J., & Herman, C. P. (1985). Dieting and bingeing: A causal analysis. *American Psychologist, 40,* 193–201.

Pyle, R. L., Mitchell, J. E., & Eckert, E. D. (1981). Bulimia: A report of 34 cases. *Journal of Clinical Psychiatry, 42,* 60–64.

Pyszczynski, T., & Greenberg, J. (1987). Self-regulatory perseveration and the depressive self-focusing style: A self-awareness theory of reactive depression. *Psychological Bulletin, 102,* 122–138.

Rosch, D. S., Crowther, J. H., & Graham, J. R. (1991). MMPI-derived personality description and personality subtypes in an undergraduate bulimic population. *Psychology of Addictive Behaviors, 5,* 15–22.

Ruderman, A. (1986). Bulimia and irrational beliefs. *Behaviour Research and Therapy, 24,* 193–197.

Schneider, J. A., O'Leary, A., & Agras, W. S. (1987). The role of perceived self-efficacy in recovery from bulimia: A preliminary examination. *Behaviour Research and Therapy, 25,* 429–432.

Schotte, D. E., Cools, J., & McNally, R. J. (1990). Film-induced negative affect triggers overeating in restrained eaters. *Journal of Abnormal Psychology, 99,* 317–320.

Schwarzenegger, A., & Hall, D. K. (1977). *Arnold: The education of a bodybuilder.* New York: Simon & Schuster.

Seligman, M. E. P. (1975). *Helplessness: On depression, development, and death.* San Francisco: Freeman.

Shafran, R., & Mansell, W. (2001). Perfectionism and psychopathology: A review of research and treatment. *Clinical Psychology Review, 21,* 879–906.

Shaw, H. E., Stice, E., & Springer, D. W. (2004). Perfectionism, body dissatisfaction, and self-esteem in predicting bulimic symptomatology: Lack of replication. *International Journal of Eating Disorders, 36,* 41–47.

Slade, P. D., & Dewey, M. E. (1986). Development and preliminary validation of SCANS: A screening instrument for identifying people at risk of developing anorexia and bulimia nervosa. *International Journal of Eating Disorders, 5,* 517–538.

Smith, G. T., Hohlstein, L. A., & Atlas, J. G. (1989, August). *Race differences in eating disordered behavior and eating-related expectancies.* Paper presented at the 97th annual convention of the American Psychological Association, New Orleans, LA.

Steenbarger, B. N., & Aderman, D. (1979). Objective self-awareness as a nonaversive state: Effect of anticipating discrepancy reduction. *Journal of Personality, 47,* 330–339.

Steiger, H., Leung, F. Y., Puentes-Neuman, G., & Gottheil, N. (1992). Psychosocial profiles of adolescent girls with varying degrees of eating and mood disturbances. *International Journal of Eating Disorders, 11,* 121–131.

Stice, E. (1998). Modeling of eating pathology and social reinforcement of the thin-ideal predict onset of bulimic symptoms. *Behaviour Research and Therapy, 36,* 931–944.

Stice, E. (2001). A prospective test of the dual-pathway model of bulimic pathology: Mediating effects of dieting and negative affect. *Journal of Abnormal Psychology, 110,* 124–135.

Stice, E., Killen, J. D., Hayward, C., & Taylor, C. B. (1998). Age of onset for binge eating and purging during late adolescence: A 4-year survival analysis. *Journal of Abnormal Psychology, 107,* 671–675.

Striegel-Moore, R. H., Silberstein, L. R., Frensch, P., & Rodin, J. (1989). A prospective study of disordered eating among college students. *International Journal of Eating Disorders, 8,* 499–509.

Tachi, T., Murakami, K., Murotsu, K., & Washizuka, T. (2001). Affective states associated with bingeing and purging behaviors in Japanese patients with bulimia nervosa. *British Journal of Medical Psychology, 74,* 487–496.

Tafarodi, R. W., & Swann, W. B., Jr. (1995). Self-liking and self-competence as dimensions of global self-esteem: Initial validation of a measure. *Journal of Personality Assessment, 65,* 322–342.

Terry-Short, L. A., Owens, G. R., Slade, P. D., & Dewey, M. E. (1995). Positive and negative perfectionism. *Personality and Individual Differences, 18,* 663–668.

Tice, D. M., Bratslavsky, E., & Baumeister, R. F. (2001). Emotional distress regulation takes precedence over impulse control: If you feel bad, do it! *Journal of Personality and Social Psychology, 80,* 53–67.

Vohs, K. D., Bardone, A. M., Joiner, T. E., Jr., Abramson, L. Y., & Heatherton, T. F. (1999). Perfectionism, perceived weight status, and self-esteem interact to predict bulimic symptoms: A model of bulimic symptom development. *Journal of Abnormal Psychology, 108,* 695–700.

Vohs, K. D., & Heatherton, T. F. (2001). Self-esteem and threats to self: Implications for self-construals and interpersonal perceptions. *Journal of Personality and Social Psychology, 81,* 1103–1118.

Vohs, K. D., Heatherton, T. F., & Herrin, M. (2001). Disordered eating and the transition to college: A prospective study. *International Journal of Eating Disorders, 29,* 280–288.

Vohs, K. D., Voelz, Z. R., Pettit, J. W., Bardone, A. M., Katz, J., Abramson, L. Y., et al. (2001). Perfectionism, body dissatisfaction, and self-esteem: An interactive model of bulimic symptom development. *Journal of Social and Clinical Psychology, 20,* 476–497.

Wilson, G. T., Brick, J., Adler, J., Cocco, K., & Breslin, C. (1989). Alcohol and anxiety reduction in female social drinkers. *Journal of Studies on Alcohol, 50,* 226–235.

Wilson, G. T., Fairburn, C. G., Agras, W. S., Walsh, B. T., & Kraemer, H. (2002). Cognitive-behavioral therapy for bulimia nervosa: Time course and mechanisms of change. *Journal of Consulting and Clinical Psychology, 70,* 267–274.

Yager, J., Landsverk, J., Edlestein, C. K., & Jarvik, M. (1988). A 20-month follow-up study of 628 women with eating disorders: II. Course of associated symptoms and related clinical features. *International Journal of Eating Disorders, 7,* 503–513.

Cognitive Vulnerability to Anorexia Nervosa

David M. Garner
River Centre Clinic
Bowling Green State University

Cristina Magana
Fresno State University

Anorexia nervosa has been a psychiatric diagnosis for many years; however, it was not until the past two decades that it commanded widespread interest in mainstream psychology, psychiatry, and allied professions (Theander, 2004). One reason for this interest is recognition of its significant health consequences. Anorexia nervosa is estimated to be the third most common chronic medical illness in girls age 15–19 (Lucas, Beard, O'Fallon, & Kurland, 1991). It is associated with significant medical complications (Becker, Grinspoon, Klibanski, & Herzog, 1999) and mortality rates exceed the expected incidence of death from all causes among women age 15–24 by 12-fold (Sullivan, 1995).

Early conceptualizations of anorexia nervosa from a cognitive perspective were based on clinical literature indicating that abnormal attitudes toward food and weight are common and persistent features in anorexia nervosa, greatly interfering with full recovery from the disorder. Dally and Gomez (1979) observed that "these attitudes are the most distressing and long-lasting features of anorexia nervosa . . . and are likely to continue or to recur in situations of crisis for many years" (pp. 134–135). Theander (1970) reported that virtually no patients in his follow-up study were free from "neurotic fixations" on body weight. Awareness of these earlier observations, as well as clinical experience, led to the proposal of an approach to cognitive behavioral therapy for anorexia nervosa (Garner & Bemis, 1982, 1985) following Beck's (1976) model for other emotional disorders.

Cognitive theories of anorexia nervosa have identified two broad types of cognitive dysfunction that can influence the onset and maintenance of the disorder. The first is the *nature and content* of maladaptive beliefs and assumptions; the second relates to *modes of information processing,* such as selective attention, perceptual distortions, confirmatory bias, and illusory correlations that maintain dysfunctional beliefs and behavior. The nature and content of beliefs can be further divided into two domains that have been of theoretical and research focus. The primary target of investigation has been beliefs and attitudes about food, shape, weight, and weight gain that are thought to be specific forms of psychopathology in anorexia nervosa. However, increasing attention has focused on core beliefs (beliefs are unconditional and nonsituation specific) and higher order belief systems reflected by low self-esteem, perfectionism, and maturity fears as potential maintaining variables in anorexia nervosa. The aim of this chapter is to selectively review research on the nature and content of maladaptive beliefs as well as possible information-processing disturbances as sources of cognitive vulnerability to anorexia nervosa.

COGNITIVE THERAPY FOR ANOREXIA NERVOSA

Initial conceptualizations of anorexia nervosa from a cognitive behavioral perspective were derived from clinical observations and adapted to address certain distinctive features of the disorder (Garner & Bemis, 1982). Some of these include idiosyncratic beliefs related to food and weight; specific reasoning errors and disturbed information processing related to the significance given to weight and shape; the role of cultural influences in the development and maintenance of beliefs about weight and shape; positive and negative cognitive reinforcement contingencies that maintain symptoms; the operation of underlying assumptions, dysfunctional self-schemas, and core beliefs (e.g., low self-esteem, self-identity, perfectionism, pursuit of asceticism, need for self-control, fears of maturity, "anorexic identity," and enteroceptive deficits); and the interaction between psychological and physical aspects of the disorder (i.e., psychological state and starvation symptoms) that make normalizing eating and body weight imperative. Important theoretical contributions were also made by Slade (1982) and Guidano and Liotti (1983) at about the same time. Slade (1982) emphasized the importance of low self-esteem and perfectionism or self-control in the maintenance of anorexia nervosa. Guidano and Liotti took a developmental perspective linking a failure to develop autonomy and self-expression in childhood to later deficits in "personal identity." Therapy is aimed at correcting these deep personal identity structures and little emphasis is placed on food, eating, and weight.

More recently, the cognitive model of anorexia nervosa has been expanded and refined with further articulation of motivational factors (Garner, Vitousek, & Pike, 1997; Garner & Rosen, 1990, 1994; Vitousek, Watson, & Wilson, 1998), information-processing errors (Cooper, 1997b; Channon, Hemsley, & de Silva, 1988; Cooper, Anastasiades, & Fairburn, 1992; Vitousek & Hollon, 1990), individual personality variables (Garner, 1991, 2004a; Vitousek & Manke, 1994), core beliefs (Cooper & Turner, 2000; Leung, Waller, & Thomas, 1999; Waller et al., 2003; Waller, Dickson, & Ohanian, 2002), self-representations (Garner & Bemis, 1985; Garner, Garfinkel, Rockert, & Olmsted, 1987; Vitousek & Ewald, 1993), interpersonal and family maintaining variables (Garner et al., 1997), and the rationale for the longer duration of therapy required to address treatment resistance, achieve an appropriate body weight, and interrupt costly relapses (Garner & Bemis, 1985; Garner et al., 1997; Pike, Loeb, & Vitousek, 1996; Vitousek, 1996). The evidence supporting a cognitive model of eating disorders has been reviewed in detail elsewhere (Cooper, 1997b; Vitousek, 1996).

This broad-based cognitive therapy for anorexia nervosa has also been applied to treatment-resistant bulimia nervosa (Garner, 1986); however, it contrasts with the well-established, time-limited, and focused approach to bulimia nervosa described by Fairburn and colleagues (Fairburn, 1981, 1985; Fairburn, Marcus, & Wilson, 1993; Fairburn et al., 1995).

RELEVANT DIAGNOSTIC ISSUES

A look at potential unique cognitive vulnerabilities to anorexia nervosa requires an understanding of the limitations imposed by the current diagnostic classification system for eating disorders. The *DSM–IV–TR* (APA, 2000) separates the two main eating disorders, anorexia and bulimia nervosa, into mutually exclusive categories based largely on the basis of a somewhat arbitrary body weight threshold (Walsh & Garner, 1997). Moreover, the *DSM–IV* approach of categorizing bulimia nervosa may require a frequency threshold for binge eating and self-induced vomiting that is overly stringent, thereby failing to adequately capture the spectrum of clinically relevant eating disorder symptoms (Sullivan, Bulik, & Kendler, 1998). There is also a danger in conceptualizing these disorders as separate entities in evaluating cognitive functioning because it is well established that some patients move between the diagnostic categories at different points in time, regardless of whether or not they have received treatment (Eddy et al., 2002; Herzog et al., 1999; Russell, 1979). Moreover, studies not only indicate similarities between anorexia and bulimia nervosa on a wide range of psychological measures, but also extraordinary heterogeneity on these same measures within each diagnostic group (Cachelin & Maher, 1998; Garner, Garner, & Rosen, 1993; Garner, Garfinkel, & O'Shaughnessy, 1985; Oliosi & Dalle Grave, 2003).

CONTEXT FOR COGNITIVE VULNERABILITY: MULTIDETERMINED MODEL OF EATING DISORDERS

The examination of cognitive vulnerability to anorexia nervosa must be placed in the broader theoretical context of the accumulating evidence that eating disorders are multidetermined and heterogeneous in nature. Most models assume that eating disorders develop and are maintained by cultural, individual (developmental, psychological, biological, and exposure to adverse life events), and familial predisposing or risk factors. As indicated in Fig. 14.1, these have been hypothesized to converge in different combinations and interactions resulting in restrictive dieting aimed at achieving a greater sense of self-control or self-worth (Garner, 1993; Garner & Garfinkel, 1980; Tylka & Subich, 2004). Once weight loss is achieved, the anorexia nervosa is maintained, in part, by the cognitive, emotional, and physical effects of "starvation symptoms" on the individual (Garner, 1997). Certain risk factors are not easily differentiated into classes of predisposing, precipitating, or perpetuating factors and the precise mechanism of action for many known risks remains elusive. The period of vulnerability for certain risk factors is fixed because of their nature (e.g., gender, ethnicity, or birth complications), whereas others may exert their influence at multiple points in the development and maintenance of

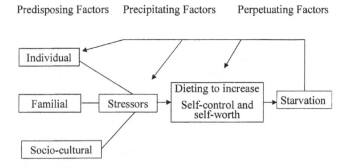

FIG. 14.1. Causal and maintaining factors in eating disorders. Adapted from "Pathogenesis of anorexia nervosa" by D. M. Garner, 1993, *The Lancet, 341*, pp. 1631–1635; and "Socio-cultural factors in the development of anorexia nervosa" by D. M. Garner and P. E. Garfinkel, 1980, *Psychological Medicine, 10*, pp. 647–656. Adapted with permission.

the disorder (e.g., family dieting or a genetic liability for perfectionism). Table 14.1 lists predisposing or risk factors that have received the most solid empirical support through both cross-sectional and longitudinal studies (Fairburn & Harrison, 2003; Garner, 1993; Jacobi, Hayward, de Zwaan, Kraemer, & Agras, 2004; Stice, 2002). This chapter focuses on a subset of risk factors relevant to cognitive vulnerability to anorexia nervosa.

CULTURE AND COGNITIVE VULNERABILITY

Cognitive functioning does not occur in a vacuum but is highly influenced by the cultural context. Of the variables identified as risk factors for anorexia nervosa, sociocultural pressures to be thin have probably received the most theoretical attention (Blowers, Loxton, Grady-Flesser, Occhipinti, & Dawe, 2003; Brown et al., 2003; Garner & Garfinkel, 1980; Garner, Garfinkel, Schwartz, & Thompson, 1980; Ghaderi, 2003; Gordon, 2001; Wardle & Watters, 2004; Wiseman, Gray, Mosimann, & Ahrens, 1992). The rise in eating disorders in Western culture has been attributed to societal modernization, gendered-linked opportunities and constraints, as well as the mass media's emphasis on ultra-thinness as a standard for beauty (Garner et al., 1980; Gordon, 2001). Eating disorders are more common in Western countries; however, increasing Westernization and globalization has been implicated in the development of eating disorders in non-Western countries (Abou-Saleh, Younis, & Karim, 1998). As young women from other more weight-tolerant cultures (e.g., Egyptian, Japanese, and Chinese) are assimilated into "thinness-conscious" Western culture, they become more fearful of fatness, and eating disorder symptoms proliferate (Dolan, 1991; A. M. Lee & S. Lee, 1996).

TABLE 14.1
Major Risk Factors Identified for Anorexia Nervosa

Risk Factors for Eating Disorders	Potency
SOCIOCULTURAL	
Living in Western Society	√√√
Sports Emphasizing Slimness	√√√
INDIVIDUAL: FIXED & BEHAVIORAL	
Female Gender	√√√
Ethnicity	√√
Higher body weight	√√√
Restrictive Dieting	√√√
High Levels of Exercise	√√
Alcohol / Drug Abuse	√

(Continued)

TABLE 14.1
(Continued)

Risk Factors for Eating Disorders	Potency
INDIVIDUAL: TRAITS / CORE BELIEFS / SCHEMAS	
Drive for Thinness	√√√
Body Dissatisfaction & Weight Concerns	√√√
Body Misperception	√
Low Self-Esteem or Ineffectiveness	√√√
Depression	√√
Perfectionism	√√√
Asceticism / Self-Sacrifice	√
Obsessive Compulsive Traits	√√√
Anxiety / Worry	√√
Interpersonal Insecurity / Alienation / Attachment Deficits	√√
Fears of Psychobiological Maturity	√
Harm-Avoidant Temperament	√
Low Interoceptive Awareness	√√
Emotional Regulation Problems (over- or under-control)	√√
Anger	√√
INDIVIDUAL: COGNITIVE PROCESSING	
Reasoning Errors	√√√
Information Processing / Attentional Bias	√√
Neuropsychological Deficits	√
GENETIC FACTORS	√√√
INDIVIDUAL DEVELOPMENTAL	
Early Childhood Feeding Problems	√
Pregnancy Complications / Premature Birth	√
Childhood Anxiety Problems	√
Childhood Obesity	√
Early Puberty	√
Age: Adolescence	√√
ADVERSE LIFE EVENTS	
Physical Abuse or Neglect	√√
Sexual Abuse	√√
Bullying and Teasing	√√
Physical Illness	√
Weight Loss in Adolescence	√√
PARENTAL RISK FACTORS	
Obesity	√
Dieting	√√
Mother with an Eating Disorder	√√√
Critical Comments about Weight	√√
High Levels of Exercise	√
High Performance Expectations	√
Over-Concern / Hypervigilance	√
Depression	√
Low Contact / Neglect / Conflict	√
Substance Misuse	√

Note. Estimate based on summary data from: Jacobi, Hayward, de Zwaan, Kraemer, and Agras (2004); Stice (2002); Fairburn and Harrison (2003). √ = Low. √√ = Medium. √√√ = High.

Pressures on women to conform to the ultra-slender body ideal of feminine beauty have intensified over the past 50 years. To illustrate this trend, Garner et al. (1980) documented the progressive decline in weights and narrowing of shapes of *Playboy* centerfolds and Miss America contestants between 1959 and 1979; there was also an increase in diet-for-weight-loss advertisements in popular women's magazines during the same time period. When evaluated against weight norms, just over 5% of female life-insurance policyholders between age 20 and 29 were as thin as the average Miss America Pageant winner between 1970 and 1978 (Garner et al., 1980). Wiseman et al. (1992) found that these trends continued over the subsequent decade.

Garner and Garfinkel (1978, 1980) reasoned that if cultural pressures to be slim and diet contribute to the expression of anorexia nervosa, then the disorder should be overrepresented in ballet students and fashion models, due to the demands to maintain a low weight to meet performance or appearance standards. In a study of 183 professional ballet students from several different schools, they found that 6.5% of the sample met rigorous diagnostic criteria for anorexia nervosa and students from the most competitive schools had the highest incidence of the disorder. Moreover, 38% of the dance sample had elevated scores on a measure of symptoms common in anorexia nervosa.

Although traditionally it was believed that eating disorders were "culture specific" to White, middle-class women (Silber, 1986), it is now well recognized that eating problems and disorders occur in minority populations. Wildes, Emery, and Simons (2001) conducted a meta-analysis of 35 studies of eating disturbance and body dissatisfaction in White and non-White populations and found that Whites experienced greater body dissatisfaction than their non-White counterparts; however, they concluded that these differences have been historically overemphasized. In a study comparing the prevalence and correlates of body dissatisfaction among White, Hispanic, and Asian sixth- and seventh-grade girls, Robinson et al. (1996) found that Hispanic girls reported significantly greater body dissatisfaction than White girls, with Asian girls in-between. However, after adjusting for body mass index (weight/height^2), normal and overweight White, Hispanic, and Asian girls reported similar levels of body dissatisfaction. Body mass index was the strongest independent predictor of increased body dissatisfaction in all three ethnic groups.

ASSESSMENT OF COGNITIVE VULNERABILITY

A central tenet of the cognitive theory of anorexia nervosa is that certain idiosyncratic self-statements, automatic thoughts, and underlying assumptions about food, eating, weight, and shape become interactive with more general core beliefs, underlying assumptions, and self-schemata. Before presenting the evidence, it is important to briefly review the major methods of assessing beliefs about weight, shape, and dieting.

Self-Report Measurement

There has been a proliferation of self-report measures of weight, shape, and eating concerns in recent years, making a full review of methods well beyond the scope of this chapter. The reader is encouraged to consult more comprehensive sources for further information (Craighead, 2002). The advantage of self-report measures is that they provide an efficient and economical means of sampling beliefs about weight and shape for clinical and research purposes. Self-report measures should not be used as the sole basis for diagnostic and treatment decisions; however, they do have advantages of economical administration and actuarial scoring. They also minimize interviewer bias and other potential threats to validity that stem from responses derived from the interaction between the interviewer and the participant. The two most widely used self-reports are the Eating Attitudes Test (Garner, Olmsted, Bohr, & Garfinkel, 1982) and the Eating Disorder Inventory (Garner, 1991, 2004a; Garner, Olmsted, & Polivy, 1983). The 26-item version of the Eating Attitudes Test (EAT-26) provides factor scores for "dieting," "bulimia and food preoccupation," and "oral control."

The Eating Disorder Inventory-3 (EDI-3; Garner, 2004a) consists of 91 items from the EDI-2 (Garner, 1991) organized onto 12 primary scales, consisting of three eating disorder–specific scales and nine scales that assess core beliefs or psychological constructs highly relevant to, but not specific to, eating disorders (see Table 14.2). The eating disorder–specific scales—Drive for Thinness, Bulimia, and Body Dissatisfaction—have been used as operational measures of eating and weight concerns in a large number of cross-sectional and longitudinal studies on cognitive vulnerability to eating disorders (Garner, 2004a; Jacobi et al., 2004). The EDI-3 Referral Form is an adaptation of these three scales, along with self-reported weight and eating symptoms, used specifically for case finding and screening for eating disorders (Garner, 2004b).

Self-report measures have several limitations. First, it has been pointed out that they are vulnerable to bias related to demand characteristics, denial, and distortion (Vitousek, Daly, & Heiser, 1991). Second, they are not geared to distinguish qualitatively different meaning systems that can be activated by the same verbal behavior. According to Teasdale and Barnard (1993), lower level beliefs (propositional) do not evoke emotion and have a much weaker effect on behavior than emotion-laden beliefs (implicational). Thus, the self-statement "I feel fat" can be a simple statement of

TABLE 14.2
Constructs Assessed by the Eating Disorder Inventory-3

Eating Disorder Inventory-3
Eating Disorder Risk Scales
Drive for thinness (DT)
Bulimia (B)
Body dissatisfaction (BD)
Psychological Scales
Low self-esteem (LSE)
Personal alienation (PA)
Interpersonal insecurity (II)
Interpersonal alienation (IA)
Interoceptive deficits (ID)
Emotional dysregulation (ED)
Perfectionism (P)
Asceticism (A)
Maturity fears (MF)
Composite Scales[1]
Eating disorder risk composite (EDRC)
Ineffectiveness composite (IC)
Interpersonal problems composite (IPC)
Affective problems composite (APC)
Overcontrol composite (OC)
General psychological maladjustment composite (GPMC)
Response Style Indicators[1]
Inconsistency (IN)
Infrequency (IF)
Negative impression (NI)

[1]Composite scales and Response Style Indicators are new to the EDI-3.

fact (propositional belief) or it can imply a self-schemata imbued with intense emotions, leading to overwhelming feelings of inadequacy (implicational belief). Finally, self-report measures cover only conscious experiences and may not be useful for examining thought processes that lie outside of immediate awareness.

Semi-Structured Interviews for Assessing Beliefs About Weight and Shape

Semi-structured interviews have the advantage of allowing the clinician to achieve greater precision in distinguishing concerns about weight and shape that are of clinical proportions from those that may not be indicative of a formal eating disorder. A number of structured interviews have been developed in recent years; however, the Eating Disorder Examination (EDE; Fairburn & Cooper, 1993) is the best validated and has generated a large body of research. It is an investigator-based semi-structured interview for assessing psychopathology specific to eating disorders. Responses are organized on four subscales (i.e., Restraint, Eating Concern, Shape Concern, and Weight Concern). The EDE has the advantages of allowing a fine-grained appraisal of the specific psychopathology of eating disorders with investigator probes to clarify the meaning behind question responses. Disadvantages of the interview include the fact that it takes an hour or more to administer, it requires a trained interviewer, and it is not suitable when anonymity or group administration is required. Also, it assesses only a narrow range of eating variables without tapping psychological constructs that have been shown to be important in the development and maintenance of eating disorders.

Unstructured Interviews

The content of structured interviews is restricted to cognitive constructs narrowly defined by the investigator. They also rely on retrospective reports that may not correspond to a moment-by-moment representation of thinking patterns or cognitive style. More unstructured methods have been proposed to capture relevant cognitive domains, as well as the valence of concerns regarding food, weight, and shape (Cooper, 1997b). Thoughts Checklists and concurrent verbalization have been used with some success (Cooper & Fairburn, 1992); however, unstructured interviews are limited by yielding data that are not as easy to analyze as standardized self-report measures. Moreover, they are time consuming, and some participants might find them to be overly intrusive.

Measures of Information Processing

Cognitive vulnerability to anorexia nervosa has also pointed to systematic errors in information processing—such as selective attention, confirmatory bias, selective memory around weight-related issues, and body-size misperception—that may play a role in maintaining symptoms in a relatively automatic manner (Cooper, 1997a; Garner & Bemis, 1982; Vitousek & Hollon, 1990). Selective information processing has been assessed in anorexia nervosa using the Stroop Color-Naming Task (1935), which involves presenting participants with cards containing words printed in different colors (see Cooper, 1997b). The instructions are to name the colors in which the words are printed while ignoring the meaning of the words. Based on information-processing theory, the premise is that there will be more color-naming interference, reflected by greater response latencies, for words that have a greater personal significance for the individual. Other methods have been used to examine selective retrieval of memory concepts related to food, body weight, and shape such as questionnaires designed to assess interpretation of ambiguous scenarios (Cooper, 1997a), essays with weight-related content (King, Polivy, & Herman, 1991), word-stem completion tasks (Hermans, Pieters, & Eelen, 1999), and electro-physiological measures such as event-related evoked potentials (Dodin & Nandrino, 2003).

Measures of Perceptual Distortion

Body-size misperception was described by Bruch (1962) as a core feature of anorexia nervosa; however, there has been controversy about whether op-erational measures of this construct assess phenomena that are "percep-tual," "conceptual," or a mixture of both (Cash & Deagle, 1997; Cash & Pruzinsky, 2002; Garner & Garfinkel, 1981). Distorted body-size perception in anorexia nervosa has been measured primarily by body-part size estima-tion (Slade & Russell, 1973) and whole-body techniques (Garner, Garfinkel, Stancer, & Moldofsky, 1976). In a meta-analysis of body image studies, Cash and Deagle (1997) found that whole-body methodologies produced larger clinical-control effect-size differences than body-part methods.

BODY IMAGE DISTURBANCE AND ANOREXIA NERVOSA

The importance of body image in anorexia nervosa is reflected in its inclu-sion in the diagnostic criteria for anorexia nervosa in the *Diagnostic and Statistical Manual of Mental Disorders* (*DSM–IV*, APA, 1994): "an intense fear of gaining weight or becoming fat, even though underweight" [APA, p. 544] and "disturbance in the way in which one's body weight or shape is experienced, undue influence of body weight or shape on self-evalu-ation, or denial of the seriousness of current low body weight" (p. 545).

   This criterion reflects the view that the body image construct is multidi-mensional, involving disturbances in cognitive-evaluative as well as in-formation-processing domains. Both forms of body image disturbance have been the subjects of extensive research using a wide range of meas-urement techniques (Cash & Deagle, 1997; Garner & Garfinkel, 1981).

   Even though there is widespread acceptance that body image is a key concept in anorexia nervosa, there have been some who have argued that it is largely culture bound and should be dropped from the current re-quired diagnostic criteria (S. Lee, 1995; Palmer, 1993). Keel and Klump (2003) concluded that cultural factors may play a greater role in the pathogenesis of bulimia than in anorexia nervosa, based on a review of historical, epidemiological, and genetic evidence. Nevertheless, reviews of cross-sectional and longitudinal research have found that body dissatisfaction and weight concerns, operationalized by various measurement techniques, are potent risk factors for the development of a continuum of disordered eating patterns, with restrictive dieting with anorexia nervosa representing the extreme (Jacobi et al., 2004; Stice, 2002).

Perceptual Body-Size Distortion

Bruch (1962) described distorted body-size perception as a core feature of anorexia nervosa. The discrepancy between the patients' mental picture of their body and their actual appearance provides compelling clinical evidence for a perceptual disturbance. In the face of obsessive focus on the body, as well as an intellectual understanding that they are horribly underweight, many anorexia nervosa patients really do appear to overestimate their body size. This remarkable clinical observation has resulted in decades of research aimed at operationally defining and studying body-size misperception in anorexia nervosa.

Clinical observations of body image disturbance in anorexia nervosa have led to at least two different operational measures of size misperception: body-part size estimation procedures that involve estimation of the width or depth of specific regions of the body (i.e., face, chest, hips, etc.), and whole-body techniques that involve the estimation of the whole-body size using a distorted image of the subject's own body. In a meta-analysis of body image studies, Cash and Deagle (1997) found that whole-body methodologies produced larger clinical control effect-size differences than body-part methods. According to this analysis, the average eating disordered patient distorts her size to a greater extent than about 73% of controls. The explanation for the modest advantage of the whole-body techniques is not clear, but may relate to the fact that these methods involve direct exposure to one's self-image rather than the more indirect estimation of the width of a particular body region. This may induce a heightened negative emotional experience related to body size and may magnify the self-size distortion. Moreover, perceptual distortion differences between eating disordered and control subjects do not seem to reflect a generalized sensory-perceptual deficit because eating disorder patients and controls do not differ in object-size appraisals (Cash & Deagle, 1997).

Smeets, Ingleby, Hoek, and Panhuysen (1999) proposed two possible explanations for observed size overestimation in anorexia nervosa. The first is that size overestimation reflects pure visual misperception. In this case, patients retrieve a fatter image of themselves from visual memory and self-estimations reflect this image. The second explanation attributes size misperception to the reconstruction of visual representations based on particular thoughts and feelings. In this case, size distortion of the visual body image is one of memory rather than of perception. The inability of anorexic patients to "perceive" themselves accurately may be related to impaired hemispheric symmetry in storing visual representations of the body or to impaired interhemispheric interaction with reduced right hemispheric updating of body image that is maintained by the left hemisphere.

In summary, in their meta-analytic review of the size estimation research, Cash and Deagle (1997) concluded that body-size overestimation tends to be "relatively weak, unstable, or nonpathognomic" among eating disorder patients (p. 177). It can be influenced by negative mood states, viewing thin images of women in the media, and perceived overeating. These findings are consistent with the understanding of body-size overestimation as a form of information-processing bias that reflects a cognitive judgment rather than a purely perceptual event (Cooper, 1997b). Epstein et al. (2001) reached this conclusion based on results from a controlled study of cognitive and perceptual variables in 20 anorexia nervosa patients. Rather than having a fixed and distorted body image, anorexia nervosa patients may have a loose, unstable, or weak mental representation of their body that is biased by reactivity to cultural ideals for beauty, as well as to cognitive and affective variables. The observation that size misperception is not unique to anorexia nervosa has led Palmer (1993) to conclude that body-size misperception should be dropped from the current diagnostic criteria for anorexia nervosa. Nevertheless, it may be premature to abandon size misperception research entirely because it has been shown to predict higher levels of psychopathology, including external loss of control, low ego strength, and higher levels of depression, introversion, anxiety, physical anhedonia, atypical thinking, eating problems, prior treatment failure, lack of clinical progress, and poor clinical outcomes in anorexia nervosa (see Cash & Pruzinsky, 2002; Thompson, 1996).

BELIEFS RELATED TO EATING, WEIGHT, AND SHAPE

Body dissatisfaction and the desire to lose weight (drive for thinness) are two of the most well-recognized cognitive precursors to dieting and the development of eating disorder symptoms in community samples of preadolescents, adolescents, and adult females (for reviews, see Cash & Deagle, 1997; Jacobi et al., 2004; Stice, 2002; Tylka, 2004). Research has shown that more than 80% of female adolescents often "feel fat" (Greenfield, Quinlan, Harding, Glass, & Bliss, 1987). Fear of fatness is common in girls as young as 6 to 10 years old, and these attitudes and behaviors escalate significantly during adolescence, particularly among those at the heavier end of the weight spectrum (Blowers et al., 2003; Button, Loan, Davies, & Sonuga-Barke, 1997; Davison, Markey, & Birch, 2000; Edlund, Halvarsson, & Sjödén, 1996).

Body dissatisfaction (weight and shape dissatisfaction) is more prevalent in girls and women than in boys and men (McCabe & Ricciardelli, 2004). In a study of 8- to 10-year-olds, Wood, Becker, and Thompson (1996) found that 55% of the girls and 35% of the boys were dissatisfied with their size. These attitudes lead to attempts to lose weight that are also associated with gender. Field and colleagues (1999) surveyed 16,000 boys and girls and reported that 44% of 14-year-old girls and 19% of the boys of the same age were trying to lose weight.

A number of prospective studies have shown that the EDI Body Dissatisfaction and Drive for Thinness scales predict the development of later serious eating disturbances. Both scales have been found to predict the development of severe eating disorder symptoms in high school girls (Killen, Taylor, Hayward, & Haydel, 1996; Leon, Fulkerson, Perry, Keel, & Klump, 1999). A 4-year prospective study of female college undergraduates found that initially high Drive for Thinness scores were related more to subsequent eating disorder symptoms than to depressed mood or ineffectiveness (Dobmeyer & Stein, 2003). In a 10-year prospective study, Joiner, Heatherton, and Keel (1997) found that the Drive for Thinness scale was a consistent, unique, and significant predictor of bulimic symptoms 10 years later, as assessed by the EDI Bulimia scale. Finally, in a 5-year prospective study of newborns and their mothers, Stice, Agras, and Hammer (1999) reported that elevated maternal Drive for Thinness, Bulimia, and Body Dissatisfaction scale scores predicted the emergence of early childhood eating disturbances.

Because the majority of prospective studies have shown that Body Dissatisfaction and Drive for Thinness scales predict restrictive dieting and "eating disorder symptoms" in nonclinical samples, it is important to establish that there is a real connection between restrictive dieting and the actual development of a clinical eating disorder. Patton, Johnson-Sabine, Wood, Mann, and Wakeling (1990) reported that the risk of developing an eating disorder is almost eight times higher in adolescent females classified as "dieters" compared to "nondieters" and, in a more recent study, "severe dieters" were shown to have an 18 times higher risk (Patton, Selzer, Caffey, Carlin, & Wolfe, 1999). Sundgot-Borgen (1994) examined risk factors for eating disorders among 522 elite athletes representing six different groups of sports and found that 117 (22.4%) were classified as "at risk" for an eating disorder, based on scores on the Drive for Thinness and Body Dissatisfaction subscales of the Eating Disorder Inventory. Of the "at-risk" athletes who participated in a clinical interview ($N = 103$), 48% met criteria for anorexia or bulimia nervosa and an additional 41% displayed significant fears of fatness and eating disorder symptoms. The prevalence of eating disorders was greatest in sports that required a thinner shape to meet performance or appearance standards. In a 2-year prospective study of ballet students, Garner et al. (1987) found that Body Dissatisfaction and Drive for Thinness were the only scales on the Eating Disorder Inventory that significantly predicted the development of anorexia nervosa and severely disordered eating patterns.

Nevertheless, understanding the role of body dissatisfaction as a risk factor for anorexia nervosa must reconcile the fact that body dissatisfaction is endemic to young women in Western culture; however, it leads to the expression of eating disorders in only a small fraction of the population. Recent longitudinal research using multivariate models has indicated a complex relationship between body dissatisfaction and various sociocultural, biological, interpersonal, personality, and affective factors that mediate variables. In a study of girls from 10 to 13 years old, Blowers et al. (2003) found that body mass had a direct association with body dissatisfaction, but a more complex model involving media pressure, internalization of the thin ideal, and social comparison improved the prediction of body dissatisfaction. This is consistent with an earlier study by Stice, Schupak-Neuberg, Shaw, and Stein (1994), who found a positive relationship between media exposure to thin ideal body stereotypes and eating disorder symptoms. The results also indicated that this effect was mediated by gender-role endorsement and internalization of the thin body ideal. In a community sample of women, Ghaderi (2003) used structural modeling analysis to develop a risk profile for disordered eating that improved the predictive power of body dissatisfaction by adding measures of low self-esteem, low perceived social support from the family, and escape-avoidance coping. Similarly, Tylka (2004) found that body surveillance, neuroticism, and having a family member or friend with an eating disorder increased the strength of the association between body dissatisfaction and eating disorder symptomatology among college women.

Other self-report measures have documented overconcern with food, weight, and shape in patients with eating disorders. For example, Cooper and Fairburn (1992) used a brief Thoughts Checklist and concurrent verbalization in a study comparing anorexia and bulimia nervosa patients with control groups on three behavioral tasks. Concurrent verbalization results indicated that the patients with eating disorders had more negative self-statements about eating, weight, and shape during the tasks than controls. Moreover, it was concluded that patients with anorexia nervosa showed more concern with eating. These concerns appeared to be qualitatively different from those of the other groups. Cooper and Turner (2000) examined assumptions and beliefs in anorexia nervosa patients, dieters, and female controls using the Eating Disorder Belief Questionnaire (Coo-

per, Cohen-Tovee, Todd, Wells, & Tovee, 1997). Results indicated that anorexia nervosa patients differed in cognitive content and scored higher on
assumptions about weight, shape, eating, and negative self-beliefs as compared to dieters and female controls. Mizes (1992) used the Anorectic
Cognitions Scale to differentiate anorexia and bulimia nervosa patients
from noneating disordered psychiatric controls. A factor analysis of this
measure yielded three meaningful cognitive constructs: perception of
weight and eating as a basis of approval from others, belief that rigid
weight and eating control is fundamental to self-worth, and rigidity of
weight and eating regulation efforts.

In summary, body dissatisfaction, drive for thinness, and other beliefs
about weight, shape, and eating should be considered potent and well-
supported sources of cognitive vulnerability to anorexia nervosa. Body
dissatisfaction and other weight-related beliefs do not uniformly lead to
restrictive dieting, and not all of those who engage in restrictive dieting
develop anorexia nervosa. Therefore, a further understanding of these
complex relationships needs to include a wide range of variables presumed to either amplify or moderate body dissatisfaction and drive for
thinness using improved measurement technology, larger sample sizes,
more powerful analytic methods (e.g., structural modeling and other
multivariate techniques), and longitudinal designs.

CORE BELIEFS, UNDERLYING ASSUMPTIONS,
AND SELF-SCHEMATA

The schematic content of self-concept deficits and the adaptive functions
they serve have been central to the cognitive conceptualization of anorexia nervosa (Garner, 1986; Garner & Bemis, 1982, 1985; Garner &
Rosen, 1990; Guidano & Liotti, 1983; Vitousek & Ewald, 1993; Vitousek &
Hollon, 1990). Vitousek and Ewald (1993) organized self-concept deficits
that are characteristic of anorexia nervosa into three broad clusters of variables: the unworthy self, the perfectible self, and the overwhelmed self.
The *unworthy self* is characterized by low self-esteem, feelings of helplessness, a poorly developed sense of identity, a tendency to seek external ver-
ification, extreme sensitivity to criticism, and conflicts over autonomy/
dependence. The second cluster, the *perfectible self*, includes perfectionism,
grandiosity, asceticism, and a "New Year's resolution" cognitive style.
The third cluster, the *overwhelmed self*, is characterized by a preference for
simplicity, a preference for certainty, and a tendency to retreat from complex or intense social environments. According to Vitousek and Ewald
(1993), these self-concept deficits are not specific to anorexia nervosa;

however, their linkage to beliefs about body weight and shape constitutes a vulnerability to this eating disorder.

Low Self-Esteem and Ineffectiveness

Bruch (1962) was the first to describe "all pervasive feelings of ineffectiveness" as a central feature in eating disorders. According to cognitive theory, anorexia nervosa is crystallized when the belief that "it is absolutely essential that I become thin" becomes inexorably tied to the regulation of self-esteem (i.e., weight, shape, or thinness) and serves "as the sole or predominant referent for inferring personal value or self-worth" (Garner & Bemis, 1982, p. 142). The main theories of anorexia nervosa have linked these cognitive variables regarding body weight, size, and shape to more general core beliefs related to the self such as guilt, poor self-esteem, and fears of biological maturity (Garner & Bemis, 1982, 1985).

Support for the role of more general negative core beliefs in anorexia nervosa comes from Clark (1992), who found that these patients express more depressive beliefs about the self and the future than controls. Marshall, Palmer, and Stretch (1993) demonstrated that anorexia nervosa patients express more negative beliefs related to guilt, self-esteem, and self-evaluation compared to normal controls.

Theoretical formulations regarding the critical role of low self-esteem in the development and maintenance of disordered eating patterns have received empirical support in a growing number of longitudinal studies of children and adolescents (Fairburn & Harrison, 2003; Garner, 1993; Jacobi et al., 2004; Quadflieg & Fichter, 2003; Steiger, Israel, Gauvin, Ng Ying Kin, & Young, 2003). Leon et al. (1999) found that low self-esteem was a significant predictor of the development of disordered eating in both girls and boys. In a 2-year prospective study, low self-esteem was a predictor of binge eating in adolescent girls (Stice, Presnell, & Spangler, 2002). Fichter, Quadflieg, and Rehm (2003) reported that low self-esteem at the beginning of treatment predicted poor outcome in a 6-year followup of anorexia nervosa patients. In a long-term outcome study of anorexia nervosa, Löwe et al. (2001) found that elevated scores on the EDI Ineffectiveness scale predicted poor outcome. Low self-esteem and frequency of maternal dieting have been found to predict dieting awareness in young girls (Hill & Pallin, 1998).

There is evidence that self-esteem is not a unitary construct; it has been conceptualized as having two distinct factors: self-liking and self-competence. In a study of female participants from a high risk population, Silvera et al. (1998) found a strong relationship between eating disorders and self-liking but not self-competence. This is in contrast to Bers and Quinlan (1992), who reported that anorexia nervosa patients scored significantly higher on a measure of perceived competence deficits compared to nonclinical and psychiatric samples.

Based on factor analytic studies of several large samples of patients with eating disorders, Garner (2004a) differentiated the "ineffectiveness" construct assessed on earlier versions of the EDI into two related constructs represented by scales on the recent revision of the instrument—the EDI-3 (Garner, 2004a). The EDI-3 Low Self-Esteem scale assesses low self-liking and the Personal Alienation scale measures a pervasive sense of emotional emptiness, aloneness, and a poor sense of self-understanding. The summed T-scores on these scales form the Ineffectiveness Composite scale (Garner, 2004a). This distinction is consistent with earlier studies using multiple measures of self-concept in anorexia nervosa. Wagner, Halmi, and Maguire (1987) compared eating disorder patients and nonclinical controls and found that the patients experienced distinct and specific difficulties in the areas of social ineffectiveness, personal independence, and self-esteem. Similarly, Butow, Beumont, and Touyz (1993) found that eating disorder patients described themselves with constructs such as feelings of inadequacy, worthlessness, and insecurity as well as a sense of social isolation.

Cooper, Todd, and Wells (1998) compared eating disorder patients with nonclinical controls using a semi-structured interview to investigate the link between negative self-evaluation and specific beliefs about weight, shape, and eating. The link between these two domains was identified, but only for the patient group. Most patients reported that they could identify specific origins for their negative self-evaluation, and these typically included teasing or criticism from family members, peers, and teachers, or excessive emphasis on food and eating at home or at school. All patients believed that dieting was a way of counteracting the negative implications associated with their self-beliefs. Assumptions about weight and shape were found to distinguish patients with anorexia nervosa, dieters, and female controls in another study by Cooper and Turner (2000) using the Eating Disorder Belief Questionnaire. They found that patients scored higher than the other two groups on assumptions about weight and shape, assumptions about eating, and negative self-beliefs, whereas the dieters scored higher than the female controls on assumptions about weight and shape. In sum, a number of different methods have provided support for the main cognitive theory of anorexia nervosa, namely that patients exhibit self-statements, automatic thoughts, and underlying assumptions that reflect undue concern with food and eating, weight, and shape.

Cooper (1997a) found that eating disorders appear to be associated with biased judgments involving the self. Patients with anorexia and bulimia nervosa were compared to female controls on questionnaires that were designed to assess interpretation of ambiguous scenarios with either a negative or positive outcome. When events had a negative outcome, the patients responded spontaneously to open-ended questions with a weight and shape interpretation. Later, in a forced-choice format, they selected the weight and shape interpretation in preference to interpretations not connected to weight and shape. In both open-ended and forced-choice format, this bias was specific to judgments involving the self. When events had a positive outcome, the bias was reversed and, in the two formats, it was found only in judgments involving others. In both cases (i.e., for negative self-referent events and for positive other-referent events), patients predicted that weight and shape explanations were more likely. Both groups of patients estimated that negative outcomes involving the self would be more costly. The patients with bulimia nervosa also estimated that positive outcomes involving the self would be more beneficial.

Perfectionism

The association between perfectionism and anorexia nervosa appears to be particularly robust. It has been found to predate the onset of the disorder (Fairburn, Cooper, Doll, & Welch, 1999), is present during the acute phase (Garner et al., 1983; Halmi et al., 2000), persists well after recovery (Bastiani, Rao, Weltzin, & Kaye, 1995; Sullivan, Bulik, Fear, & Pickering, 1998; Srinivasagam et al., 1995; Sutandar-Pinnock et al., 2003), runs in families (Woodside et al., 2002), and generally predicts poor outcome (Bizeul, Sadowsky, & Rigaud, 2001; Löwe et al., 2001; Sutandar-Pinnock et al., 2003). Perfectionism was commonly considered to be characteristic of the restricting type of anorexia nervosa (Casper, 1990; Strober, 1980); however, studies comparing the different types of the disorder have shown that the Perfectionism scale of the EDI is elevated in the binge-eating/purging type, along with other indicators of severity of the disorder (Garner, Garner, & Rosen, 1993; Halmi et al., 2000).

The structure of perfectionism has been examined and found to be multidimensional in several studies. Joiner and Schmidt (1995) used a confirmatory factor analysis (CFA) of the EDI Perfectionism scale to demonstrate that the items on this scale are best represented by a multidimensional factor structure with three EDI Self-Oriented Perfectionism (EDI-SOP) items and three EDI Socially Prescribed Perfectionism (EDI-SPP) items. Similar dimensions to perfectionism were proposed by Hewitt and Flett (1991). The multidimensional model of perfectionism was extended by Sherry, Hewitt, Besser, McGee, and Flett (2004), who used CFA and structural equation modeling (SEM) to support a two-factor model defined by three EDI-SOP and three EDI-SPP items. Using data from a sample of male and female university students, they found this model to provide a better fit for the data than a unidimensional model.

The EDI-SOP and EDI-SPP were independently related to eating disorder symptoms. For women, they found that the interaction between EDI-SOP and EDI-SPP significantly predicted eating disorder symptoms, and a greater level of EDI-SPP increased the impact of EDI-SOP on eating disorders. Even though the EDI-SOP and EDI-SPP dimensions were strongly intercorrelated, it was stressed that not distinguishing these items from each other would suppress independent information from each dimension and interactive information between both dimensions. Sherry, Hewitt, Besser, McGee, and Flett (2004) suggested that the SOP and SPP Perfectionism factors provide a measure to test competing theories regarding the relative impact of the self-oriented "clinical perfectionism" concept proposed by Shafran, Cooper, and Fairburn (2002) or socially prescribed perfectionism, as proposed by Bruch (1982). A study of paired and unpaired twins by Tozzi et al. (2004) supported the multidimensional conceptualization of perfectionism and found evidence of heritability for all three subscales of the Multidimensional Perfectionism Scale (Frost, Marten, Lahart, & Rosenblate, 1990) with the greatest heritability associated with the "concern with mistakes" scale.

Obsessionality

Even after recovery from the disorder, many anorexia nervosa patients remain rigid, perfectionistic, and obsessional (Casper, 1990; Strober, 1980). As many as 69% of restricters and 44% of the binging/purging anorexia nervosa subgroups have a concurrent diagnosis of obsessive-compulsive disorder (OCD; Halmi et al., 1991). Using the Multidimensional Personality Questionnaire, Casper (1990) found that restricting anorexia nervosa patients were particularly prone to self-control, behavioral constraint, inhibition of emotionality, and conscientiousness. These traits were present when patients were actively symptomatic with their disorder as well as when recovered. These results are consistent with other studies, using the Tridimensional Personality Questionnaire (Cloninger, Przybeck, & Svrakic, 1991), indicating that restricting anorexia nervosa patients are inhibited, overcontrolled, perfectionistic, and obsessional (Brewerton, Hand, & Bishop, 1993; Casper, Hedeker, & McClough, 1992; Srinivasagam et al., 1995). Importantly, restricting anorexia nervosa patients do not seem to have the types of obsessional target symptoms (e.g., compulsive checking or sexual obsessions) that are commonly reported for people with ego-dystonic OCD. Rather, the obsessive-compulsive symptoms in anorexia nervosa tend to focus on the obsessive need for order, symmetry, exactness, and arranging (Matsunaga et al., 1999; Srinivasagam et al., 1995). Wade, Bulik, Neale, and Kendler (2000) reported a modest correlation in the genetic liabilities for anorexia nervosa and major depression, suggesting a genetic liability that predisposes an individual to both disorders.

There is evidence of a genetic contribution to cognitive vulnerability expressed in terms of personality and temperamental traits such as obsessionality, perfectionism, rigidity, harm avoidance, and depression (Bulik, Sullivan, Weltzin, & Kaye, 1995; Enoch et al., 1998; Wade et al., 2000).

Asceticism

Asceticism can be expressed through dieting as a form of purification, thinness as virtue, and fasting as an act of penitence. Rejection of food or "oral self-restraint" may be part of a more general theme of renunciation of physical gratification described in anorexia nervosa (Rampling, 1985). This may take the form of purposeful sleep deprivation, self-inflicted pain through cutting or picking at skin to the point of bleeding, purging, standing for long periods, exercising for atonement, and generally avoiding pleasure. Some clinicians have observed a shift in the psychopathology of eating disorders over the past several decades where "ascetic motives" for weight loss have been replaced by the "drive for thinness" as the most common motivational theme. In a study of restricting anorexia nervosa patients who were assessed at the beginning of inpatient treatment and again 6 months later, Fassino et al. (2001) found that the EDI-2 Asceticism scale predicated poor response to treatment. The Asceticism scale has been preserved on the revised EDI-3 based on factor analytic studies of multiple samples of eating disorder patients (Garner, 2004a).

Interoceptive Deficits

Confusion and mistrust related to affective and bodily functioning have been repeatedly described as an important characteristic of those who develop eating disorders. Bruch (1962) was the first to suggest that a "lack of interoceptive awareness" is central to the understanding of eating disorders. Interoceptive deficits, as measured by the EDI Interoceptive Awareness subscale, have been shown to predict poor prognosis in patients with anorexia nervosa in long-term follow-up studies (Bizeul et al., 2001; Löwe et al., 2001). This scale has been refined on the revised EDI-3 and its replacement, the Interoceptive Deficits scale, has improved psychometric qualities (Garner, 2004a).

Poor Impulse Control

For more than 20 years, variations in impulse control have been described as a cognitive style that differentiates subgroups of eating disorder patients. Patients with bulimic symptoms (bulimia nervosa and the binge-eating/purging subtypes) have been characterized as emotionally labile and impulsive in contrast to restricting anorexia nervosa patients who tend to be more emotionally inhibited and obsessional (Casper, Eckert, Halmi, Goldberg, & Davis, 1980; Garfinkel, Moldofsky, & Garner, 1980). Toner, Garfinkel, and Garner (1987) used the Matching Familiar Figures Test (MFFT; Kagan, Rosman, Day, Albert, & Phillips, 1964) to compare the cognitive style of bulimic and nonbulimic patients along the impulsive-reflective dimension and found that the bulimic anorexia nervosa patients made significantly more errors and had significantly longer response latencies compared to restricting anorexia nervosa patients. Kaye, Bastiani, and Moss (1995) also used the MFFT and found that restricting anorexia nervosa patients had longer latencies but did not differ in errors compared to a small group of bulimia nervosa patients. Thus, these studies indicate that the relatively slow and accurate cognitive style of restricting patients is consistent with the clinical observation of these patients as being reflective and careful in analyzing new information. This is in contrast to bulimic patients who tend to be cognitively more impulsive in their approach to problem-solving tasks.

Although there are diagnostic subgroup differences on these variables, it is important to emphasize that there is extraordinary heterogeneity of the impulsivity trait within each diagnostic subgroup (Garner, 2004a; Garner, Olmsted, & Garfinkel, 1985). Moreover, both impulsive and compulsive traits can both occur in the same patient, regardless of diagnostic subgroup (Favaro & Santonastaso, 1998, 1999; Steiger et al., 2003).

Maturity Fears

Crisp (1965, 1997) proposed that the central cognitive vulnerability in anorexia nervosa relates to psychobiological maturity associated with an adult weight. According to this view, weight loss becomes the mechanism for avoiding adolescent turmoil, conflicts, and developmental expectations because it results in a return to prepubertal appearance and hormonal status.

Elevated scores on the EDI Maturity Fears scale have been found to predict poor outcome in several studies of anorexia nervosa. In a 6-month follow-up of restricting anorexia nervosa patients, Fassino et al. (2001) found that Maturity Fears predicted a poor outcome. Carter, Blackmore, Sutandar-Pinnock, and Woodside (2004) compared relapsed and non-relapsed anorexia nervosa patients with a mean survival time of 18 months and found significant group-by-time interaction for the Maturity Fears and other EDI subscales. Both relapsed and nonrelapsed groups showed a significant reduction in Maturity Fears from admission to discharge, but scores increased significantly from discharge to follow-up among relapsed patients. Thus, fears of psychobiological maturity may reflect cognitive vulnerability to anorexia nervosa, but the evidence is weak at this time.

Core Beliefs Assessed by the Young Schema Questionnaire (YSQ)

Leung, Waller, and Thomas (1999) used the Young Schema Questionnaire (YSQ; Young, 1994) to compare restricting and binge-eating/purging anorexia nervosa patients with bulimia nervosa patients and normal controls. They found eating disorder diagnostic subgroups were similar on core beliefs measured by YSQ subscales and that all eating disorder groups scored higher than controls on 15 out of 16 YSQ subscales. Thus, certain core beliefs are clearly associated with eating disorders; however, those assessed by the YSQ do not appear to meaningfully differentiate between diagnostic subgroups. In a subsequent study of the relationship between the YSQ and the EDI-2 scales, Waller et al. (2002) found that "unrelenting standards" beliefs of the YSQ were associated with the Interoceptive Awareness and Impulse Regulation subscales of the EDI-2. The abandonment, emotional inhibition, mistrust/abuse, and social isolation core beliefs measured by the YSQ had the most consistent links to the EDI-2 psychological scales. They found there were no associations with the EDI-2 subscales and dependence/incompetence beliefs, but that emotional inhibition was associated with a wide range of EDI-2 psychological scales. Their findings supported a multidetermined and multidimensional view of the underlying causal and maintenance factors involved in eating disorders, which is compatible with theoretical and clinical suggestions that core beliefs should be treated as central triggers for eating disturbance. Thus, the treatment of eating disorders may depend on addressing unconditional core beliefs as well as cognitions and attitudes, such as low self-esteem and perfectionism, which have a more immediate link to eating disorders.

Waller et al. (2003) established a link between anger and unhealthy core beliefs measured by the YSQ in a comparison between 140 women with eating disorders and 50 nonclinical female college students. The women with eating disorders had higher levels of state anger and anger suppression, especially when they exhibited bulimic symptoms. Although unhealthy core beliefs were associated with higher levels of trait anger in both groups, the association with anger suppression occurred only in the clinical group. This is consistent with Garner (2004a), who found that that hostility on the SCL-90 had significant and robust correlations with all eating and noneating-related scales (except Maturity Fears) on the EDI-3. This was the only external measure in the EDI-3 validation study to have high correlations across the entire range of scales measuring very different psychological domains. This suggests that anger, both expressed and suppressed, is a core belief that needs to be the focus of treatment in anorexia nervosa.

Selective Information Processing

Reasoning errors such as dichotomous thinking, poor tolerance for ambiguity, selective abstraction, personalization, superstitious thinking, magnification, and overgeneralization have been observed clinically in anorexia nervosa and specific therapeutic strategies have been suggested to correct them (Garner & Bemis, 1982, 1985). Systematic cognitive distortions in the processing and interpretation of events (e.g., selective attention, confirmatory bias, and selective memory around weight-related issues) may play a role in maintaining symptoms in a relatively automatic manner (Garner & Bemis, 1982; Vitousek & Hollon, 1990).

Selective information processing has been assessed in anorexia nervosa using the Stroop Color-Naming Task (Stroop, 1935), which involves presenting participants with cards containing words printed in different colors. The instructions are to name the colors in which the words are printed while ignoring the meaning of the words. Based on information-processing theory, the premise is that there will be more color-naming interference, reflected by greater response latencies, for words that have a greater personal significance for the individual. Channon et al. (1988) were the first to use a modified version of the Stroop test to compare anorexia nervosa patients and nonclinical controls on six color-naming tasks. Results indicated that anorexic patients were more preoccupied with food than nonclinical controls by being slower to color-name food and body words as compared to control conditions and control subjects.

Cooper and colleagues (Cooper & Fairburn, 1992; Cooper & Todd, 1997) conducted a series of studies using dieters with a history of eating disorders, dieters without a history of eating disorders, patients with anorexia nervosa, patients with bulimia nervosa, and nonclinical controls. Cooper and Fairburn (1992) found that normal dieters were similar to nonclinical controls by failing to show selective processing of information related to eating, shape, and weight. However, patients with eating disorders and dieters with a history of eating disorders showed selective attention for eating, shape, and weight concerns. Cooper and Fairburn included eating, weight, and shape concerns within the same card; therefore, it is not possible to determine differences within eating, weight, and shape concerns. In a subsequent study, Cooper and Todd (1997) separated the three areas of concern by Stroop card and found that both bulimic and anorexic patients showed selective attention for eating and weight. However, anorexic patients also showed selective processing of information related to shape.

Perpiña, Hemsley, Treasure, and de Silva (1993) used a modified version of the Stroop test to investigate the selective processing of food and body-size information, comparing anorexic and bulimic patients to controls on categorical (diagnosis) or dimensional criteria (restraint or Drive for Thinness), or both. The Drive for Thinness subscale of the EDI (Garner, 1991) was used to measure weight and shape concerns and the Restraint Scale (Herman & Polivy, 1980) was used to differentiate between restrained and unrestrained eaters. Using the categorical approach, they found that clinical groups were slower than controls in color-naming body and food words. Perpiña et al. reported that anorexic patients differed with controls in processing food terms, suggesting they are more concerned with eating; however, bulimic patients differed with controls in processing body terms, suggesting they were more concerned with weight and appearance. Using the dimensional approach, they showed that a high Drive for Thinness was associated with slower processing of body-related but not food-related terms, whereas high restraint was associated with slower processing of both food- and body-related terms. This suggested that restraint and Drive for Thinness dimensions indicate a different concern about food and body, respectively. When combining categorical and dimensional approaches, they found differences among the four groups in the food but not the body sets, possibly indicating that the control group might have contained a large section of restrained eaters. Their results suggested that eating disorder patients and some controls show a selective processing of information related to food and body, which is shared by some control subjects who are restrained eaters.

Huon (1995) reviewed the use of the Stoop test and questioned the reliability of these equivocal findings. Although the studies appear to suggest that people with eating disorders show selective bias toward concerns of food, weight, and shape, the results are tenuous given the variability in the employment of the Stroop task. Methodological limitations have included failing to match control and experimental groups by age, not including salient experimental groups such as dieters, combining food and shape words in a single target Stroop card, failing to counterbalance the presentation of the Stroop cards in order to minimize practice effects or boredom, including different amounts of words per card, and failing to use semantically related words on the control cards in order to minimize Stroop interference.

Rieger et al. (1998) also criticized the Stroop methodology as a relatively weak test of attention bias and offered a visual probe detection task as an alternative. This procedure involves displaying two words, one above the other, followed by a visual probe shown in the same location as

one of the word stimuli along with instructions to signal detection of the
target word as soon as possible. These researchers noted that subjects with
eating disorders tended to direct their attention away from stimulus
words connoting a thin physique and toward words representing a large
physique. The study authors argued that if individuals with eating disorders are indeed more likely to attend to information consistent with fatness and ignore information consistent with thinness, then this attentional
effect may serve to maintain concerns about body weight and shape, even
in the presence of contradictory evidence.

Selective Memory: Access and Retrieval

The Stroop tasks in anorexia nervosa indicate that memory concepts related to food, weight, and shape may be more accessible and more easily
primed. Other methods have examined selective retrieval of memory concepts related to food, body weight, and shape. King et al. (1991) studied
selective memory by presenting anorexia nervosa patients and other comparison groups with an essay containing food and weight items, as well as
neutral items, and then asking participants to reproduce the essay as completely as possible. The anorexia nervosa patients recalled more weight-
related items than neutral items.

   Hermans et al. (1999) measured both accessibility and retrievability in
anorexia nervosa and control subjects by using tests of implicit memory
(word-stem completion) as the measure of accessibility and explicit memory (cued recall) as the measure of retrievability. Subjects were presented
with a series of 64 words divided into both anorexia-related and anorexia-
unrelated categories. The anorexia-unrelated words consisted of those
with positive, negative, and neutral affective ratings in order to control for
the effect that emotional state may have on response latencies (a potential
problem with the Stroop or other memory tests). Arguably, anorexia
nervosa patients could be more threatened by food, weight, and shape-
related stimuli and this may account for longer response latencies (Vitousek & Hollon, 1990).

   Vartanian, Polivy, and Herman (2004) discussed their recent work using the Implicit Association Test (IAT; Greenwald, McGhee, & Schwartz,
1998) and found that certain food- and weight-related attitudes and behaviors were supported by implicit cognitions. In certain domains, they
found that the IAT and explicit measures appeared to assess the same underlying construct, whereas in other domains the IAT could reflect
learned associations that had not necessarily been internalized as personal
beliefs or attitudes. They pointed out that implicit cognition measures
could provide access to thoughts and schemas that play a role in influencing feelings and behavior. Although implicit cognitions are considered to

be relatively resistant to change, two studies have shown that repeatedly paired categories of stimuli could apparently change underlying implicit associations (Karpinski & Hilton, 2001). Vartanian et al. (2004) concluded that implicit tests might be useful when there is reason to doubt self-report validity—due to possible misrepresentation of thoughts, feelings, and behavior—and provide important information about treatment progress. In this respect, implicit tests could also be helpful in corroborating self-reports in cases where involuntary hospitalization is sought.

Vartanian et al. (2004) also described using the IAT to examine the connection between implicit and explicit attitudes toward food and weight, and proposed that the difference observed between restrained and unrestrained eaters in explicit attitudes toward body fat reflected a difference in the internalization or self-relevance of the thinness ideal. Restrained eaters had both explicit and implicit negative attitudes toward fatness and positive attitudes toward thinness, and reported engaging in behaviors that were consonant with those attitudes. However, unrestrained eaters had implicit negative attitudes toward fatness but did not report parallel explicit attitudes and behaviors. This suggested that even though most people have negative attitudes toward body fat, only restrained eaters have internalized these negative attitudes as self-relevant. Therefore, incorporating implicit measures might help to isolate components of body dissatisfaction that contribute to disordered eating. Because body dissatisfaction is associated with relapse among bulimia nervosa patients, Vartanian et al. (2004) suggested that if body dissatisfaction is supported by implicit cognitive processes, then patients who terminate treatment after demonstrating changes in their explicit attitudes toward body shape without experiencing a corresponding change in their implicit cognitions may be at increased risk for relapse.

Hermans et al. (1999) reasoned that if anorexia nervosa is positively associated with higher accessibility of anorexia-related words, as suggested by Stroop tasks, then this should be reflected in more word-stem completions for anorexia-related words as compared to nonanorexia-related words. Results showed a strong bias toward explicit memory for anorexia-related words for patients with anorexia nervosa but not for nondieting controls. There was no evidence for a similar bias in implicit memory.

Meyer, Waller, and Watson (2000) assessed the processing speed of self-directed threat words among a nonclinical female sample after interstimulus delay intervals (ISI) of different durations. They found that, regardless of eating psychopathology levels, the women were slower to respond to threats that had a longer ISI than those having a shorter ISI, and more bulimic women were particularly slow to respond to self-directed threats following a 1,500-ms interval. These results suggested that during the early stages of processing, the defense process does not limit the amount of focus onto the threat schemata; however, at 1,500-ms ISI, the defense mechanism restricts the amount of focus of those with more bulimic attitudes, resulting in decreased processing speed. However, after the 2,000-ms interval, they found the cognitive defense process was no longer effective. Meyer et al. stated that the amount of time an individual has to process threat cues appeared to be crucial, based on different response times for different ISI durations. This has important methodological implications, given that threat detection techniques do not account for temporal factors. Meyer et al. pointed out that effective eating disorder treatment may need to focus on altering patient reaction to self-directed ego threats or teach more appropriate coping mechanisms.

Lovell, Williams, and Hill (1997) also identified support for selective attention among anorexics, bulimics, and recovered anorexics indicating that a cognitive bias may persist even when recovery is achieved. Using an emotional Stroop task, they reported that women with bulimia nervosa and women who had recovered from anorexia nervosa were more distracted by shape concerns than women who had recovered from bulimia and nonclinical samples.

In summary, data from the Stroop and memory recall tasks provide some support for the idea that anorexia nervosa patients have a cognitive bias toward food, weight, and shape information that may play a role in the development and maintenance of the disorders. The findings can be understood in terms of a model in which food and weight concerns become reciprocally and dynamically linked within the memory structures of the patient with anorexia nervosa (Hermans et al., 1999; King et al., 1991; Vitousek & Hollon, 1990). Hermans et al. (1999) hypothesized a process by which the conscious ruminations about appearance, food, and weight act as "mnemonic cues" to retrieve and activate weight-related self-schemata. This process involves "the formation of associative links that lead to higher probabilities of activation of the characteristic concerns about shape and weight and their relation to self-worth" (pp. 198–199) that serve to maintain anorexia nervosa.

Convergent Evidence From Electrophysiological Methods

It has been hypothesized that body image disturbance may be due to localized brain dysfunction associated with diminished ability to recognize and integrate certain nonverbal stimuli (Kinsbourne & Bemporad, 1984). Bradley et al. (1997) found changes in EEG event-related potentials during perceptual-cognitive tasks supporting the hypothesis of a right hemispheric dysfunction in anorexia nervosa that persisted with weight gain. These findings led to the prediction that anorexia nervosa patients would have difficulty in sensory integration tasks involving spatial orientation because they involve the right hemisphere to a greater extent (Grunwald et al., 2001). Grunwald et al. (2001) tested function by comparing anorexia nervosa patients and controls in their ability to reproduce the structure of symbols on paper after exploring their sunken reliefs with both hands and with eyes closed. The patient reproductions were poorer in quality than controls and unchanged by weight gain. Moreover, analysis of spectral EEG power during the symbol reproduction task showed significant group differences indicative of dysfunction in somatosensory integration processing of the right parietal cortex.

Dodin and Nandrino (2003) used electrophysiological indices for testing the ability of anorexic subjects to filter out irrelevant stimuli in controlled information-processing tasks, specifically the recognition of simple and complex body images and geometrical shapes. Anorexic patients were found to have larger P300 amplitudes and longer P300 latencies for frequent stimuli, regardless of task complexity. The authors explained that the nonspecific hyperarousal in anorexia nervosa and a relative inability to filter out irrelevant stimuli led to a saturation of the patients' working memory.

In summary, there are a number of different methods that have provided support for the main cognitive theory of anorexia nervosa, namely, that patients exhibit self-statements, automatic thoughts, and underlying assumptions that reflect undue concern with food and eating, weight and shape. Future directions for research are refinement of self-report and less structured measures so they tap conceptual domains that distinguish anorexia nervosa from other eating disorders, and isolating important aspects of these beliefs that may be more closely linked to the development and maintenance of eating disorders.

Cognitive Vulnerability and Starvation Symptoms

Food intake varies markedly from day to day and the human organism generally compensates with ease to temporary decrements in energy balance in response to a range of internal and external events. However, consistent negative energy balance, leading to sustained weight suppression, challenges biologic systems responsible for the homeostatic regulation of body weight (Keesey, 1993). One of the most important advancements in understanding anorexia nervosa has been recognition of the profound cognitive and emotional effects of starvation, as well as differentiation of these from primary eating disorder symptoms. Individuals exposed to sustained caloric restriction and weight loss can experience symptoms such as depression, anxiety, obsessionality, irritability, labile moods, feelings of inadequacy, fatigue, food preoccupations, poor concentration, social withdrawal, and the urge to binge eat. These symptoms were dramatically illustrated in a well-known "starvation" study of normal volunteers who lost an average of 25% of their former body weight in 6 months of sustained calorie restriction (Garner, 1997). Many of the starvation-induced symptoms observed in this study took many months to resolve, even after body weight had returned to normal levels. There are a number of important ways in which these symptoms can maintain anorexia nervosa. Delayed gastric emptying can make the anorexia nervosa patient, already sensitive to slight increases in weight, experience postprandial bloating (S. Lee, 1993). The tendency to engage in binge eating, particularly during the weight regain process, causes guilt, which can lead to compensatory symptoms such as vomiting. Starvation-induced obsessionality, depression, emotional sensitivity, and social isolation can aggravate preexisting emotional disturbance.

Cognitive vulnerability to anorexia nervosa can be understood in the broad theoretical context of eating disorders as multidetermined and heterogeneous in nature. Most models assume that eating disorders develop and are maintained by cultural, individual (developmental, psychological, biological, and exposure to adverse life events), and familial predisposing or risk factors. Assessment of cognitive vulnerability in anorexia nervosa has included self-report measures, semi-structured interviews, unstructured interviews, and measures of information processing including perceptual distortion. Body dissatisfaction, drive for thinness, and other beliefs about weight, shape, and eating are well-supported sources of cognitive vulnerability to anorexia nervosa. Because these beliefs do not uniformly lead to the expression of the disorder, a complete account of the pathogenesis anorexia nervosa requires expanding the focus of research to include the predisposition toward a range of core beliefs, psychological domains, information-processing styles, as well as other risk and protective factors using improved measurement technology, larger sample sizes, and powerful analytic methods.

REFERENCES

Abou-Saleh, M. T., Younis, Y., & Karim, L. (1998). Anorexia nervosa in an Arab culture. *International Journal of Eating Disorders, 23*, 207–212.

American Psychiatric Association (APA). (1994). *Diagnostic and statistical manual of mental disorders (DSM–IV)*. Washington, DC: American Psychiatric Press.

American Psychiatric Association (APA). (2000). *Diagnostic and statistical manual of mental disorders (DSM–IV–TR)*. Arlington, VA: American Psychiatric Publishing, Inc.

Bastiani, A. M., Rao, R., Weltzin, T., & Kaye, W. H. (1995). Perfectionism in anorexia nervosa. *International Journal of Eating Disorders, 17*, 147–152.

Beck, A. T. (1976). *Cognitive therapy and the emotional disorders.* New York: International Universities Press.

Becker, A. E., Grinspoon, S. K., Klibanski, A., & Herzog, D. B. (1999). Eating disorders. *New England Journal of Medicine, 340,* 1092–1098.

Bers, S. A., & Quinlan, D. M. (1992). Perceived-competence deficit in anorexia nervosa. *Journal of Abnormal Psychology, 101,* 423–431.

Bizeul, C., Sadowsky, N., & Rigaud, D. (2001). The prognostic value of initial EDI scores in anorexia nervosa patients: A prospective follow-up study of 5–10 years. Eating Disorder Inventory. *European Psychiatry, 16,* 232–238.

Blowers, L. C., Loxton, N. J., Grady-Flesser, M., Occhipinti, S., & Dawe, S. (2003). The relationship between sociocultural pressure to be thin and body dissatisfaction in preadolescent girls. *Eating Behaviors, 4,* 229–244.

Bradley, S. J., Taylor, M. J., Rovet, J. F., Goldberg, E., Hood, J., Wachsmuth, R., Azcue, M. P., & Pencharz, P. B. (1997). Assessment of brain function in adolescent anorexia nervosa before and after weight gain. *Journal of Clinical and Experimental Neuropsychology, 19,* 20–33.

Brewerton, T. D., Hand, L. D., & Bishop, E. R. (1993). The Tridimensional Personality Questionnaire in eating disorder patients. *International Journal of Eating Disorders, 14,* 213–218.

Brown, L. S., Waller, G., Meyer, C., Bamford, B., Morrison, T., & Burditt, E. (2003). Socially driven eating and restriction in the eating disorders. *Eating Behaviors, 4,* 221–228.

Bruch, H. (1962). Perceptual and conceptual disturbances in anorexia nervosa. *Psychosomatic Medicine, 24,* 187–194.

Bruch, H. (1982). Anorexia nervosa: Therapy and theory. *American Journal of Psychiatry, 139,* 1531–1538.

Bulik, C. M., Sullivan, P. F., Weltzin, T. E., & Kaye, W. H. (1995). Temperament in eating disorders. *International Journal of Eating Disorders, 17,* 251–261.

Butow, P., Beumont, P., & Touyz, S. (1993). Cognitive processes in dieting disorders. *International Journal of Eating Disorders, 14,* 319–329.

Button, E. J., Loan, P., Davies, J., & Sonuga-Barke, E. J. (1997). Self-esteem, eating problems, and psychological well-being in a cohort of schoolgirls aged 15–16: A questionnaire and interview study. *International Journal of Eating Disorders, 21,* 39–47.

Cachelin, F. M., & Maher, B. A. (1998). Restrictors who purge: Implications of purging behavior for psychopathology and classification of anorexia nervosa. *Eating Disorders, 6,* 51–63.

Carter, J. C., Blackmore, E., Sutandar-Pinnock, K., & Woodside, D. B. (2004). Relapse in anorexia nervosa: A survival analysis. *Psychological Medicine, 34,* 671–679.

Cash, T. F., & Deagle, E. A., III. (1997). The nature and extent of body-image disturbances in anorexia nervosa and bulimia nervosa: A meta-analysis. *International Journal of Eating Disorders, 22,* 107–125.

Cash, T. F., & Pruzinsky, T. (2002). *Body image: A handbook of theory, research, and clinical practice.* New York: Guilford.

Casper, R. C. (1990). Personality features of women with good outcome from restricting anorexia nervosa. *Psychosomatic Medicine, 52,* 156–170.

Casper, R. C., Eckert, E. D., Halmi, K. A., Goldberg, S. C., & Davis, J. M. (1980). Bulimia. Its incidence and clinical importance in patients with anorexia nervosa. *Archives of General Psychiatry, 37,* 1030–1034.

Casper, R. C., Hedeker, D., & McClough, J. F. (1992). Personality dimensions in eating disorders and their relevance for subtyping. *Journal of the American Academy of Child and Adolescent Psychiatry, 31,* 830–840.

Channon, S., Hemsley, D., & de Silva, P. (1988). Selective processing of food words in anorexia nervosa. *British Journal of Clinical Psychology, 27,* 259–260.

Clark, D. A. (1992). Depressive, anxious and intrusive thoughts in psychiatric inpatients and outpatients. *Behaviour Research and Therapy, 30,* 93–102.

Cloninger, C. R., Przybeck, T. R., & Svrakic, D. M. (1991). The Tridimensional Personality Questionnaire: U.S. normative data. *Psychological Reports, 69*, 1047–1057.

Cooper, M. (1997a). Bias in interpretation of ambiguous scenarios in eating disorders. *Behaviour Research and Therapy, 35*, 619–626.

Cooper, M. J. (1997b). Cognitive theory in anorexia nervosa and bulimia nervosa: A review. *Behavioural and Cognitive Psychotherapy, 25*, 113–145.

Cooper, M. J., Anastasiades, P., & Fairburn, C. G. (1992). Selective processing of eating-, shape-, and weight-related words in persons with bulimia nervosa. *Journal of Abnormal Psychology, 101*, 352–355.

Cooper, M., Cohen-Tovee, E., Todd, G., Wells, A., & Tovee, M. (1997). The Eating Disorder Belief Questionnaire: Preliminary development. *Behaviour Research and Therapy, 35*, 381–388.

Cooper, M., & Fairburn, C. G. (1992). Selective processing of eating, weight, and shape-related words in patients with eating disorders and dieters. *British Journal of Clinical Psychology, 31*, 363–365.

Cooper, M., & Todd, G. (1997). Selective processing of three types of stimuli in eating disorders. *British Journal of Clinical Psychology, 36*, 279–281.

Cooper, M. J., Todd, G., & Wells, A. (1998). Content, origins, and consequences of dysfunctional beliefs in anorexia nervosa and bulimia nervosa. *Journal of Cognitive Psychotherapy: An International Quarterly, 12*, 213–230.

Cooper, M., & Turner, H. (2000). Brief report: Underlying assumptions and core beliefs in anorexia nervosa and dieting. *British Journal of Clinical Psychology, 39*, 215–218.

Craighead, L. (2002). Obesity and eating disorders. In M. M. Antony & D. H. Barlow (Eds.), *Handbook of assessment and treatment planning for psychological disorders* (pp. 300–340). New York: Guilford.

Crisp, A. H. (1965). Clinical and therapeutic aspects of anorexia nervosa: Study of 30 cases. *Journal of Psychosomatic Research, 9*, 67–78.

Crisp, A. H. (1997). Anorexia nervosa as flight from growth: Assessment and treatment based on the model. In D. M. Garner & P. E. Garfinkel (Eds.), *Handbook of treatment for eating disorders* (pp. 248–277). New York: Guilford.

Dally, P. I., & Gomez, I. (1979). *Anorexia nervosa.* London: Henemann.

Davison, K. K., Markey, C. N., & Birch, L. L. (2000). Etiology of body dissatisfaction and weight concerns among 5-year-old girls. *Appetite, 35*, 143–151.

Dobmeyer, A. C., & Stein, D. M. (2003). A prospective analysis of eating disorder risk factors: Drive for thinness, depressed mood, maladaptive cognitions, and ineffectiveness. *Eating Behaviors, 4*, 135–147.

Dodin, V., & Nandrino, J.-L. (2003). Cognitive processing of anorexic patients in recognition tasks: An event-related potentials study. *International Journal of Eating Disorders, 33*, 299–307.

Dolan, B. (1991). Cross-cultural aspects of anorexia nervosa and bulimia: A review. *International Journal of Eating Disorders, 10*, 67–79.

Eddy, K. T., Keel, P. K., Dorer, D. J., Delinsky, S. S., Franko, D. L., & Herzog, D. B. (2002). Longitudinal comparison of anorexia nervosa subtypes. *International Journal of Eating Disorders, 31*, 191–201.

Edlund, B., Halvarsson, K., & Sjödén, P. (1996). Eating behaviours and attitudes to eating, dieting, and body image in 7-year-old Swedish girls. *European Eating Disorders Review, 4*, 40–53.

Enoch, M. A., Kaye, W. H., Rotondo, A., Greenberg, B. D., Murphy, D. L., & Goldman, D. (1998). 5-Ht2A promoter polymorphism 1438GA, anorexia nervosa, and obsessive-compulsive disorder. *Lancet, 351*, 1785–1786.

Epstein, J., Wiseman, C. V., Sunday, S. R., Klapper, F., Alkalay, L., & Halmi, K. A. (2001). Neurocognitive evidence favors "top down" over "bottom up" mechanisms in the pathogenesis of body size distortions in anorexia nervosa. *Eating and Weight Disorders, 6,* 140–147.

Fairburn, C. G. (1981). A cognitive-behavioral approach to the management of bulimia. *Psychological Medicine, 141,* 631–633.

Fairburn, C. G. (1985). Cognitive-behavioral treatment for bulimia. In D. M. Garner & P. E. Garfinkel (Eds.), *Handbook of psychotherapy for anorexia nervosa and bulimia* (pp. 160–192). New York: Guilford.

Fairburn, C. G., & Cooper, Z. (1993). Eating Disorder Examination (12th edition). In C. G. Fairburn & G. T. Wilson (Eds.), *Binge eating: Nature, assessment, and treatment* (pp. 317–360). New York: Guilford.

Fairburn, C. G., Cooper, Z., Doll, H. A., & Welch, S. L. (1999). Risk factors for anorexia nervosa: Three integrated case control comparisons. *Archives of General Psychiatry, 56,* 468–476.

Fairburn, C. G., & Harrison, P. J. (2003). Eating disorders. *Lancet, 361,* 407–416.

Fairburn, C. G., Marcus, M. D., & Wilson, G. T. (1993). Cognitive behavior therapy for binge eating and bulimia nervosa: A comprehensive treatment manual. In C. G. Fairburn & G. T. Wilson (Eds.), *Binge eating: Nature, assessment, and treatment* (pp. 361–404). New York: Guilford.

Fairburn, C. G., Norman, P. A., Welch, S. L., O'Connor, M. E., Doll, H. A., & Peveler, R. C. (1995). A prospective study of outcome in bulimia nervosa and the long-term effect of three psychological treatments. *Archives of General Psychiatry, 52,* 304–312.

Fassino, S., Abbate, D. G., Amianto, F., Leombruni, P., Garzaro, L., & Rovera, G. G. (2001). Nonresponder anorectic patients after 6 months of multimodal treatment: Predictors of outcome. *European Psychiatry, 16,* 466–473.

Favaro, A., & Santonastaso, P. (1998). Impulsive and compulsive self-injurious behavior in bulimia nervosa: Prevalence and psychological correlates. *Journal of Nervous and Mental Diseases, 186,* 157–165.

Favaro, A., & Santonastaso, P. (1999). Different types of self-injurious behavior in bulimia nervosa. *Comprehensive Psychiatry, 40,* 1–5.

Fichter, M. M., Quadflieg, N., & Rehm, J. (2003). Predicting the outcome of eating disorders using structural equation modeling. *International Journal of Eating Disorders, 34,* 292–313.

Field, A. E., Camargo, C. A., Jr., Taylor, C. B., Berkey, C. S., Frasier, A. L., Gillman, M. W., et al. (1999). Overweight, weight concerns, and bulimic behaviors among girls and boys. *Journal of the American Academy of Child and Adolescent Psychiatry, 38,* 754–760.

Frost, R. O., Marten, P., Lahart, C., & Rosenblate, R. (1990). The dimensions of perfectionism. *Cognitive Therapy and Research, 13,* 449–468.

Garfinkel, P. E., Moldofsky, H., & Garner, D. M. (1980). The heterogeneity of anorexia nervosa. *Archives of General Psychiatry, 37,* 1036–1040.

Garner, D. M. (1986). Cognitive therapy for bulimia nervosa. *Annals of Adolescent Psychiatry, 13,* 358–390.

Garner, D. M. (1991). *Eating Disorder Inventory–2 professional manual.* Odessa, FL: Psychological Assessment Resources.

Garner, D. M. (1993). Pathogenesis of anorexia nervosa. *The Lancet, 341,* 1631–1635.

Garner, D. M. (1997). Psychoeducational principles in treatment. In D. M. Garner & P. E. Garfinkel (Eds.), *Handbook of treatment for eating disorders* (pp. 145–177). New York: Guilford.

Garner, D. M. (2004a). *Eating Disorder Inventory–3 professional manual.* Odessa, FL: Psychological Assessment Resources.

Garner, D. M. (2004b). *Eating Disorder Inventory–3 referral form.* Odessa, FL: Psychological Assessment Resources.

Garner, D. M., & Bemis, K. M. (1982). A cognitive-behavioral approach to anorexia nervosa. *Cognitive Therapy and Research, 6,* 123–150.

Garner, D. M., & Bemis, K. M. (1985). Cognitive therapy for anorexia nervosa. In D. M. Garner & P. E. Garfinkel (Eds.), *Handbook of psychotherapy for anorexia nervosa and bulimia* (pp. 107–146). New York: Guilford.

Garner, D. M., & Garfinkel, P. E. (1978). Sociocultural factors in anorexia nervosa. *Lancet, 2,* 674.

Garner, D. M., & Garfinkel, P. E. (1980). Socio-cultural factors in the development of anorexia nervosa. *Psychological Medicine, 10,* 647–656.

Garner, D. M., & Garfinkel, P. E. (1981). Body image in anorexia nervosa: Measurement, theory and clinical implications. *International Journal of Psychiatry in Medicine, 11,* 263–284.

Garner, D. M., Garfinkel, P. E., & O'Shaughnessy, M. (1985). The validity of the distinction between bulimia with and without anorexia nervosa. *American Journal of Psychiatry, 142,* 581–587.

Garner, D. M., Garfinkel, P. E., Rockert, W., & Olmsted, M. P. (1987). A prospective study of eating disturbances in the ballet. *Psychotherapy and Psychosomatics, 48,* 170–175.

Garner, D. M., Garfinkel, P. E., Schwartz, D. M., & Thompson, M. M. (1980). Cultural expectations of thinness in women. *Psychological Reports, 47,* 483–491.

Garner, D. M., Garfinkel, P. E., Stancer, H. C., & Moldofsky, H. (1976). Body image disturbances in anorexia nervosa and obesity. *Psychosomatic Medicine, 38,* 327–336.

Garner, D. M., Garner, M. V., & Rosen, L. W. (1993). Anorexia nervosa "restricters" who purge: Implications for subtyping anorexia nervosa. *International Journal of Eating Disorders, 13,* 171–185.

Garner, D. M., Olmsted, M. P., Bohr, Y., & Garfinkel, P. E. (1982). The Eating Attitudes Test: Psychometric features and clinical correlates. *Psychological Medicine, 12,* 871–878.

Garner, D. M., Olmsted, M. P., & Garfinkel, P. E. (1985). Similarities among bulimic groups selected by different weights and weight histories. *Journal of Psychiatric Research, 19,* 129–134.

Garner, D. M., Olmsted, M. P., & Polivy, J. (1983). Development and validation of a multidimensional Eating Disorder Inventory for anorexia nervosa and bulimia. *International Journal of Eating Disorders, 2,* 15–34.

Garner, D. M., & Rosen, L. W. (1990). Anorexia nervosa and bulimia nervosa. In A. S. Bellack, M. Hersen, & A. E. Kazdin (Eds.), *International handbook of behavior modification and therapy* (2nd ed., pp. 805–817). New York: Plenum.

Garner, D. M., & Rosen, L. W. (1994). Aggressive and destructive behavior in eating disorders. In M. Hersen, R. Ammerman, & L. Sisson (Eds.), *Handbook of aggressive and destructive behavior in psychiatric patients* (pp. 409–428). New York: Plenum.

Garner, D. M., Vitousek, K., & Pike, K. (1997). Cognitive-behavioral therapy for anorexia nervosa. In D. M. Garner & P. E. Garfinkel (Eds.), *Handbook of treatment for eating disorders* (pp. 94–144). New York: Guilford.

Ghaderi, A. (2003). Structural modeling analysis of prospective risk factors for eating disorder. *Eating Behaviors, 3,* 387–396.

Gordon, R. (2001). Eating disorders East and West: A culture-bound syndrome unbound. In M. Nasser, M. Katzman, & R. Gordon (Eds.), *Eating disorders and cultures in transition* (pp. 1–16). New York: Taylor & Francis.

Greenfield, D., Quinlan, D. M., Harding, P., Glass, E., & Bliss, A. (1987). Eating behavior in an adolescent population. *International Journal of Eating Disorders, 6,* 99–111.

Greenwald, A. G., McGhee, D. E., & Schwartz, J. L. (1998). Measuring individual differences in implicit cognition: The Implicit Association Test. *Journal of Personality and Social Psychology, 74,* 1464–1480.

Grunwald, M., Ettrich, C., Assmann, B., Dahne, A., Krause, W., Busse, F., & Gertz, H. J. (2001). Deficits in haptic perception and right parietal theta power changes in patients with anorexia nervosa before and after weight gain. *International Journal of Eating Disorders, 29,* 417–428.

Guidano, V. F., & Liotti, G. (1983). *Cognitive processes and emotional disorders: A structural approach to psychotherapy*. New York: Guilford.

Halmi, K. A., Eckert, E., Marchi, P., Sampugnaro, V., Apple, R., & Cohen, J. (1991). Comorbidity of psychiatric diagnoses in anorexia nervosa. *Archives of General Psychiatry, 48*, 712–718.

Halmi, K. A., Sunday, S. R., Strober, M., Kaplan, A., Woodside, D. B., Fichter, M., Treasure, J., Berrettini, W. H., & Kaye, W. H. (2000). Perfectionism in anorexia nervosa: Variation by clinical subtype, obsessionality, and pathological eating behavior. *American Journal of Psychiatry, 157*, 1799–1805.

Herman, P. C. P., & Polivy, J. (1980). Restrained eating. In A. J. Stunkard (Ed.), *Obesity* (pp. 208 225). Philadelphia: Saunders.

Hermans, D., Pieters, G., & Eelen, P. (1999). Implicit and explicit memory for shape, body weight, and food-related words in patients with anorexia nervosa and nondieting controls. *Journal of Abnormal Psychology, 107*, 193–202.

Herzog, D. B., Dorer, D. J., Keel, P. K., Selwyn, S. E., Ekeblad, E. R., Flores, A. T., Greenwood, D. N., Burwell, R. A., & Keller, M. B. (1999). Recovery and relapse in anorexia and bulimia nervosa: A 7.5-year follow-up study. *Journal of the America Academy of Child and Adolescent Psychiatry, 38*, 829–837.

Hewitt, P. L., & Flett, G. L. (1991). Dimensions of perfectionism in unipolar depression. *Journal of Abnormal Psychology, 100*, 98–101.

Hill, A. J., & Pallin, V. (1998). Dieting awareness and low self-worth: Related issues in 8-year old girls. *International Journal of Eating Disorders, 24*, 405–413.

Huon, G. F. (1995). The Stroop Color-Naming Task in eating disorders: A review of the research. *Eating Disorders: The Journal of Treatment and Prevention, 3*, 124–132.

Jacobi, C., Hayward, C., de Zwaan, M., Kraemer, H. C., & Agras, W. S. (2004). Coming to terms with risk factors for eating disorders: Application of risk terminology and suggestions for a general taxonomy. *Psychological Bulletin, 130*, 19–65.

Joiner, T. E., Jr., Heatherton, T. F., & Keel, P. K. (1997). Ten-year stability and predictive validity of five bulimia-related indicators. *American Journal of Psychiatry, 154*, 1133–1138.

Joiner, T. E., Jr., & Schmidt, N. B. (1995). Dimensions of perfectionism, life stress, and depressed and anxious symptoms: Prospective support for diathesis-stress but not specific vulnerability among male undergraduates. *Journal of Social and Clinical Psychology, 14*, 165–183.

Kagan, J., Rosman, B. L., Day, D., Albert, J., & Phillips, W. (1964). Information processing in the child: Significance of analytic reflective attitudes. *Psychological Monographs, 78*, 1–37.

Karpinski, A., & Hilton, J. L. (2001). Attitudes and the Implicit Associations Test. *Journal of Personality and Social Psychology, 81*, 774–788.

Kaye, W. H., Bastiani, A. M., & Moss, H. (1995). Cognitive style of patients with anorexia nervosa and bulimia nervosa. *International Journal of Eating Disorders, 18*, 287–290.

Keel, P. K., & Klump, K. L. (2003). Are eating disorders culture-bound syndromes? Implications for conceptualizing their etiology. *Psychological Bulletin, 129*, 747–769.

Keesey, R. E. (1993). Physiological regulation of body energy: Implications for obesity. In A. J. Stunkard & T. A. Wadden (Eds.), *Obesity: Theory and therapy* (2nd ed., pp. 77–96). New York: Raven.

Killen, J. D., Taylor, C. B., Hayward, C., & Haydel, K. F. (1996). Weight concerns influence the development of eating disorders: A 4-year prospective study. *Journal of Consulting and Clinical Psychology, 64*, 936–940.

King, G. A., Polivy, J., & Herman, C. P. (1991). Cognitive aspects of dietary restraints: Effects on person memory. *International Journal of Eating Disorders, 10*, 313–321.

Kinsbourne, M., & Bemporad, B. (1984). Lateralization of emotion: A model and the evidence. In N. A. Fox & J. R. Davidson (Eds.), *The psychobiology of affective development* (pp. 259–291). Hillsdale, NJ: Lawrence Erlbaum Associates.

Lee, A. M., & Lee, S. (1996). Disordered eating and its psychosocial correlates among Chinese adolescent females in Hong Kong. *International Journal of Eating Disorders, 20,* 177–183.

Lee, S. (1993). Gastric emptying and bloating in anorexia nervosa. *British Journal of Psychiatry, 162,* 128–129.

Lee, S. (1995). Self-starvation in context: Towards a culturally sensitive understanding of anorexia nervosa. *Social Science and Medicine, 41,* 25–36.

Leon, G. R., Fulkerson, J. A., Perry, C. L., Keel, P. K., & Klump, K. L. (1999). Three to four year prospective evaluation of personality and behavioral risk factors for later disordered eating in adolescent girls and boys. *Journal of Youth and Adolescence, 28,* 181–196.

Leung, N., Waller, G., & Thomas, G. (1999). Core beliefs in anorexic and bulimic women. *Journal of Nervous and Mental Disease, 187,* 736–741.

Lovell, D. M., Williams, J. M. G., & Hill, A. B. (1997). Selective processing of shape-related words in women with eating disorders and those who have recovered. *British Journal of Clinical Psychology, 36,* 421–432.

Löwe, B., Zipfel, S., Buchholz, C., Dupont, Y., Reas, D. L., & Herzog, W. (2001). Long-term outcome of anorexia nervosa in a prospective 21-year follow-up study. *Psychological Medicine, 31,* 881–890.

Lucas, A. R., Beard, C. M., O'Fallon, W. M., & Kurland, L. T. (1991). 50-year trends in the incidence of anorexia nervosa in Rochester, Minn.: A population-based study. *American Journal of Psychiatry, 148,* 917–922.

Marshall, P. D., Palmer, R. L., & Stretch, D. (1993). The description and measurement of abnormal beliefs in anorexia nervosa: A controlled study. *International Journal of Methods in Psychiatric Research, 3,* 193–200.

Matsunaga, H., Kiriike, N., Iwasaki, Y., Miyata, A., Yamagami, S., & Kaye, W. H. (1999). Clinical characteristics in patients with anorexia nervosa and obsessive-compulsive disorder. *Psychological Medicine, 29,* 407–414.

McCabe, M. P., & Ricciardelli, L. A. (2004). Body image dissatisfaction among males across the lifespan: A review of past literature. *Journal of Psychosomatic Research, 56,* 675–685.

Meyer, C., Waller, G., & Watson, D. (2000). Cognitive avoidance and bulimic psychopathology: The relevance of temporal factors in a nonclinical population. *International Journal of Eating Disorders, 27,* 405–410.

Mizes, J. S. (1992). Validity of the Mizes Anorectic Cognitions Scale: A comparison between anorectics, bulimics and psychiatric controls. *Addictive Behaviours, 17,* 283–289.

Oliosi, M., & Dalle Grave, R. (2003). A comparison of clinical and psychological features in subgroups of patients with anorexia nervosa. *European Eating Disorders Review, 11,* 306–314.

Palmer, R. L. (1993). Weight concern should not be a necessary criterion for the eating disorders: A polemic. *International Journal of Eating Disorders, 14,* 459–465.

Patton, G. C., Johnson-Sabine, E., Wood, K., Mann, A. H., & Wakeling, A. (1990). Abnormal eating attitudes in London schoolgirls—A prospective epidemiological study: Outcome at twelve months follow-up. *Psychological Medicine, 20,* 383–394.

Patton, G. C., Selzer, R., Caffey, C., Carlin, J. B., & Wolfe, R. (1999). Onset of adolescent eating disorders: A prospective epidemiological study: Outcome at twelve month follow-up. *Psychological Medicine, 20,* 383–394.

Perpiña, C., Hemsley, D., Treasure, J., & de Silva, P. (1993). Is selective information processing of food and body words specific to patients with eating disorders? *International Journal of Eating Disorders, 14,* 359–366.

Pike, K. M., Loeb, K., & Vitousek, K. (1996). Cognitive-behavioral therapy for anorexia nervosa and bulimia nervosa. In J. K. Thompson (Ed.), *Body image, eating disorders, and obesity: An integrative guide for assessment and treatment* (pp. 253–302). Washington, DC: American Psychological Association.

Quadflieg, N., & Fichter, M. M. (2003). The course and outcome of bulimia nervosa. *European Child and Adolescent Psychiatry, 12*, 99–109.

Rampling, D. (1985). Ascetic ideals and anorexia nervosa. *Journal of Psychiatric Research, 19*, 89–94.

Rieger, E., Schotte, D. E., Touyz, S. W., Beumont, P. J., Griffiths, R., & Russell, J. (1998). Attentional biases in eating disorders: A visual probe detection procedure. *International Journal of Eating Disorders, 23*, 199–205.

Robinson, T. N., Killen, J. D., Litt, I. F., Hammer, L. D., Wilson, D. M., Haydel, K. F., Hayward, C., & Taylor, C. B. (1996). Ethnicity and body dissatisfaction: Are Hispanic and Asian girls at increased risk for eating disorders? *Journal of Adolescent Health, 19*, 384–393.

Russell, G. F. M. (1979). Bulimia nervosa: An ominous variant of anorexia nervosa. *Psychological Medicine, 9*, 429–448.

Shafran, R., Cooper, Z., & Fairburn, C. G. (2002). Clinical perfectionism: A cognitive-behavioural analysis. *Behaviour Research and Therapy, 40*, 773–791.

Sherry, S. B., Hewitt, P. L., Besser, A., McGee, B. J., & Flett, G. L. (2004). Self-oriented and socially prescribed perfectionism in the Eating Disorder Inventory Perfectionism subscale. *International Journal of Eating Disorders, 35*, 69–79.

Silber, T. J. (1986). Anorexia nervosa in Blacks and Hispanics. *International Journal of Eating Disorders, 5*, 121–128.

Silvera, D. H., Bergersen, T. D., Bjorgum, L., Perry, J. A., Rosenvinge, J. H., & Holte, A. (1998). Analyzing the relation between self-esteem and eating disorders: Differential effects of self-liking and self-competence. *Eating and Weight Disorders, 3*, 95–99.

Slade, P. D. (1982). Towards a functional analysis of anorexia nervosa and bulimia nervosa. *British Journal of Clinical Psychology, 21*, 167–179.

Slade, P. D., & Russell, G. F. M. (1973). Awareness of body dimension in anorexia nervosa: Cross-sectional and longitudinal studies. *Psychological Medicine, 3*, 188–199.

Smeets, M. A. M., Ingleby, J. D., Hoek, H. W., & Panhuysen, G. E. M. (1999). Body size perception in anorexia nervosa: A signal detection approach. *Journal of Psychosomatic Research, 46*, 465–477.

Srinivasagam, N. M., Kaye, W. H., Plotnicov, K. H., Greeno, C., Weltzin, T. E., & Rao, R. (1995). Persistent perfectionism, symmetry, and exactness after long-term recovery from anorexia nervosa. *American Journal of Psychiatry, 152*, 1630–1634.

Steiger, H., Israel, M., Gauvin, L., Ng Ying Kin, N. M., & Young, S. N. (2003). Implications of compulsive and impulsive traits for serotonin status in women with bulimia nervosa. *Psychiatry Research, 120*, 219–229.

Stice, E. (2002). Risk and maintaining factors for eating pathology: A meta-analytic review. *Psychological Bulletin, 128*, 825–848.

Stice, E., Agras, W. S., & Hammer, L. D. (1999). Risk factors for the emergence of childhood eating disturbances: A five-year prospective study. *International Journal of Eating Disorders, 25*, 375–387.

Stice, E., Presnell, K., & Spangler, D. (2002). Risk factors for binge eating onset in adolescent girls: A 2-year prospective investigation. *Health Psychology, 21*, 131–138.

Stice, E., Schupak-Neuberg, E., Shaw, H. E., & Stein, R. I. (1994). Relation of media exposure to eating disorder symptomatology: An examination of mediating mechanisms. *Journal of Abnormal Psychology, 103*, 836–840.

Strober, M. (1980). Personality and symptomatological features in young, non-chronic anorexia nervosa patients. *Journal of Psychosomatic Research, 24*, 353–359.

Stroop, J. R. (1935). Studies of interference in serial verbal reactions. *Journal of Experimental Psychology, 18*, 643–662.

Sullivan, P. F. (1995). Mortality in anorexia nervosa. *American Journal of Psychiatry, 152*, 1073–1074.

Sullivan, P. F., Bulik, C. M., Fear, J. L., & Pickering, A. (1998). Anorexia nervosa: A 12-year follow-up study. *American Journal of Psychiatry, 155*, 934–946.

Sullivan, P. F., Bulik, C. M., & Kendler, K. S. (1998). Genetic epidemiology of binging and vomiting. *British Journal of Psychiatry, 173*, 75–79.

Sundgot-Borgen, J. (1994). Eating disorders in female athletes. *Sports Medicine, 17*, 176–188.

Sutandar-Pinnock, K., Woodside, D. B., Carter, J. C., Olmsted, M. P., & Kaplan, A. S. (2003). Perfectionism in anorexia nervosa: A 6–24-month follow-up study. *International Journal of Eating Disorders, 33*, 225–229.

Teasdale, J. D., & Barnard, P. J. (1993). *Affect, cognition, and change: Re-modelling depressive thought*. Hillsdale, NJ: Lawrence Erlbaum Associates.

Theander, S. (1970). Anorexia nervosa. A psychiatric investigation of 94 female patients. *Acta Psychiatrica Scandanavia, Supplementum, 214*, 1–194.

Theander, S. S. (2004). Trends in the literature on eating disorders over 36 years (1965–2000): Terminology, interpretation and treatment. *European Eating Disorders Review, 12*, 4–17.

Thompson, J. K. (1996). *Eating disorders, obesity, and body image: A practical guide to assessment and treatment*. Washington, DC: American Psychological Association.

Toner, B. B., Garfinkel, P. E., & Garner, D. M. (1987). Cognitive style of patients with bulimic and diet-restricting anorexia nervosa. *American Journal of Psychiatry, 144*, 510–512.

Tozzi, F., Aggen, S. H., Neale, B. M., Anderson, C. B., Mazzeo, S. E., Neale, M. C., & Bulik, C. M. (2004). The structure of perfectionism: A twin study. *Behavior Genetics, 34*, 483–494.

Tylka, T. L. (2004). The relation between body dissatisfaction and eating disorder symptomatology: An analysis of moderating variables. *Journal of Counseling Psychology, 51*, 178–191.

Tylka, T. L., & Subich, L. M. (2004). Examining a multidimensional model of eating disorder symptomatology among college women. *Journal of Counseling Psychology, 51*, 314–328.

Vartanian, L. R., Polivy, J., & Herman, C. P. (2004). Implicit cognitions and eating disorders: Their application in research and treatment. *Cognitive and Behavioral Practice, 11*, 160–167.

Vitousek, K. M. (1996). The current status of cognitive-behavioral models of anorexia nervosa and bulimia nervosa. In P. M. Salkovskis (Ed.), *Frontiers of cognitive therapy* (pp. 383–418). New York: Guilford.

Vitousek, K. M., Daly, J., & Heiser, C. (1991). Reconstructing the internal world of the eating-disordered individual: Overcoming distortion in self-report. *International Journal of Eating Disorders, 10*, 647–666.

Vitousek, K. M., & Ewald, L. S. (1993). Self-representation in eating disorders: A cognitive perspective. In Z. Segal & S. Blatt (Eds.), *The self in emotional disorders: Cognitive and psychodynamic perspectives* (pp. 221–257). New York: Guilford.

Vitousek, K. M., & Hollon, S. D. (1990). The investigation of schematic content and processing in eating disorders. *Cognitive Therapy and Research, 14*, 191–214.

Vitousek, K. M., & Manke, F. (1994). Personality variables and disorders in anorexia nervosa and bulimia nervosa. *Journal of Abnormal Psychology, 103*, 137–147.

Vitousek, K., Watson, S., & Wilson, G. T. (1998). Enhancing motivation for change in treatment-resistant eating disorders. *Clinical Psychology Review, 18*, 391–420.

Wade, T. D., Bulik, C. M., Neale, M., & Kendler, K. S. (2000). Anorexia nervosa and major depression: Shared genetic and environmental risk factors. *American Journal of Psychiatry, 157*, 469–471.

Wagner, S., Halmi, K. A., & Maguire, T. V. (1987). The sense of personal ineffectiveness in patients with eating disorders: One construct or several? *International Journal of Eating Disorders, 4*, 495–505.

Waller, G., Babbs, M., Milligan, R., Meyer, C., Ohanian, V., & Leung, N. (2003). Anger and core beliefs in the eating disorders. *International Journal of Eating Disorders, 34*, 118–124.

Waller, G., Dickson, C., & Ohanian, V. (2002). Cognitive content in bulimic disorders: Core beliefs and eating attitudes. *Eating Behaviors, 3*, 171–178.

Walsh, B. T., & Garner, D. M. (1997). Diagnostic issues. In D. M. Garner & P. E. Garfinkel (Eds.), *Handbook of treatment for eating disorders* (2nd ed., pp. 25–33). New York: Guilford.

Wardle, J., & Watters, R. (2004). Sociocultural influences on attitudes to weight and eating: Results of a natural experiment. *International Journal of Eating Disorders, 35,* 589–596.

Wildes, J. E., Emery, R. E., & Simons, A. D. (2001). The roles of ethnicity and culture in the development of eating disturbance and body dissatisfaction: A meta-analytic review. *Clinical Psychology Review, 21,* 521–551.

Wiseman, C. V., Gray, J. J., Mosimann, J. E., & Ahrens, A. H. (1992). Cultural expectations of thinness in woman: An update. *International Journal of Eating Disorders, 11,* 85–89.

Wood, K., Becker, J., & Thompson, J. (1996). Body image dissatisfaction in pre-adolescent children. *Journal of Applied Developmental Psychology, 98,* 93–96.

Woodside, D. B., Bulik, C. M., Halmi, K. A., Fichter, M. M., Kaplan, A., Berrettini, W. H., Strober, M., Treasure, J., Lilenfeld, L., Klump, K., & Kaye, W. H. (2002). Personality, perfectionism, and attitudes toward eating in parents of individuals with eating disorders. *International Journal of Eating Disorders, 31,* 290–299.

Young, J. E. (1994). *Cognitive therapy for personality disorders: A schema focused approach* (2nd ed.). Sarasota, FL: Professional Resource Press.

Cognitive Vulnerability to Eating Disorders: An Integration

Pamela K. Keel
University of Iowa

Within the *Diagnostic and Statistical Manual* (4th ed.; *DSM–IV*) definitions of anorexia nervosa (AN) and bulimia nervosa (BN), one cognitive symptom is shared: the undue influence of weight and/or shape on self-evaluation (APA, 2000). As discussed in chapters 13 and 14, the cognitive imperative for both AN and BN is to control body weight or shape. The consequence of a failure to do so is a devaluation of the self. However, in understanding cognitive vulnerability to eating disorders, the distinction between etiological risk factor and symptom arises. Is it fair to conclude that overconcern with weight and shape represents a cognitive vulnerability factor when overconcern is part of the phenomenon for which it is supposed to increase risk? Leon, Keel, Klump, and Fulkerson (1997) addressed this question by noting that some risk factors may differ from the phenomenon they predict by degree rather than quality. Indeed, longitudinal research by Killen et al. (1996) demonstrated that weight concerns prospectively predicted development of bulimic symptoms in high school girls after controlling for levels of bulimic symptoms at baseline. Although stating that weight and shape concerns increase risk for disorders characterized by weight and shape concerns may seem tautological, there is merit in exploring the nature of these cognitive factors as has been done by Abramson and her colleagues (Bardone, Vohs, Abramson, Heatherton, & Joiner, 2000; Vohs, Bardone, Joiner, Abramson, & Heatherton, 1999; Vohs et al., 2001). Such work has revealed why weight and shape concerns contribute to the development of eating disorders in only a minority of women who wish to lose weight.

Although body dissatisfaction is normative for women (Striegel-Moore, Silberstein, & Rodin, 1986), not all women with eating disorders report body dissatisfaction (Cash & Deagle, 1997). If attempts to control the body are successful, then individuals with eating disorders can, and do, derive satisfaction from this achievement. However, many individuals are unable to attain the ideal they set for themselves or their goals become increasingly thinner as they lose weight. In both cases, they are left with a discrepancy between their actual and ideal body. In anorexia nervosa (AN), this can lead to increasingly severe measures to restrict food intake resulting in a state of starvation. In bulimia nervosa (BN), this leads to a paradoxical situation in which individuals who are attempting to restrict their food intake binge eat and then use inappropriate compensatory behavior to avoid weight gain. One question that arises is, why can some individuals restrict their food intake and achieve weight loss while others cannot? In addition to the similarities in cognitive vulnerability to AN and BN, are there differences in cognitive vulnerability that account for the disparate consequences of the disorders on body weight? In order to answer these questions, this chapter reviews the cognitive vulnerabilities that appear to be shared between these syndromes as well as those that appear to be unique.

SHARED COGNITIVE VULNERABILITIES

Both AN and BN are characterized by a set of cognitive distortions that include dichotomous thinking (Peterson & Mitchell, 2001) and selective abstraction (Beck, 1970), among others. Dichotomous thinking is expressed in many of the features common to both eating disorders. For example, foods become classified as either "good" or "bad." Similarly, individuals categorize their pattern of eating as either "good" or "bad." Dichotomous thinking can be seductive for individuals in significant distress because it simplifies the world tremendously. Research has demonstrated that when individuals experience increased stress, their ability to handle complex information diminishes (Vedhara, Hyde, Gilchrist, Tyrtherleigh, & Plummer, 2000). Unfortunately, dichotomous thinking lacks flexibility and does not adapt to changes in context. For example, losing weight is "good" and gaining weight is "bad" even when weight loss becomes dangerous.

Dichotomous thinking is also characteristic of the personality style of perfectionism. Anything that is not perfect (i.e., lacking any flaws) is worthless. Unfortunately, viewing the world in this way increases the probability of failure to nearly 1.0. For the binge eater, eating one cookie is as bad as eating an entire box, so there is no reason to stop eating once a dietary transgression occurs. Thus, the failure to control food intake according to rigidly held rules results in loss of control over eating. For a patient with AN, perfectionism can be the overriding theme in life. Rooms must be clean, books must be in alphabetical order, and objects must be arranged just so (Halmi et al., 2000). The body becomes another object that must be perfect, and perfection is defined by specific weight and shape criteria. As suggested in the example given for AN, perfectionism may be more accurately considered a personality style than a cognitive feature. However, because personalities shape the way that people perceive and think about their environments, a perfectionist personality contributes to cognitive rigidity and selective abstraction.

Cognitive rigidity in individuals with eating disorders reveals itself as a certain perseverative approach to problems. In the case of a patient with AN, there is the rigidly held belief that weight loss will achieve happiness and freedom from fears of becoming fat. However, as patients lose more and more weight, they tend to become more depressed and more terrified of weight gain. For patients with BN, they often come into treatment with the hope of eliminating binge eating episodes so that they can successfully lose weight through dieting. Dieting is rarely viewed as the problem. So both groups of patients engage in a behavior motivated to achieve a specific end, and the exact opposite result occurs. However, these individuals do not reevaluate the efficacy of their behaviors according to the consequences, they simply persist with the belief that somehow they just have not done enough or just have not done it right. Cognitive rigidity has also been observed on neuropsychological testing in patients with the restricting subtype of AN and, unlike some forms of cognitive impairment in AN, it has been uncorrelated with starvation (Fassino et al., 2002).

Selective abstraction occurs when a part comes to stand for the whole. This is particularly likely to occur among perfectionists because if something would be perfect if not for one specific flaw, then this one flaw carries an undue amount of importance in evaluating the worth of the whole. For example, a woman with AN may be able to acknowledge that she is not fat in several areas of her body (e.g., shoulders and arms) and may even express the desire to build muscle mass in her upper body. However, if she sees fat on her thighs, this one region of her body carries the evaluation of her whole body as "too fat," despite her emaciation. Similarly, a patient with BN may describe himself as a vegetarian who believes it is wrong to eat animals because he has eliminated meat from his diet. However, he will ignore his consumption of fast food hamburgers during binge eating episodes. In this case, selective abstraction provides a "moral" justification for dietary rules that may increase risk of binge eating episodes.

Thus, rather than feeling good about both small and large successes, the cognitive distortions of people with eating disorders leave them vulnerable to suffer innumerable failures in terms of their eating, their bodies, and their lives. Patients with eating disorders are at increased risk for depression and anxiety disorders because of these cognitive features. The extent to which general dysphoria gets funneled into dissatisfaction with weight or shape has been proposed as an etiological factor for the development of bulimia nervosa (Keel, Mitchell, et al., 2001), and longitudinal work suggests that negative affect (the tendency to experience depression and anxiety) increases risk of developing eating disorders (Leon, Fulkerson, Perry, Keel, & Klump, 1999; Stice, 2001). For adolescents, controlling weight and shape may seem like a manageable solution to alleviate distress; however, for many, it becomes a trap. A vicious cycle develops in which general threats to self-evaluation are funneled into a need to obtain or maintain a specific body weight or shape, and the few successes and numerous failures to control body weight and shape negatively influence self-evaluation.

DISTINCT COGNITIVE VULNERABILITIES

Although experts in the field of eating disorders have argued that AN and BN share a common set of cognitive vulnerabilities, there is evidence for differences between the two eating disorders. First, cross-cultural research points to a nonfat phobic form of AN (Keel & Klump, 2003; Lee, Ho, & Hsu, 1993). Conversely, when BN is found in a non-Western context, it is accompanied by body image disturbance (Keel & Klump, 2003). Second, as is pointed out by Garner and Magana (chap. 14, this vol.), the empirical support for the cognitive model of BN is far greater than that for AN. Third, cognitive behavioral therapy has demonstrated significantly greater efficacy in the treatment of BN than in the treatment of AN (Keel & Haedt, in press; Peterson & Mitchell, 1999; Shafran, Keel, Haedt, & Fairburn, in press). Although some of these patterns can be explained by the lower prevalence rate of AN relative to BN (and thus greater difficulty in conducting adequately powered studies of AN), some of these patterns may reveal the extent to which the cognitive models discussed earlier have significantly greater relevance for understanding vulnerability to BN than AN.

Vohs et al. (1999, 2001) and Bardone et al. (2000) demonstrated that perfectionism, perceived weight status, and self-esteem interact to predict the future development of bulimic symptoms. Although individuals with AN are perfectionists, sometimes perceive themselves to be overweight (despite being underweight), and can suffer from low self-esteem, it seems that these factors do not lead to bulimic symptoms among those with the restricting subtype of AN. This suggests that one or more of these variables or their interactions perform differently among women with the restricting subtype of AN. The most obvious candidate is perceived weight status. Although a great deal of attention has been given to the misperception of weight by women with AN, most women with AN are aware that they are successful in their attempts to lose weight (Cash & Deagle, 1997). Thus, unlike women with BN, they might experience self-efficacy in their ability to reduce their weight. Interestingly, women with the binge/purge subtype of AN tend to be objectively heavier (although still underweight) compared to women with the restricting subtype of AN (Eddy et al., 2002). There are two possible interpretations of this difference. First, women with AN binge/purge subtype gain weight as a result of their binge eating behavior, and this causes them to weigh more than women with AN restricting subtype. Second, women with AN binge/purge subtype are less successful in losing weight, develop decreased self-efficacy, and fall into the same pattern demonstrated for women who develop bulimic symptoms at normal weight.

As noted in the introduction, AN and BN share the cognitive symptom of undue influence of weight and shape on self-evaluation—this symptom appears among the diagnostic criteria for both disorders. However, for BN, this is a required symptom. For AN, this is one of several possible expressions of the cognitive processes that identify patients with AN. Individuals with AN can have any of the following: "Disturbance in the way in which one's body weight or shape is experienced, undue influence of body weight or shape on self-evaluation, *or* denial of the seriousness of the current low body weight" (APA, 2000, p. 589, emphasis added). This list suggests that there can be greater heterogeneity in the cognitive features that make up AN as compared to BN. Although the first two symptoms center on concerns about weight or shape, the third is a bit different. It focuses on what Rieger, Touyz, Swain, and Beumont (2001) referred to as "ego-syntonic emaciation." Unlike the fear of gaining weight or becoming fat, the absence of concern over low weight occurs cross-culturally and cross-historically (Keel & Klump, 2003). Further, this symptom belongs to a larger cognitive aspect that differs markedly between the syndromes—the extent to which the symptoms are experienced as ego-syntonic versus ego-dystonic.

Patients with AN tend to be characterized by not viewing their eating disorder as a problem. They are most often brought to medical attention by a family member, friend, or school official. In fact, the key symptom of AN is "refusal" to maintain a minimally normal weight for height. So, by definition, patients with AN are actively engaged in continuing their eating disorder and can be quite resistant to treatment. Among patients treated for BN, most have sought treatment on their own. Interestingly, epidemiologic data suggest that most women who suffer from BN in the community never seek treatment (Fairburn, Welch, Norman, O'Connor, & Doll, 1996). So the apparent differences between AN and BN might be diminished if the comparison were between groups ascertained through the community rather than through treatment settings. However, the difference between groups in a treatment setting seems consistent with the symptom presentation. Both groups are attempting to restrict food intake in order to control body weight. Thus, refusing to maintain a normal body weight is consistent with this motivation. Conversely, binge eating episodes are not. Although this cognitive difference in experience of the eating disorder may be more of a result of eating disorder symptoms than an aspect of the cognitive vulnerability for developing the eating disorder, it likely impacts the maintenance of symptoms and treatment response.

Differences in impulse control have been implicated in explaining why some women who restrict their food intake successfully reach very low weights whereas others develop binge eating. On neuropsychological assessments, individuals with bulimic symptoms demonstrated significantly greater impulsivity compared to controls (Ferraro, Wonderlich, & Jocic, 1997), and impulsiveness has been implicated specifically for the symptom of binge eating across eating disorder subtypes (Keel, 2003). As reviewed by Garner and Magana (chap. 14, this vol.), starvation produces several changes in biological and cognitive function. One effect is increased preoccupation with food and eating. Yet, individuals with the restricting subtype of AN appear to be able to suppress impulses to eat. This suggests that they are able to exert a significant level of cognitive control over their behaviors. Although this may be thought of colloquially as "will power," this does not seem to be an accurate characterization because much of this control comes from fear of eating (Strober, 2004). In this way, patients with restricting AN resemble patients with OCD. However, instead of having obsessions concerning fear of contamination by germs, patients fear contamination by food. Fassino et al. (2002) reported that the cognitive impairments demonstrated by women with the restricting subtype of AN were similar to those found in neuropsychological tests of patients with OCD. Imaging studies have demonstrated that the neurological response to high fat food resembles that to disgusting things among patients with AN (Treasure, 1998). Although this could be characterized as an affective response to food and eating, it is accompanied by a cognitive framework in which food, calories, and fat are dangerous elements that should be avoided. Interestingly, these cognitions seem to be less culture-bound than those concerning weight or shape (Keel & Klump, 2003). Thus, fears of becoming fat may be a feature of AN in a culture that idealizes thinness and denigrates fatness, but it may be an idiom of distress for a more general cognitive vulnerability to developing AN.

Another factor that differs between women with AN and women with BN is age of onset, and this results in developmental differences in cognitive vulnerabilities (Keel, Leon, & Fulkerson, 2001). AN tends to develop during puberty. Conversely, BN tends to develop toward the end of adolescence when girls are approaching young adulthood. In addition to differences in developmental milestones at these times in the life span, peri-puberty and late adolescence are characterized by different levels of cognitive development (Eckstein & Shemesh, 1992). Our work (Keel, Fulkerson, & Leon, 1997) and the work of others (Gralen, Levine, Smolak, & Murnen, 1990) suggest that girls' body image tends to be more related to their actual body size at younger ages. There is a more concrete basis for their evaluations of their weight satisfaction and attempts to alter their weight. Conversely, as girls mature, they develop a more abstract basis for evaluating their body image, and actual body weight becomes a weak predictor of weight satisfaction or attempts to alter weight (Leon et al., 1999). Similarly, Vohs et al. (1999) reported that increases in bulimic symptoms from end of high school to freshman year of college was predicted, in part, by their *perceived* weight status, and actual BMI had no significant influence.

Among individuals who perceive themselves to be overweight, dieting institutes cognitive control over eating and disrupts awareness of actual hunger and satiety signals (Polivy & Herman, 1985). This cognitive control is very vulnerable to cognitive disinhibitors. An example was given earlier in this chapter. If a person tells herself that no cookies are allowed but finds herself in a situation where she eats a single cookie, this will serve as a cognitive disinhibitor. The rule has been broken so there is no reason not to eat all of the cookies before resuming the "no cookie" rule the next morning. This hypothesis has received a great deal of empirical support in both longitudinal studies demonstrating that dieters are eight times more likely to develop an eating disorder than nondieters (Patton, Johnson-Sabine, Wood, Mann, & Wakeling, 1990) and experimental work demonstrating that restrained eaters eat more than unrestrained eaters only when they have been exposed to a cognitive disinhibitor (Ruderman, 1986). However, Stice (2001) suggested that dieting does not necessarily lead to binge eating.

TREATMENT IMPLICATIONS

To the extent that the cognitive vulnerabilities for BN have been well researched and are fairly precisely defined, cognitive behavioral treatment for BN has demonstrated efficacy (Keel & Haedt, in press; Peterson & Mitchell, 1999; Shafran et al., in press). Conversely, evidence for the efficacy of cognitive behavioral approaches in AN has been sparse (Keel & Haedt, in press; Peterson & Mitchell, 1999; Shafran et al., in press). Some of this may be due to genuine differences between the disorders and some of it may be attributable to the greater challenge of conducting controlled treatment trials for AN than BN. However, even in naturalistic studies, individuals with AN tend to require a great deal more treatment, including inpatient treatment, than individuals with BN (Keel et al., 2002; Striegel-Moore, Leslie, Petrill, Garvin, & Roseneck, 2000), and women with AN tend to have lower and slower recovery as compared to women with BN (Herzog et al., 1999).

For BN, the recommended treatment is cognitive behavioral therapy (CBT) (Keel & Haedt, in press; Peterson & Mitchell, 1999; Shafran et al., in press). The behavioral aspects of treatment tend to focus on self-monitoring, establishing a regular pattern of eating (discussing the role of dieting in triggering binge eating), coming up with alternatives to binge eating, stimulus control, and contingency management. Cognitive aspects include identifying problems, alternative responses to problems, and anticipating consequences, identifying and restructuring maladaptive cognitions, and addressing underlying beliefs (Fairburn, 1984; Peterson & Mitchell, 2001). For example, if a patient with BN insists upon weighing *exactly* 125 pounds, the normalcy of small weight fluctuations, sources of weight fluctuations (other than fat), and the impossibility of remaining at exactly 125 pounds are discussed, and the patient is encouraged to allow a *range* of acceptable weights. Another treatment that has demonstrated efficacy in the treatment of BN is interpersonal therapy (IPT) (Fairburn et al., 1995). IPT does not focus on eating behaviors or weight and shape-related cognitions. Instead, it focuses on interpersonal relationships. Although this treatment does have demonstrated efficacy, it appears to be associated with a slower rate of recovery than CBT (Fairburn et al., 1995). Finally, behavioral therapy (BT) has demonstrated efficacy for BN. Most studies suggest that treatment response does not differ between BT and CBT in patients with BN (Keel & Haedt, in press; Shafran et al., in press). However, some data suggest greater maintenance of improvements in CBT as compared to BT (Fairburn et al., 1995). Thus, for BN, the best treatment directly addresses cognitive distortions thought to underlie the development and maintenance of the disorder.

For AN, treatments with the greatest empirical support are more eclectic. For example, a promising form of treatment for AN is a family-based treatment (Eisler et al., 2000; Le Grange, 1999; Lock & Le Grange, 2001). This treatment represents a significant departure from historical approaches to the treatment of AN in which "parentectomies" were actively promoted and experts felt that family and friends made "the worst attendants" (Gull, 1874). However, patients with AN tend to be younger than patients with BN, and they are most often brought into therapy by family members (rather than being self-referred). So family therapy has been an aspect of AN treatment for a long time. Earlier treatments tended to view the expression of AN as a symptom of problems in the family system, and the family was "the patient" in past treatments of AN (Minuchin, Rosman, & Baker, 1978). Current approaches enlist family as members of the treatment team and have demonstrated efficacy in randomized controlled trials (Keel & Haedt, in press; Shafran et al., in press).

The differences in treatment approaches for AN and BN partially reflect the differences in medical risks associated with the disorders, developmental differences related to age differences between patient groups, but also potentially etiological differences in their cognitive vulnerabilities. Whereas the most efficacious treatment for BN focuses on the exact cognitions that are implicated in its etiology, the most efficacious treatment for AN has a much broader focus.

DIRECTIONS FOR FUTURE RESEARCH

Fairburn, Cooper, and Shafran (2002) proposed a new transdiagnostic cognitive behavioral therapy for eating disorders based on the model that AN and BN share the same underlying cognitive vulnerability—the overimportance of shape and weight. This could represent the first direct test of this model of shared cognitive vulnerability. If the treatment works equally well in women of normal and below normal body weight (i.e., there is no association between treatment response and body mass index, BMI, with an adequate range of BMI), then this research will have supported the presence of shared cognitive vulnerabilities. If, like previous research, treatment outcome and recovery differ markedly based on body weight, then modifications to the model will be necessary. The direction of these modifications can be obtained through a series of alternative hypotheses.

One possibility is that AN and BN do share the same underlying cognitive vulnerabilities, but the presence of low weight in AN makes it more difficult to address these. Starvation is known to alter cognitive processes and lead to even greater rigidity and tendency to think in concrete terms. So, even if both disorders are caused by the same cognitive features, the symptoms of one may make treatment more difficult. This alternative hypothesis could be tested by examining the association between weight and cognitive deficits on neuropsychological assessments and using cognitive deficits as a covariate in examining the association between BMI and treatment response.

A second possibility is that cognitive vulnerability to AN is closer to that for OCD than that for BN. Strober (2004) proposed that liability for extreme fear conditioning may represent the underlying vulnerability for AN. Applying pathological fear conditioning as a novel paradigm for examining AN, Strober indicated specific hypotheses that could be empirically tested. Specifically, Strober posited that weight-recovered AN patients, as compared to controls, would demonstrate increased speed in acquiring conditioned fears, delayed extinction of conditioned fears, and differential patterns of activation in the amygdala during fear conditioning.

A third possibility is that AN has a completely unique set of cognitive vulnerabilities. The emphasis on weight phobia to explain the symptoms of AN may represent a historically and ethnically specific idiom of distress (Lee et al., 1993) or a culturally meaningful explanation for behaviors for which the true causes are poorly understood (Keel & Klump, 2003). Researchers working within the United States (Banks, 1992; Katzman & Lee, 1997) and Canada (Steiger, 1993) have similarly acknowledged that the motivations behind self-starvation are not limited to concerns about weight and shape. This work points to an area in need of further investigation: What are the cognitive vulnerabilities to AN that reside outside of the usual suspects of weight and shape concerns? Unfortunately, limited empirical data provide insight into this question. Most prospective risk factor research predicts the more heterogeneous category of disordered eating rather than specific eating disorders, and there is reason to believe that women with AN do not self-report their symptoms in large epidemiological studies (Whitehouse, Cooper, Vize, Hill, & Vogel, 1992). Thus, the low base rate of AN relative to BN or EDNOS, as well as a tendency for individuals with AN to avoid self-identification, make it difficult to examine cognitive vulnerability factors specific for this disorder. Thus, additional studies designed to simply describe and characterize cognitive features of AN would represent a significant contribution.

Individuals with AN and BN share a set of cognitive distortions that seem to be important in maintaining their disorders. However, several factors suggest that unique cognitive vulnerabilities may exist for these syndromes. Given the strength of cognitive research for BN, and the shortage of cognitive research for AN, possible future directions for AN research were introduced. Studies utilizing neuropsychological assessment and imaging techniques may improve the description and characterization of cognitive vulnerabilities for AN as well as extend what is already known for BN.

REFERENCES

American Psychiatric Association. (2000). *Diagnostic and statistical manual of mental disorders* (4th ed., text rev.). Washington, DC: American Psychiatric Association.

Banks, C. G. (1992). "Culture" in culture-bound syndromes: The case of anorexia nervosa. *Social Science Medicine, 34,* 867–884.

Bardone, A. M., Vohs, K. D., Abramson, L. Y., Heatherton, T. F., & Joiner, T. E. (2000). The confluence of perfectionism, body dissatisfaction, and low self-esteem predicts bulimic symptoms: Clinical implications. *Behavior Therapy, 31,* 265–280.

Beck, A. T. (1970). *Depression: Causes and treatment.* Philadelphia: University of Pennsylvania Press.

Cash, T. F., & Deagle, E. A., III. (1997). The nature and extent of body-image disturbances in anorexia nervosa and bulimia nervosa: A meta-analysis. *International Journal of Eating Disorders, 22,* 107–125.

Eckstein, S. G., & Shemesh, M. (1992). The rate of acquisition of formal operational schemata in adolescence: A secondary analysis. *Journal of Research in Science Teaching, 29,* 441–451.

Eddy, K. T., Keel, P. K., Dorer, D. J., Delinsky, S. S., Franko, D. L., & Herzog, D. B. (2002). A longitudinal comparison of anorexia nervosa subtypes. *International Journal of Eating Disorders, 31,* 191–201.

Eisler, I., Dare, C., Hodes, M., Russell, G., Dodge, E., & Le Grange, D. (2000). Family therapy for adolescent anorexia nervosa: The results of a controlled comparison of two family interventions. *Journal of Child Psychology and Psychiatry, 41,* 727–736.

Fairburn, C., Cooper, Z., & Shafran, R. (2002, April). *A new "transdiagnostic" cognitive behavioral treatment for eating disorders.* Workshop given at the International Conference on Eating Disorders, Boston, MA.

Fairburn, C. G. (1984). Cognitive-behavioral treatment for bulimia. In D. M. Garfinkel & P. E. Garner (Eds.), *Handbook of psychotherapy for anorexia nervosa and bulimia* (pp. 160–192). New York: Guilford.

Fairburn, C. G., Norman, P. A., Welch, S. L., O'Connor, M. E., Doll, H. A., & Peveler, R. C. (1995). A prospective study of outcome in bulimia nervosa and the long-term effects of three psychological treatments. *Archives of General Psychiatry, 52,* 304–312.

Fairburn, C. G., Welch, S. L., Norman, P. A., O'Connor, M. E., & Doll, H. A. (1996). Bias and bulimia nervosa: How typical are clinic cases? *American Journal of Psychiatry, 153,* 386–391.

Fassino, S., Piero, A., Daga, G. A., Leombruni, P., Mortara, P., & Rovera, G. G. (2002). Attentional biases and frontal functioning in anorexia nervosa. *International Journal of Eating Disorders, 31,* 274–283.

Ferraro, F. R., Wonderlich, S., & Jocic, Z. (1997). Performance variability as a new theoretical mechanism regarding eating disorders and cognitive processing. *Journal of Clinical Psychology, 53,* 117–121.

Gralen, S. J., Levine, M. P., Smolak, L., & Murnen, S. K. (1990). Dieting and disordered eating during early and middle adolescence: Do the influences remain the same? *International Journal of Eating Disorders, 9,* 501–512.

Gull, W. W. (1874). Anorexia nervosa (apepsia hysterica, anorexia hysterica). *Transactions of the Clinical Society of London, 7,* 22–28.

Halmi, K. A., Sunday, S. R., Strober, M., Kaplan, A., Woodside, D. B., Fichter, M., Treasure, J., Berretini, W. H., & Kaye, W. H. (2000). Perfectionism in anorexia nervosa: Variation by clinical subtype, obsessionality, and pathological eating behavior. *American Journal of Psychiatry, 157,* 1799–1805.

Herzog, D. B., Dorer, D. J., Keel, P. K., Selwyn, S. E., Ekeblad, E. R., Flores, A. T., Greenwood, D. N., Burwell, B. A., & Keller, M. B. (1999). Recovery and relapse in anorexia nervosa and bulimia nervosa: A 7.5 year follow-up study. *Journal of the American Academy of Child and Adolescent Psychiatry, 38,* 829–837.

Katzman, M. A., & Lee, S. (1997). Beyond body image: The integration of feminist and transcultural theories in the understanding of self starvation. *International Journal of Eating Disorders, 22,* 385–394.

Keel, P. K. (2003). Validity of categorical distinctions for eating disorders: From disorders to symptoms. In M. Maj, K. Halmi, J. J. Lopez-Ibor, & N. Sartorius (Eds.), *Evidence and experience in psychiatry: Vol. 6. Eating disorders* (pp. 52–54). Chichester, England: Wiley.

Keel, P. K., Dorer, D. J., Eddy, K. T., Delinsky, S. S., Franko, D. L., Blais, M. A., Keller, M. B., & Herzog, D. B. (2002). Predictors of treatment utilization among women with anorexia and bulimia nervosa. *American Journal of Psychiatry, 159,* 140–142.

Keel, P. K., Fulkerson, J. A., & Leon, G. R. (1997). Disordered eating precursors in pre- and early adolescent girls and boys. *Journal of Youth and Adolescence, 26,* 203–216.

Keel, P. K., & Haedt, A. (in press). Empirically supported psychosocial interventions for eating disorders and eating problems. *Journal of Clinical Child and Adolescent Psychology.*

Keel, P. K., & Klump, K. L. (2003). Are eating disorders culture-bound syndromes? Implications for conceptualizing their etiology. *Psychological Bulletin, 129,* 747–769.

Keel, P. K., Leon, G. R., & Fulkerson, J. A. (2001). Vulnerability to eating disorders in childhood and adolescence. In R. E. Ingram & J. M. Price (Eds.), *Vulnerability to psychopathology* (pp. 389–411). New York: Guilford.

Keel, P. K., Mitchell, J. E., Davis, T. L., & Crow, S. J. (2001). Relationship between depression and body dissatisfaction in women diagnosed with bulimia nervosa. *International Journal of Eating Disorders, 30,* 48–56.

Killen, J. D., Taylor, C. B., Hayward, C., Haydel, K. F., Wilson, D. M., Hammer, L., Kraemer, H., Blair-Greiner, A., & Strachowski, D. (1996). Weight concerns influence the development of eating disorders: A 4-year prospective study. *Journal of Consulting and Clinical Psychology, 64,* 936–940.

Le Grange, D. (1999). Family therapy for adolescent anorexia nervosa. *Journal of Clinical Psychology, 55,* 727–739.

Lee, S., Ho, T. P., & Hsu, L. K. (1993). Fat phobic and non-fat phobic anorexia nervosa: A comparative study of 70 Chinese patients in Hong Kong. *Psychological Medicine, 23,* 999–1017.

Leon, G. R., Fulkerson, J. A., Perry, C. L., Keel, P. K., & Klump, K. (1999). Three to four year prospective evaluation of personality and behavioral risk factors for later disordered eating in adolescent girls and boys. *Journal of Youth and Adolescence, 28,* 181–196.

Leon, G. R., Keel, P. K., Klump, K. L., & Fulkerson, J. A. (1997). The future of risk factor research in understanding the etiology of eating disorders. *Psychopharmacology Bulletin, 33,* 405–411.

Lock, J., & Le Grange, D. (2001). Can family based treatment of anorexia nervosa be manualized? *Journal of Psychotherapy Practice and Research, 10,* 253–261.

Minuchin, S., Rosman, B. L., & Baker, L. (1978). *Psychosomatic families: Anorexia nervosa in context.* Cambridge, England: Harvard University Press.

Patton, G. C., Johnson-Sabine, E., Wood, K., Mann, A. H., & Wakeling, A. (1990). Abnormal eating attitudes in London schoolgirls: A prospective epidemiological study—outcome at twelve month follow-up. *Psychological Medicine, 20,* 383–394.

Peterson, C. B., & Mitchell, J. E. (1999). Psychosocial and pharmacological treatment of eating disorders: A review of research findings. *Journal of Clinical Psychology, 55,* 685–697.

Peterson, C. B., & Mitchell, J. E. (2001). Cognitive-behavioral therapy for eating disorders. In J. E. Mitchell (Ed.), *The outpatient treatment of eating disorders. A guide for therapists, dietians, and physicians* (pp. 144–167). Minneapolis: University of Minnesota Press.

Polivy, J., & Herman, C. P. (1985). Dieting and binge eating: A causal analysis. *American Psychologist, 40,* 193–201.

Rieger, E., Touyz, S. W., Swain, T., & Beumont, P. J. V. (2001). Cross-cultural research on anorexia nervosa: Assumptions regarding the role of body weight. *International Journal of Eating Disorders, 29,* 205–215.

Ruderman, A. J. (1986). Dietary restraint: A theoretical and empirical review. *Psychological Bulletin, 99,* 247–262.

Shafran, R., Keel, P. K., Haedt, A., & Fairburn, C. G. (in press). Psychological treatments for eating disorders. In K. Halmi & U. Schmidt (Eds.), *Cambridge handbook of effective treatments in psychiatry, eating disorders.*

Steiger, H. (1993). Anorexia nervosa: Is it the syndrome or the theorist that is culture- and gender-bound? *Transcultural Psychiatric Research Review, 30,* 347–358.

Stice, E. (2001). A prospective test of the dual-pathway model of bulimic pathology: Mediating effects of dieting and negative affect. *Journal of Abnormal Psychology, 110,* 124–135.

Striegel-Moore, R. H., Leslie, D., Petrill, S. A., Garvin, V., & Roseneck, R. A. (2000). One-year use and cost of inpatient and outpatient services among female and male patients with an eating disorder: Evidence from a national database of health insurance claims. *International Journal of Eating Disorders, 27,* 381–389.

Striegel-Moore, R. H., Silberstein, L. R., & Rodin, J. (1986). Toward an understanding of risk factors for bulimia. *American Psychologist, 41,* 246–263.

Strober, M. (2004). Pathological fear conditioning and anorexia nervosa: On the search for novel paradigms. *International Journal of Eating Disorders, 35,* 504–508.

Treasure, J. (1998, November). *Imaging emotion in anorexia nervosa.* Paper presented at the Eating Disorders Research Society annual meeting, Cambridge, MA.

Vedhara, K., Hyde, J., Gilchrist, I. D., Tyrtherleigh, M., & Plummer, S. (2000). Acute stress, memory, attention and cortisol. *Psychoneuroendocrinology, 25,* 535–549.

Vohs, K. D., Bardone, A. M., Joiner, T. E., Abramson, L. Y., & Heatherton, T. F. (1999). Perfectionism, perceived weight status, and self-esteem interact to predict bulimic symptoms: A model of bulimic symptom development. *Journal of Abnormal Psychology, 108,* 695–700.

Vohs, K. D., Voelz, Z. R., Pettit, J. W., Bardone, A. M., Katz, J., Abramson, L. Y., Heatherton, T. F., & Joiner, T. E. (2001). Perfectionism, body dissatisfaction, and self-esteem: An interactive model of bulimic symptom development. *Journal of Social and Clinical Psychology, 20,* 476–497.

Whitehouse, A. M., Cooper, P. J., Vize, C. V., Hill, C., & Vogel, L. (1992). Prevalence of eating disorders in three Cambridge general practices: Hidden and conspicuous morbidity. *British Journal of General Practice, 42,* 57–60.

Author Index

419

E

Subject Index

A

Abuse, *see* Childhood maltreatment
Affective structures and attachment disruption, 81–82
Agoraphobia, *see* Panic disorder
Analogue research, 19–20
Anorexia nervosa, 365–394, *see also* Eating disorders
  and asceticism, 385
  assessment of cognitive vulnerability to, 371–375
  and ballet dancers, 371
  and body dissatisfaction and drive for thinness, 377–380
  and body image disturbance, 375–377, 392
  cognitive theories of, 366–367, 381
  and core beliefs, 387–388
  and culture, 369, 371, 375, 379
  diagnostic issues associated with, 367–368
  and ethnicity, 371
  and impulse control, 385–386
  and information processing, 388–393
  and interoceptive deficits, 385
  maintenance of, 366, 392, 394
  and maturity fears, 386–387
  mortality rate of, 365

  and the multidetermined model of eating disorders, 368–369
  and obsessionality, 384–385
  and perfectionism, 383–384
  prevalence of, 265
  resemblance to OCD, 410
  risk factors for, 369–370
  and self-concept deficits, 380–381
  and self-esteem, 381–383
  and starvation symptoms, 393–394
  treatment of, 366–367, 387, 411–413
Anxiety disorders, 175–203, 303–322, *see also* specific anxiety disorders *and* Cognitive Vulnerability to Anxiety Project
  cognitive vulnerability to
    and cognitive overload, 184–185
    cognitive style associated with, *see* Looming maladaptive style (LMS)
    common factors of, 176–178
    development of, 186–187, 312–313
    and disorder specific factors, 178
    and issues in conceptualization of, 303–304
    and the looming vulnerability model of anxiety (LVM), 178–180, 192–193, 199–201, 311, *see also* Looming maladaptive style (LMS)